HYPNOTHERAPY
OF WAR NEUROSES

A CLINICAL PSYCHOLOGIST'S CASEBOOK

By

JOHN G. WATKINS, Ph.D.

ASSOCIATE PROFESSOR OF PSYCHOLOGY
STATE COLLEGE OF WASHINGTON.
FORMERLY CHIEF CLINICAL PSYCHOLOGIST
WELCH CONVALESCENT HOSPITAL
DAYTONA BEACH, FLORIDA

THE RONALD PRESS COMPANY ⨳ NEW YORK

To

THE MANY VETERANS

WHOSE WOUNDS, THOUGH REAL, ARE INVISIBLE

PREFACE

This is a report of psychotherapy done by the author in the neuro-psychiatric division of an Army convalescent hospital during the recent war. The men whose treatment is described in the case studies were combat veterans who had broken under the stress of war, men needing individual therapy to get them well.

These patients received individualized attention in a Special Treatment Company. They differed widely in native abilities, education, and social background. What they had in common was that all had become neurotically ill during their Army service and that hypnosis was used as an integral part of their treatment.

The cases have been selected from a much larger number in order to illustrate the different forms which war neurosis—the "shellshock" of 1918—may take and the variations of therapeutic attack which were necessary to bring about improvement. These case reports are presented for their interest to other clinicians and as an aid to the professional student who wishes to learn hypnotherapy.

The cases are introduced by a brief account of the nature and purposes of wartime psychotherapy, the theoretical basis of the author's work, and the nature and practical application of hypnotherapeutic techniques.

Although this book is directed in general to clinical psychologists, psychiatrists, and students in these specialties, some of the materials in it should be of interest to those from related disciplines such as general medicine, education, sociology, and anthropology.

JOHN G. WATKINS

Pullman, Washington
October, 1949.

v

ACKNOWLEDGMENTS

To credit adequately each individual whose cooperation and assistance helped in producing this work would be an impossible task. Services were rendered by many of the patients and staff members of Welch Hospital, including members of the secretarial staff who donated extra time to copy the first drafts of the manuscript.

Throughout almost the entire period covered by the cases, Sergeant Henry P. Lampman acted as Psychiatric Social Worker for the Company. His untiring and skillful therapeutic efforts on behalf of the patients won the respect and admiration of patients and staff alike. His use of progressive relaxation and non-directive therapy was closely coordinated with the hypnotherapy. His insight and tactful contact were often crucial in turning a case in a favorable direction. The writer feels privileged to have had his assistance in the handling of these cases.

Among the Army doctors to whom the author is indebted, special acknowledgment is made to Major Lawrence J. Roose, MC, Battalion Psychiatrist. Major Roose served with the writer in Company F, later becoming Clinical Director for the Neuropsychiatric Division of the Hospital, and made many therapeutic suggestions in the treatment of the cases described.

Special thanks are likewise due to Major Norman R. Shulack, MC, Psychiatrist, who first as Battalion Commander and later as Director of the Neuropsychiatric Division provided the encouragement, facilities, and medical backing which made possible the hypnotherapeutic activities in Company F. During the last half of the period Lieutenant Millard B. McGee, MC, served as Psychiatrist for Company F. The writer is very grateful for his assistance and close collaboration in the handling of the cases. His personal support and constructive review of the early drafts of the manuscript provided a great stimulus for the furtherance of this work.

Finally, the writer wishes to give special thanks to his wife, Doris, for her steady support and help in the revision of the manuscript, retyping of the text, and editing and correcting of proof.

J. G. W.

CONTENTS

PART I

Military Neuroses

PART II

Hypnotherapy

PART III

Individual Case Studies

PART IV

The Hypnoanalytic Treatment of an Entrenched Phobia

PART V

Evaluation

PART I

MILITARY NEUROSES

CHAPTER 1

INTRODUCTION

Shell shock or battle neurosis was first recognized as a major combat problem in the first World War. Our veterans' hospitals still contain many chronic, uncured cases from that war. The advent of the recent war with its increase of bombs as well as shells brought, as had been expected, a larger number and proportion of neuropsychiatric (NP) casualties. This increase was even greater than anticipated. A flood of incapacitated men poured to the rear, while facilities and personnel for treating them proved highly inadequate.

Battle Neurosis in the Second World War

A neurosis may look like an organic illness, but it isn't. Furthermore, it requires special methods of treatment. The neuroses are extremely complex illnesses and among the most difficult to cure. Studies in the etiology and therapy of nervous maladjustments have been made by psychoanalysts, psychiatrists, and psychologists. Yet, even before the war, when cases were much less numerous and the specialist could spend almost unlimited time with each individual, therapy was unsure and "cures" were problematical. No rapid method of therapy had been developed. Not only did clinicians differ in their points of view and approach to treatment, but there was also wide disagreement on diagnosis and diagnostic terminology. Thus, during the war the greatest number of casualties was occurring in an area in which medical science had made the least advance.

To meet this problem the United States Army, somewhat belatedly, mustered all the psychiatrically and psychologically trained personnel available, and professional literature was widely disseminated among these specialists, who served within the medical corps under command of the Surgeon General's Office. Considerable latitude for research was granted. As a result, new therapeutic methods and procedures were developed. Advances were made in both drug therapies and psychotherapies. In many cases, a startling remission of symptoms occurred. First-aid treatments improved to the point that a large number of neurotic casualties could be immediately saved

3

and returned to combat duty after a few days (Grinker and Spiegel, 1944 [1]).

Still others seemed to develop a chronicity in their symptoms. Months after their breakdown they continued to be ill, exhibiting little or no improvement in spite of a wide variety of treatments. These cases were evacuated to the United States. They ultimately reached a convalescent hospital for extended treatment preparatory to re-entrance on limited duty or discharge to civilian life. It is with these cases that this book is concerned—the neuroses that were tough and unresponsive to superficial treatments.

We shall be concerned with the "whys" and with the "What can be done about it?" in the treatment of battle neurosis. Why does George continue to remain ill months after hospitalization, while his buddy, Bill, is well enough in a few days to return to the line? They both had the same amount of service and spent the same period of time under heavy combat conditions. They looked equally healthy, and both appeared in the same good physical condition on previous medical examinations. Yet, Bill is back fighting, while George seems hopelessly ill. He is depressed and "blue." He "knows" that he will "never be any good any more," and he is worried that he may commit suicide or go insane. Why?

If we could find out "why," there was still the question, "What can we do about it?" How could George's condition be improved? Perhaps the psychiatrist would recommend an analysis. This might indeed do the job and untangle George's badly scrambled nervous system. Still, there was no certainty that it would, and an analysis would cost George or his parents several thousands of dollars. It might take years. Few there were who could afford an analysis, and fewer who were prepared to treat those who could. The crying need of the time was for a quicker method of therapy which could show a reasonable percentage of success—one that required only a few weeks, not years.

Need for New Methods in Psychotherapy

The psychoanalytic approach to treatment is generally recognized as the most successful therapy for deep-seated neuroses. The traditional techniques of psychoanalysis, however, are so time-consuming as to preclude their use in the vast majority of cases. Psychoanalysts themselves have recognized this limitation to their method and some

---

[1] Dates following names identify entries in the Bibliography.

have eagerly experimented with possible short cuts (Ferenczi, 1928). Unfortunately many other analysts have taken the conservative viewpoint that no substantial, enduring alterations in personality structure can be achieved without the time-consuming working-through of neurotic resistances by the traditional methods developed by Freud. They have written off the therapeutic successes achieved by Stekel (1926, 1927) through brief, active analytic methods as superficial and as "a quick relief from symptoms and not attempting a cure of the underlying pathologic process" (Oberndorf, 1948).

Stekel, a student and associate of Freud who became a dissenter from the strict Freudian approach, wrote (1949) that he was convinced that "Freud's psychoanalysis may become detrimental to the patient if it extends over several years," and that "the most orthodox Freudians will realize the disproportion between effort and result." Recent trends in psychotherapy have tended to bear out Stekel's prediction. There is today considerable interest in developing brief, active methods of treatment. Coincidentally there are many who do not hold to the pessimistic belief that enduring results can be secured only by long, time-consuming procedures. Among the analytic group this experimental viewpoint seems to be following two lines of approach.

In Chicago a group of analysts (Alexander and French, 1946) has been developing a flexible therapeutic plan which replaces the daily analytic sessions with meetings at less frequent intervals, determined by the current tactics of treatment and following a more active manipulation and interpretation of transference reactions. They report generally favorable results in cases treated for brief periods ranging from one to sixty-five sessions. Considering that traditional analysis usually requires a minimum of at least two hundred sessions, this is indeed a great saving in time.

The other approach to treatment which attempts to achieve results in a brief period is through the use of hypnosis. There appears to be growing a new interest in using the hypnotic technique, not only as it has been traditionally employed but also in conjunction with other therapeutic methods, including psychoanalysis (Wolberg, 1945; Brenman and Gill, 1947).

Use of Hypnosis in Relieving Neurotic Symptoms

In this book some brief methods of treatment are described which owe their time-saving contribution to their integration with the hypnotic process. Between the past rejection of hypnosis by many therapists (because simple, direct suggestion under hypnosis does not permanently cure) and the advanced reintegrative techniques of the psychoanalyst lies an intermediate field. In this area psychiatrists and clinical psychologists can utilize hypnotherapeutic methods to effect *reasonably permanent* symptomatic relief. They make no attempt to rebuild the patient's basic personality structure but are content within the space of a few sessions to relax, if not resolve, a few of the major unconscious conflicts and to strengthen the ego so that it can handle the remainder without excessive anxiety and suffering. It is in this area that this work hopes to make its contribution.

Plan of This Book

In this book we will first make a brief survey of the usual group and "educative" therapies employed in Welch and other military hospitals in order to describe the background and "climate" in which hypnotherapy was practiced by the author.

We will then turn to an objective conceptualization of neuroses, their structure and treatment. This brief theoretical outline serves to give purpose to the various therapeutic tactics that were employed in the treatment of the cases described thereafter. It indicates the general frame of reference which acted as a guide to the therapy.

This treatment might be called "analytic-type" because it is psychoanalytically oriented and has borrowed heavily from Freudian theory and practice. However, it is not psychoanalysis, as it has also departed widely from this theory both in techniques and in the psychological definition of many of its terms. At the risk of oversimplification, but in the interests of a better understanding by the lay patient, this theory has been diagrammatically presented with the simplest and fewest number of factors possible. This scheme or analogy was found very useful in bringing the patient to an intellectual understanding of his disorder as one of the steps in attaining deeper insights. The aim in developing this concrete analogy has not been to improve dynamic theory but to offer a practical working formula to the practicing psychotherapist.

The particular contribution in this book lies, it is believed, in the fact that the therapy represents an amalgamation of concepts and practices from three widely differing schools. In the classical psychiatric literature, psychoanalytic theory, hypnosis, and motivational psychology have been largely divorced from one another. The psychoanalysts first began with hypnosis and then later rejected it, while studies in motivational psychology have been made largely by psychologists rather than by medical men. The point of view presented here is eclectic. It prefers a therapy that will work (regardless of how many disciplines it must borrow from) to any neat, theoretical system.

In reviewing various therapeutic tactics, we will consider the use and misuse of hypnosis, the reasons why it was prematurely rejected, and the apparent slowness in its full development. The actual methods used for inducing trance will also be discussed for the benefit of those professional psychiatrists and psychologists who wish to utilize it in their therapy or research. Nonprofessional people are warned against tinkering with hypnosis. There are certain dangers involved which will be brought out in the course of the discussion.

The cases which will be presented illustrate different types of neuroses and the therapy applied. These histories have been selected for their interest both as types of neurosis and as illustrations of therapeutic technique. No attempt has been made to select only those in which "cures" or symptomatic relief were effected. In the large majority there appears to have been a considerable improvement in the patient. If it were not so, there would be no justification for the writing of this book. Of course, only a fraction of the total number of cases receiving therapy in the Special Treatment Company could be so described.

The hypnoanalysis of a deep-seated neurosis presented at the end of the book describes the rather extended treatment of a case in which a number of advanced and complex methods were employed. Some unusual results occurred which may stimulate further research and study.

General implications and findings from the case studies are integrated in the final summary chapter, which is intended to contribute to a better understanding of the problems of neurosis and the development of better methods of treating these disorders.

CHAPTER 2

PSYCHOTHERAPY IN A MILITARY SETTING

Army Background of Psychoneurotic Cases

The cases to be described in this book were all treated at Welch Convalescent Hospital. Patients arrived at this installation after having been evacuated from combat theaters to the United States. Each patient had passed through a number of hospitals and had received a variety of treatments before reaching Welch Hospital. NP treatment was undertaken with a knowledge of, and allowance for, any existing or pre-existing organic pathology. This was the end of the line. At this point the final therapeutic effort within the military service was made and the decision was taken as to whether the soldier was to be returned to duty, usually in a limited capacity, or be given a medical discharge (CDD) to civilian life.

In order that the special treatment problems posed in the handling of these soldiers may be clear to the reader, a brief résumé of the typical patient's recent history previous to his arrival at this installation is in order.

The typical patient had developed a psychoneurosis after a period of service in a combat area. Among the patients were men from the Anzio Beachhead, from Cassino, from St. Lô, from the Battle of the Bulge, and from other well-known battlefields of the second World War.

Their first treatment had been evacuation from combat. In each division there was a rest area some distance behind the lines. Many men would respond to a few days of relaxation, especially if their cases had been promptly noted. This, of course, had nothing to do with the predisposing factors but relieved the system from the continual stress of combat. The normally well-adjusted individual might improve rapidly. His body was no longer being submitted to a constant barrage of shells, noises, groans of the dying, sights of mutilated men, and the constant alertness of a "kill or be killed" soldier. The regenerative forces within the body were able to cope with the anxiety created. With a few days of rest and sleep the soldier appeared to be completely recovered. Sometimes medicinal sedation was prescribed if the patient could not sleep or rest.

However, though greatly improved by this rest, the soldier was not necessarily "cured." He could not then return for another three months of the same combat. The stress he had endured and the anxiety developed in his body had left their mark. He probably could not "take" as much as when he first entered battle even though he looked perfectly well. A few more weeks of the same kind of severe duty and he might return to the aid station in a more severe anxiety state which would last longer.

Treatment in Rear-Echelon Hospitals

If it appeared that he was too severely disabled to improve greatly from a few days' rest, he was evacuated to the rear, to a hospital equipped to give more intensive and longer treatment. If his disorder was a reactive depression, he might be given shots of insulin to increase the metabolic processes, or his anxiety might be relieved by a narcosynthetic treatment with sodium amytal or sodium pentothal (Grinker and Spiegel, 1944). Under a barbiturate narcosis, material which had been repressed might emerge. Pentothal, commonly called "walkie-talkie" by the soldiers, seemed to have the effect of bursting "the dam of the unconscious." The patient was able to re-enact scenes involving great emotional stress, to relive painful combat experiences and to recall periods during which he was amnesic. This was called *abreaction*. It is a form of "getting it off your chest." The repressed conflict, like an infected boil, is "lanced" and the repressed pathogenic material released.

This procedure proved especially effective with acute cases. Sometimes the pentothal would relieve the anxiety, disclose the source of guilt in the depressed patient, or enable the hysteric to regain use of his paralyzed limb, stuttering voice, or impaired eyesight. Often though, the predisposing factors in the patient had been so strong or the significances so deep that he lost his symptoms only while under the influence of the drug. When he awakened they returned. The symptoms might or might not be cleared up after repeated use of the drug. In cases like this, deeper and more intensive psychotherapy was required.

In addition to these drug treatments the hospitals in the rear echelon usually had a well-planned program of activities, athletics, recreation, movies, and reading, all designed to "get his mind off it" and to provide a stable environment in which the natural forces of recovery might have the greatest opportunity to operate. Psychologically important at this time were letters from home, good buddies, and sympathetic and understanding doctors and nurses. Perhaps after several weeks or months of reconditioning of this type the patient had improved enough so that he could be returned to limited service behind the lines. There he could be of military value yet not be subjected to the extreme stress of battle. If this could not be done, he had to be evacuated to the States for longer convalescent treatment.

The more severe the breakdown, the farther back from the combat zone he was sent. And conversely, the farther removed he was from the battle area, the less chance there was of reconditioning him for combat again. If he could be revived in the rest area and returned in a few days, he might continue to give valuable service as a fighting soldier. After a few months away from combat, however, in the rear-echelon hospital, it became almost impossible to send him back to battle. By the time he had been evacuated to the United States he had developed intensive antagonism and resistance to any type of further military service and thought only in terms of going home to civilian life.

During his stay in these hospitals every possible ego-building therapy was tried. Constructive and creative activities were emphasized. He was encouraged to paint, model, or build something in an arts and crafts shop. Occupational therapy is a special form of arts and crafts work in which skilled therapists prescribe types of interesting activities which develop not only the weakened spirit but also the weakened muscles in the paralyzed arm or leg of the hysteric (War Department, 1944). Confidence in his own accomplishments and achievements sometimes worked wonders. A neurotic soldier might lose a great deal of anxiety and make considerable progress because he found he could fashion a bracelet for his wife or girl friend.

Still another type of treatment which was found effective in many cases was that of *progressive relaxation* (Jacobson, 1938; Fink, 1943). Here the patient was taught how to relax completely one set of muscles after another, until his entire body was free of tension and he could easily go to sleep. This kind of treatment was found especially useful with severe anxiety states, although it was also used effectively with other types of neuroses.

All these therapies are valuable. They are often called *superficial,* not because they are ineffective, but because they concentrate on freeing the man from the stress that started in battle and was being continued almost as a habit. These superficial treatments do not attempt to deal with the patient's unconscious conflicts. They are more directly related to his immediate environment. As such they are more suitable for group application, the type of approach which necessarily must be followed with the vast majority of Army cases. This eclectic ego-building is the essential feature in the psychobiological concept of treatment as developed by Adolf Meyer (Lief, 1948).

Procedure in Welch Hospital

Our typical patient, therefore, arrived at Welch Hospital with a well-structured neurosis which had successfully defied many previous treatment efforts over an interval of from three months to a year. His motivation was only in terms of return home, and he was usually embittered by his frequent military transfers from one hospital to another. He nearly always exhibited strong hostility to the Army and to any further therapy. Often, indeed, he had not received thorough and competent treatment. Inefficiency and incompetent personnel are too common in a large wartime Army to require any explanation or apology. However, much of his bitterness was related to displaced guilt reactions over his inability to remain with his outfit in combat.

After reaching Welch Hospital the patient was assigned through a receiving company to activities involving psychiatric, physical, and dental examinations with diagnosis and classification, accompanied by orientation into the activities of the post and his future role. Following this he was assigned to a treatment company for a period of from six weeks to several months during which his treatment included group therapy, recreational and educational activities, physical exercise, and sometimes individual psychotherapy. The companies (with the exception of the Special Treatment Company) averaged 100 to 125 men each during peak load and were staffed by a psychiatrist, a clinical psychologist, and one or two psychiatric social workers. At the termination of his stay, the decision as to his disposition was made by the psychiatrist of his company, and his orders, either return to duty or discharge to civilian life, were cut accordingly.

Within the Hospital the more difficult cases which did not respond to group treatment were referred by their psychiatrists to Company F, the Special Treatment Company. Here their cases were considered for suitability for the types of individual therapy offered in this Company. If the therapists in Company F felt that the case merited such attention, and the case was treatable by their methods, the patient was accepted and his transfer was accordingly made. At times especially problematic cases were directly assigned to the Company even though prognosis was questionable. The main types of treatment utilized in the Company were narcosynthesis, hypnotherapy, and progressive relaxation. However, the size of the group was not permitted to exceed twenty to thirty, so that time would be available for individual help.

Before turning to the consideration of individual cases, we shall in the next few chapters briefly examine psychotherapeutic theory and techniques which were utilized in the rehabilitation of these soldiers. This will give purpose and substance to the verbatim reports of treatment sessions and enable the reader to evaluate more critically the degree of success which was achieved.

CHAPTER 3

THEORETICAL BASES OF TREATMENT

Equilibrium in Human Beings

A brief theoretical consideration of the structure of the human organism is most helpful in aiding the psychotherapist to understand and effectively treat neurotic disorders. The total human being might be considered as a dynamic system of equilibrium. Forces from his environment stimulate him, and forces within him are initiated to respond. There is a constant interplay of energy. Basically, he is composed of matter and energy. As an interesting analogy which may help in understanding neuroses we might think of the body—organs, glands, and tissues—as being the "matter" side of him and his mind as being the "energy" side of him. Mind thus becomes the total of all energy distribution within the body.[1]

As the changing demands of environmental forces press in one form or another on the organism, it alters and adjusts its disposition of energies in order to maintain its own existence and integrity as a unit. On a simpler scale, we might think of the candle flame which adjusts and alters its shape as the various gusts of wind strike it, but clings tenaciously to its existence as a system of equilibrium and flattens down very low before it can be entirely blown out. Let us consider the human organism as a vastly more complex machine, with the nervous system as the channel through which the interplay of controlling energies takes place.

Since there is a continual drive for equilibrium—not a static, but a dynamic equilibrium—any upsetting forces tend to be met by counterforces. This conflict disturbs the entire balance of the system. It may result in pain or distress in any part of the body. The new condition may be necessary to maintain the essential integrity of the system of equilibrium. Hence, until the original upsetting force is understood and dealt with, the person continues in a state of illness— he maintains symptoms.

Of many of these interchanges of energy within the body we are aware—our thoughts, feelings, attitudes, emotions, wishes, etc., but

---

[1] We do not imply here any psychic dualism. In fact the physicist tends to consider energy and matter reducible to the same elementary forces. So likewise, we may think of mind as being "body-in-action."

13

only a small part of these are conscious. Under the surface there is a vast reservoir of ideas, experiences, memories, impulses, motives, attitudes, emotions, and wishes of which the person is not aware. In fact there are probably many more in his unconscious [2] than in his conscious. All these represent energy interplay within him. They may have and do have a tremendous effect in determining his behavior. That is why no person's actions are 100 per cent predictable. Only a small part of his motives and ideas are known, either to himself or to others.

In this unperceived realm of interaction disturbances can create such an imbalance in the system's equilibrium as to bring about severe surface changes: abnormal fears, abnormal behavior, and various symptoms of illness. Hence, a person can become ill, not only because tissue has been damaged, but also because energy dispositions within the body have become upset and scrambled. The upsetting forces can originate (and often do) below the threshold of consciousness.

The symptoms of a functional illness may appear at the place of a previous organic injury, masquerading as a recurrence of that earlier disability (Scott and Mallinson, 1944), or they may come out in some entirely different spot in the body. Three soldiers with almost identical backgrounds, moreover, may respond to the same exploding shell with three different sets of symptoms. One may become paralyzed, another blind, and the third suffer stomach pains. The secret as to just why the imbalance of the system took one form rather than another lies in that deeper region of consciousness which is not available to the eye under ordinary conditions.

This book will be concerned with certain submarine methods, certain diving-bell techniques by which we can penetrate a little further down into the unconscious personality and gain information which will aid us in understanding and treating better the functional disorder.

Freud's Theory of Neurosis

The first effective theory of neuroses was formulated by the founder of psychoanalysis, Sigmund Freud (1938). His work stands as a foundation for psychotherapy. Other systems of treatment have been devised, and many of his followers have altered his original con-

---

2 Some psychologists may object to the use of the words *unconscious* and *conscious* as nouns. They are employed this way for convenience and because they can be more easily grasped than by engaging in niceties of controversial theory. Actually, the writer does not conceive of *the unconscious* as a place or thing, but rather as a descriptive adjective applied to those behavior patterns and processes, either potential or kinetic, which when activated are *not perceived* by the individual.

cepts. Yet he did develop the basic ideas on which modern psychiatric treatment rests.

Briefly, he conceived of the human mind as being composed of the *Super-Ego,* one's conscience or higher unconscious motives; the *Id,* one's primitive unconscious drives; and the *Ego* or one's ability to carry out his purposes. In the unconscious, according to Freud, there is a constant battle between the Super-Ego and the Id for control of the Ego. In other words, one's better and higher nature is unconsciously struggling with one's primitive impulses. Of this struggle we are not generally aware, but the conflict creates anxiety. Since anxiety is painful, our Ego erects defenses against it. These frequently are compromises between the Super-Ego and the Id in the form of neurotic symptoms. Thus, a paralyzed hand may be the body's compromise between an overwhelming but unconscious impulse to kill one's father or wife (the Id) and an equally strong motive force from the Super-Ego which condemns the impulse. Since it would even be wrong to think about this, the conflict is repressed and is carried on at an unconscious or subliminal level. The struggle of forces underneath disturbs the surface only in the form of the paralyzed hand. The purpose of psychoanalysis is to uncover the conflict and resolve it. *Analysis* became the process of breaking down one resistance after another, of digging into the unconscious and developing insight.

Throughout this book the terms *Ego, Super-Ego,* and *Id* are used. For the benefit of those readers schooled in the theories of objective psychology some clarification is desirable. These concepts are not treated here as innate factors or mystical entities. Rather they are used as convenient terms to represent various general principles governing mental behavior.

For example, the Super-Ego stands for certain habits of thought and action, both conscious and unconscious, which have been acquired by the individual during his social growth. It represents behavior patterns, taught to the person by society, which involve subordination of the individual's pleasure impulses to the welfare of others. It includes those standards of conduct, generally unconscious, which have been established in the socialized person, whose objective is the welfare of the group over that of the individual. The Super-Ego behaves like an internalized parent which renders moral judgments on the individual's behavior.

Likewise, the Id becomes an over-all designation for the more personal or pleasure-seeking drives of the organism, especially those which run counter to the best interests of society. Psychoanalytic theory conceives of the Id drives as being unconscious, and there is nothing in current psychological theory which insists that an organism is always aware of its motives. So we here interpret the Id loosely as a name for those drives within us, generally unconscious, which seek as their object of satisfaction the personal pleasure of the individual at the expense of society.

The Ego then becomes the sum total of the organism's energies and aptitudes—its ability to maintain its integrity as a unit and successfully adjust to internal and environmental demands.

The explanations of Super-Ego, Id, and Ego given above are not in the classical psychoanalytic tradition. Rather they are an attempted reconciliation of Freudian concepts with the principles of present-day objective psychology.

It will be noted that Freud's theory can be reconciled in principle with that of systemic imbalances developed in the earlier part of this chapter. In both there is a conflict and disturbing forces which are unconscious or unperceived. In both, the external manifestations of this conflict become, either through compromise or through resolution of the conflict of forces, the neurotic symptoms. And in both, effective treatment must be concerned with the underlying conflict of unconscious drives rather than with the surface symptoms, the paralyses, headaches, intestinal distress, etc.

The foregoing review of some of the terms used in the Freudian theory of neuroses is not intended to be exhaustive. The reader who desires a statement of psychoanalytic principles is referred to Fenichel (1945). Simplification and concrete analogies for therapeutic theory are used here because the writer feels that a practical liaison must be achieved between the theoreticians and the practicing therapists. Many physicians and psychologists operate without a basic framework of purpose for their professional activities. Their therapy lacks strategical plan and becomes a kind of pragmatic opportunism. On the other hand, the scientific theorist often becomes so involved in controversies over definitional niceties that he fails to reach the suffering patient, a person more often of average intelligence, who can achieve insight only if he is taught the dynamics behind his symptoms in simple, clear, and objective terms.

Pattern of Neurotic Development and Types of Neurosis

Neurotic sickness follows a formula: *Predisposition plus stress equals neurosis.* Predisposition cocks the mechanism and stress pulls the trigger.

By *predisposition* we mean all the past factors in the patient's life, whether he bit his fingernails or was enuretic when young, whether he had many phobias, was a product of a happy or a broken home, had a normal or a distorted sex life, had good relations with parents, siblings, friends, school, etc. In short, predisposition can include about everything that has happened to a person since birth plus any weaknesses or strengths he inherited from Dad, who was a successful businessman, or Grandma, who had nervous fits.

Stress means the environmental pressure on the potential neurotic at the time of and immediately preceding his breakdown. Was he in combat three days or three months? Was he subjected to heavy shelling, or did he have a rear-echelon job? Was he severely worried over family problems or not? The formula seems to be quite simple: The more positive predisposing factors you have, the less stress you can stand. Some men developed a severe neurosis immediately after saying "I do" at the induction station. Others, with more normal adjustment experiences and fewer neuropathic traits, could stand up under months of severe combat. Every person has his breaking point. No matter how stable you are, or think you are, if enough stress is placed on you, you too will find yourself a neuropsychiatric casualty. The only reason there are more in the Army in wartime is that the stress is greater. But nobody, soldier or civilian, is immune.

Although there are many variations of neurosis, combat break-downs usually tend to divide themselves into certain types. The most common is the *anxiety reaction*. In this the patient suffers from tremors, sleeplessness, battle dreams which become nightmares and awaken him, and headaches. He may develop nausea, anorexia, or stomach pains. He may become constipated or diarrhetic. He jumps at loud noises and is very irritable toward the doctor or even his buddies. Sometimes he develops pains in various parts of his body, especially in the back.

In a variation of this anxiety state the patient may develop what is termed a *reactive depression.*[3] This commonly occurs when he has been removed from combat and hospitalized for some minor wound. As the wound heals, apathy, gloom, depression, and hostility begin to appear. The patient has to be rehospitalized as a neuro-psychiatric case. Cases of depression generally have as their basis repressed feelings of guilt or hostility. The patient feels guilty because he killed an enemy soldier, guilty because he did not or could

---

[3] This is now called *neurotic depressive reaction* in War Department Technical Bulletin, Medical 203 (1946), a revised classification of psychiatric disorders.

not save a buddy in a crucial situation, guilty that he didn't do his best, guilty that he has left his buddies back there still fighting, etc.

The next most common clinical syndrome is *hysteria.* This generally takes the form of very specific and observable symptoms. In the pure case there is little anxiety evident because all the anxiety is centered in the symptom—it is "converted" into the disability such as a paralyzed leg or arm, stuttering, amnesia, blindness, or deafness. So the illness is usually called *conversion hysteria.*[4] It is important to remember that the Ego has erected the symptom as a defense against anxiety, or has converted the nervous energies that would be used in anxiety into maintaining the symptom. Thus if one removes the symptom from an hysteric without resolving the causes of his illness, the inner conflicts, one may release a great deal of anxiety. Then the patient, minus his stutter or paralyzed leg, develops an anxiety reaction like that previously described. This point will become more evident in the case descriptions.

Another form which neurosis may take is called an *obsessive-compulsive reaction.*[5] The patient in this type may be obsessed with various strong fears such as a fear of the dark, a fear of high places, a fear of crowds, etc. Sometimes these fears are so strong as to be quite disabling. One patient's fear of crowds made it impossible for him to go to the movies. On the other hand anxiety in the patient may be fixated or structured in some compulsive actions. He may be unusually fastidious about his personal appearance and may prescribe for himself a daily ritual of behavior for every situation he meets. Another patient may wash his hands twenty or thirty times a day and become most upset if he is unable to perform this ritual in the self-prescribed manner. Still another may develop an overpowering urge to have a strong, beautiful body and exercise every day for several hours lifting weights and developing strength.

Although the cases described in this book became ill largely because of the severe stress of combat, the same symptoms are often seen in civilian neuroses. We will be concerned here largely with these three major types of neurosis: anxiety reaction, conversion hysteria, and obsessive-compulsive reaction. These do not, of course,

---

4 In War Department Technical Bulletin, Medical 203, this has been divided into *conversion reactions,* covering the physical symptoms such as spastic conditions, paralyses, blindness, etc., and *dissociative reactions,* which include the more strictly behavioral deviations such as amnesia, fugue, and somnambulism.

5 War Department Technical Bulletin, Medical 203, distinguishes between those obsessive fears or ungovernable impulses from within which it classifies under *Obsessive-Compulsive Reactions,* and fears of external phenomena such as the dark, high places, foreigners, etc., which it terms *Phobic Reactions.* These latter probably are manifest symbols of some inner unacceptable impulse.

represent all forms of neurotic illness. Very few cases, moreover, can be easily classed as purely one or the other. Thus, an hysteric may have both anxiety features and obsessive symptoms. Most patients, however, are usually centered in one or the other form of neurosis.

Relation of Neurotic to Normal Behavior

Many persons in reading about neuroses are dismayed to find these patients showing behavior traits similar to their own. Here we come to a very fundamental fact about these illnesses. The psychoneurotic is merely exhibiting to an extreme degree traits, behavior, and symptoms which are common to all of us. But he has been under great stress, and he probably had stronger predisposition. These two (stress and predisposition) reacting together have developed his weaknesses to such a marked degree as to make them painful and incapacitating. All illness and health, especially in the functional field, is a matter of degree. Psychological distress can range from the mildest maladjustments, unhappiness in work or misunderstandings between husband and wife, to the severe crippling disorder of a paralyzed hysteric doomed to a life of wheel-chair invalidism. Where the line between mere maladjustment and neurotic illness lies nobody can say.

Basic Mechanism of Neurosis

In helping patients to achieve insight into their disorders a simple gadget, constructed of wood, proved to be very useful. Complex theory may often be best explained by homely analogies which are within the grasp of every patient. In this device the relations of symptoms, dynamics, motivation, conscious, unconscious, insight, and therapy could be objectively and simply demonstrated. If diagrammatic devices representing forces in personality help in the understanding of the professional psychologist (Lewin, 1938), how much more they might be employed to aid the understanding of the patient who is accustomed to think in terms of concrete objects rather than of abstract forces.

Following is a brief sample of the type of explanation used with this device as it was actually presented in group therapy sessions with patients.

Look at Figure 1. It is a gadget consisting of a baseboard and another board hinged to it leaning slightly backwards. Notice that on

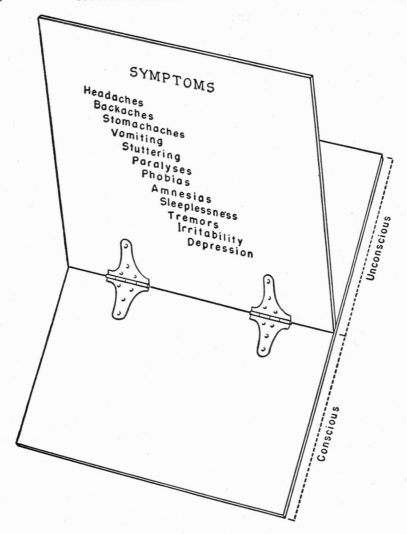

Figure 1. The Neurotic Illness as Seen by the Patient

the upright hinged board we have the *symptoms:* headaches, backaches, stomachaches, vomiting, stuttering, paralyses, phobias, etc. Now let us suppose you are looking at this contrivance from directly in front. You notice that the board with the symptoms on it stands up, and you wonder why it doesn't collapse. Why doesn't it fall over backwards? You surmise that something behind, which you can't see, must be holding it up. And you're right. In the neurosis something behind is holding up and maintaining the symptoms. But you can't see what that something is because it's unconscious. Both the patient and the doctor can see, feel, or otherwise perceive the symptoms or external manifestations of the illness. But as yet neither of them knows what is holding up these symptoms.

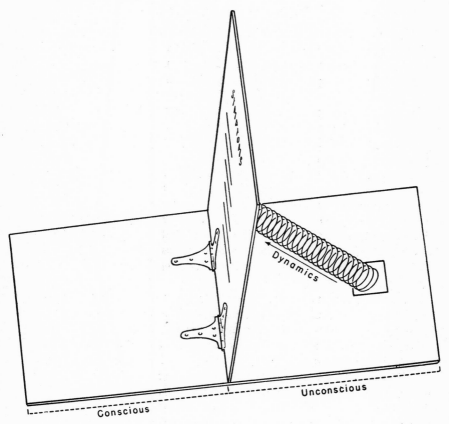

Figure 2.   The Neurotic Illness as Understood by the Therapist

Now let us take a side view of this contrivance. In Figure 2 we notice that a coil spring on which is inscribed the word *Dynamics* is preventing the symptoms from collapsing. In the person, that spring stands for the resultant of certain unconscious forces. As long as it is there the symptoms will be held up, and the patient will be ill. Remember that he sees this contrivance or neurotic mechanism from the front, as in Figure 1, even though the doctor may be permitted the side view of Figure 2.

But what would happen to the symptoms if the doctor were to take hold of that spring, dynamics, and pull it out from behind the upright board so the patient can see it? Then the symptoms have nothing left to hold them up. They collapse. That's just what happens in a neurosis when the therapist is able to extract the dynamics or roots of the illness out of the patient's unconscious mind and make them conscious.

At this point it was usually desirable to discuss the nature of resistances and the many ways they could manifest themselves. This gave the patients some concept of the difficulty involved in "extracting unconscious dynamics" and bringing about insight.

One of the first stages of insight is the admission by the patient that his illness is psychogenic and not somatogenic in origin. Most neurotic patients as their first line of defense will resist accepting a psychological etiology of their disability. An appreciation of this point is a basic part of the treatment.

We must go back to our concept of the organism as a dynamic system of equilibrium to explain the therapeutic nature of the patient's thoroughgoing acceptance of the fact that he has a neurosis. The resultant of all the forces has been integrated into a stream flowing in a certain direction—the direction of setting up and maintaining neurotic symptoms. This pattern or configuration of forces (*Gestalt*) is in the direction of illness. It is represented by the dynamics spring in Figure 2.

When the patient gains an important insight, he has changed the equilibrium of these internal forces—he has weakened the power of that dynamics spring. The energy streams of his body have been diverted; a new configuration or Gestalt must be set up, and a new type of dynamic equilibrium established. This means a fundamental modification in the energy dispositions within his body. In the case of acceptance of the true nature of his illness this new pattern will have basically changed the streams in the direction of discarding the symptoms and of getting well. The remarkable alteration which comes over a patient when he quits fighting, grasps and integrates a fundamental insight is often amazing. It is only in this change of condition and its reflection in his personality and attitude structure that the therapist can sense whether the new insight has been deeplying or superficial, genuine or only apparent.

Finally, after the evidence that there is no organic pathology present (or at least not enough to account for the distress) becomes overwhelming and respect for the therapist and his counsel gets sufficiently strong, the patient accepts. His Ego becomes strong enough to recognize the fact that he really is a neurotic—the first line is broken. This is no knockout, but at least round one in the battle for health has been won.

Further Mechanisms Operating in Neurotic Illness

What next? Now can we extract the dynamics spring and tell him that he fears the dark because as a child he developed a great unconscious fear of his father—that for him it is his father out in the dark he is afraid of because he, himself, had an unconscious incestuous desire towards his mother? Or can we tell him that his back pains are punishment for not doing all his duty the way he unconsciously thinks he should in battle? Or can we tell him that his vomiting is a rejection of sexuality because unconsciously as a child he came to believe that babies entered people through the mouth? Why, of course not. He would tell us we were crazy. No, even though all those factors were true (and sometimes the real dynamics are even more fantastic), we can't tell the patient outright what they are and expect to get anything but rejection. He has to arrive at true insight gradually. It is too big a shock for him to try to digest this all at once. It brings on more anxiety than he can handle.

So even if we as therapists know the real trouble, the patient must be gradually and patiently led to the roots of his difficulties. In the process of doing this he will put up almost every imaginable defense. He will have an excuse, a rationalization, another reason for not accepting each new concept. He will forget to come for appointments. He will misunderstand questions asked him by the therapist. He will start out upon a significant trend and then block, stop, and insist that his thoughts have nothing to do with his illness. To a significant suggestion he will respond with, "I've thought that through carefully, and it doesn't have any bearing on my problem." He' fails to realize that "thinking through" by himself has little value. A man cannot discover *unconscious* conflicts by himself, unassisted, merely by "thinking it through." His unaided thinking goes round and round like a lost man in the woods walking in circles, never discovering the real difficulty. The only ideas he has to work with are the conscious ones, and they aren't the ones that are causing the trouble. A neurotic will go through the most remarkable set of mental squirmings, twistings, dodgings, and rationalizing to escape facing a pertinent insight. Yet except for his illness he may be a highly intelligent person, even brilliant.

One senses that the patient is not free. It is as if some diabolical genie had established itself within the person of the neurotic patient and so completely taken over the functions of that individual that he is forced constantly to work against his own interests. The genie resists being dragged out of his lair like a tapeworm and uses all the resources of the person to maintain his entrenched position, while the helpless patient, like the slave laborer in Nazi Germany, must say and do that which continues his own enslavement. The genie's reactions, thoughts, desires, and attitudes will be sincerely and honestly offered to the therapist by the patient as his own.

The neurosis in its second, third, and fourth lines of defense will continue to employ the same "mother-bird and nest" technique of distracting his attention away from the real problem over and over again. An intelligent patient will make rapid strides forward, however, if he can be made to see that *the more resistance he naturally feels towards accepting a concept or idea, the more likely it is that the idea is approaching close to the true heart of his illness.* It is commonly noted that a person teased about a weakness he obviously does not have is not much disturbed. But toss a verbal dart in the direction of a true flaw in his make up and watch him bristle up and protest. Often the more nearly the therapist comes to uncovering the real difficulty, the more abusive the patient will be toward him.

The problem of uncovering dynamics and integrating them into the patient's conscious mind is truly an arduous task. The therapist must fight at every step of the way the very person whom he is trying to help, while that party is putting up a terrific struggle to prevent the very thing that will cure him. He, as the unwitting ally of his own enemy, helps the genie, neurosis, to retreat in depth from one line of defense to the next, through many points of resistance. And only when that ultimate layer of resistance is pierced does the patient become a completely free man. True, he gets a little better with each bit of territory liberated, and he may be able to control and successfully repress his symptoms when part of the battle is won. Then he gets relief from the illness, and we say that a *symptomatic cure* has been achieved.

Let us consider once more our diagrams as used to explain to the patient the forces in his neurosis. It *is* true that if we can extract those dynamics from the unconscious and make them conscious *and accepted,* the symptoms will disappear and the patient will get well. However, we must now add a few complicating factors which may still impede recovery even if true insight is secured. Let us construct another diagram picture. In Figure 3 the dynamics spring has been removed from behind the board, but the symptoms can't collapse because another spring is holding them up. We have put it in back,

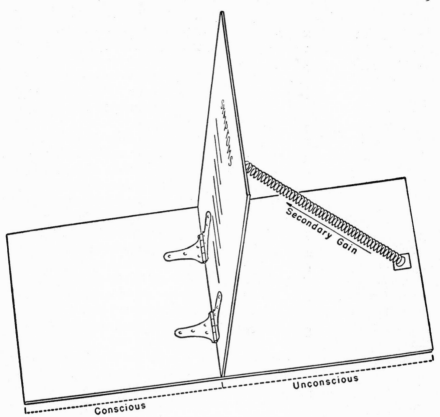

Figure 3. Neurotic Illness Maintained by Secondary Gain After Removal
of Dynamics

on the unconscious side of the figure, but this force, called the
secondary gain, can be either conscious or unconscious. Whether
pulling from in front (conscious) or pushing from behind (unconscious), it still operates as a force opposing the collapse of the
symptoms.

It works somewhat like this. The stress of combat has tripped
off a number of basic childish insecurities in a patient, setting up a
functional stutter and epigastric pain. He has been removed from
the fighting and hospitalized. While he is convalescing he gradually
comes to recognize that getting well means going back into combat.
Now here is a strong motive for not getting well. If he consciously
wants to be a good soldier his repressing mechanism will again come

to his aid. He just won't recognize or "see" the nature of this new motive. He may become very angry if we try to call it to his attention. "What are you trying to do, call me a goldbrick? If I was well I'd like to go right back and fight with my old outfit." Of course the point is that he isn't well. And if this secondary gain is strong whether conscious or unconscious, he isn't going to get well even if the dynamics have been resolved and consciously accepted. This secondary gain factor may be conscious if the patient doesn't have a high conscience or strong Super-Ego, but unconscious if he does.

Nothing succeeds like success, conscious or unconscious. So if he is kept out of combat because of this secondary gain, inevitably he soon notices that the other men who stay sick get to return to the United States. Again the therapist's job is complicated. Regardless of insight and understanding, rest, convalescence, progressive relaxation, games and entertainment, he still doesn't get well. This is not malingering. But now it is the motivation of the unrecognized and unadmitted secondary gain which is maintaining the symptoms.

Then when the patient returns to a convalescent hospital in the United States he finds that those who get well go back to limited duty, and those who stay sick are discharged to civilian life. So another secondary gain is established and takes over the maintaining of the symptoms.

Furthermore, since the patient has repressed this motive, he may develop guilt feelings about it. The Super-Ego, like the stern, just father, will see the nature of this factor and condemn it, and although the patient himself can't recognize what the trouble is, he will feel a sense of depression. His Super-Ego will have compromised by permitting the secondary gain to continue operating but extracting from the patient a punishment in the form of another symptom—depression.

Here's why one patient gets well and another doesn't under the same treatment. The second has never been able to adjust to military service as well as the first. One of those unconscious inner significances or meanings is for him a stronger-than-normal desire to escape from the rigorous discipline of service. Accordingly, ordinary treatment is ineffective, and he doesn't get well.

So he is discharged as a neuropsychiatric casualty and goes home. Now does he get well? Many do. Others don't. When he arrives back in the old home town he finds that because he was discharged for medical reasons the government will pay him a pension. *But he will cease to get this pension if he gets well.* Now a new secondary gain pushes against that set of symptoms and keeps them from collapsing. And if this can't be relinquished he may be a chronic invalid the rest of his life. He is being paid for being sick.

It is estimated that the average chronic NP casualty of the first World War has cost the taxpayers of this country about $30,000 to maintain through veterans' treatment (Appel, 1944). For the man with an organic service-connected disability, pensions are a just reward from a grateful country. But for the NP casualty they may become the very thing which will keep him half a man, a chronic suffering invalid as long as he lives.

Other secondary gains which can maintain the symptoms are the ability of the sick man to have others in the family wait on him, the gain of dodging arduous work, of being praised and well thought of for returning as a "wounded veteran." Even the demanding and securing of concessions from one's spouse because of a disability can easily become chronic. It is a cruel woman indeed who expects her poor, sick, hero-veteran husband to get out and mow the lawn.

Thus, the symptom which originally started in some unconscious conflict, the dynamics, continues because of the secondary gain it gives the patient. All this is unconscious. No malingering is involved. The patient sincerely believes that he cannot work, assume responsibilities, or have sexual relations because he is sick. The therapist knows that, because the patient cannot adjust to the work, responsibilities, or marital relations, he becomes and remains ill.

One other factor can be placed in our diagram picture of a neurotic mechanism, the counter-motivation to the secondary gain, the *Desire-to-Get-Well*. It might be likened to another spring pushing in the opposite direction to the secondary gain spring—that is in the direction of collapsing the symptoms board. It too can be either conscious or unrecognized. If it is strong enough it can overcome the secondary gain spring. The symptoms fall, and the person gets well.

If this desire-to-get-well becomes very strong it can not only overbalance the resistance of the secondary gain but also flatten the dynamics spring and push the symptoms down. This leaves the coiled dynamics spring still there, or as we might put it, the predisposing factors untouched. Under new stress in civilian life, the dynamics may be strong enough to push back the symptoms, and the person has a relapse. This is commonly the case in chronic neuroses where a superficial therapy has brought about an apparent cure.

One other adjustment needs to be made in the picture of a neurotic mechanism. We have used the term *dynamics* in a plural sense. Yet in Figure 2 it was portrayed as a single supporting spring. It would be more correct to visualize it as a bundle of springs. Seldom is in-

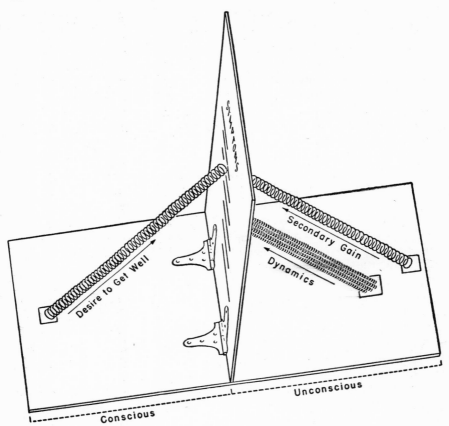

Figure 4. The Neurotic Illness as It Is Viewed for Treatment

sight complete involving the total removal of this force. Rather, insight comes in small pieces as neurotic resistances are penetrated. Each advance in understanding represents the removal of an individual spring from the bundle, thus weakening the total force maintaining the symptoms.

In Figure 4 we see the entire neurotic mechanism as it can be used to explain to the lay patient the various factors involved in keeping him sick. The clues to getting well boil down to two basic ones: "Uncover Dynamics—Motivate to Get Well." When the unconscious dynamics have been disclosed and integrated into the patient's consciousness, and when the drive to get well is greater than the motivation to remain sick, the symptoms will collapse, and the patient will recover.

In group therapy sessions discussions revolving about this simple diagrammatic explanation of a neurosis were found to help greatly in orienting the patient toward his role in treatment. Through devices of this type his understanding could objectively comprehend the forces which prevented his recovery and grasp the essentials which were needed to initiate the beginnings of insight.

CHAPTER 4

STRATEGY AND TACTICS

Predisposition plus stress equals neurosis. This is *the diagnostic formula.* It has already been discussed. A similar *formula for the therapeutic situation* might be written as follows: *Motivation plus insight equals cure.* Let us briefly consider the two basic terms of this latter proposition.

A motive is like a reservoir of force within us. It directs our activities and energies into channels designed to accomplish its purpose, and its directing influence can be unconscious as well as perceived. A motive can make us sick or well. Basically, when boiled down to the very roots, that's all a neurosis is—a sickness brought on and maintained by certain unconscious motives which find in the symptoms their satisfaction. Hence, the patient's motivational system must be made to work for us in getting him well instead of keeping him sick.

Of first importance is the patient's desire to get well. Some may ask, "Doesn't he always want to get well?" Yes, of course he does. But that's one of the fundamental points about a person's unconscious; two completely incompatible bedfellows can sleep side by side in it. He can both want to and not want to at the same time. The society of ideas and motives in our unconscious is chaotic, primitive, and illogical. We can like and dislike, or love and hate a person at the same time (Menninger, K. A. and Menninger, J. L. 1942).

Now concerning a soldier in the Army you can be sure that most of all he wants to go home. For months he's been dreaming about "the little woman," the "kids," his home, peace, and security, if that's what is waiting back there for him—and his plans to have those things if he's still unmarried. If he is quite young, it may be Mother and Dad and the old homestead. Anything which helps him to get home is OK. He'll cooperate with you. Anything which is likely to prevent it evokes from him noncooperation and antagonism. So that's the first axiom in trying to help him. If getting well means going home, he'll get well, but if getting well means returning to duty you'll find it very tough trying to treat him. This was the general experience of most therapists in Army hospitals (Levin, 1945).

Decision as to Disposition

During the early part of 1945 the trend in the convalescent hospitals was to return men to limited duty. The doctor found himself on the other side of the fence from the patient. The patient criticized the installation and its service, found fault with the doctors and "cussed" the medical treatment. It was a bitter battle, and cures were the exception rather than the rule. Every man knew that getting too well meant back to duty, and no matter how altruistic, patriotic, and well-meaning he was, this situation exerted terrific pressure on him. Over and over again one heard the same story. "Doc, I don't mind going back to duty if I could only get well." Consciously these soldiers meant that. But the "Doc" knew that they weren't getting well because improving ran counter to their entire motivational stream. Their bodies had reacted to the stress of Army life by breaking down into a neurotic illness. Could anyone expect that the promise of more of the very thing which broke them down was going to make them well? One could almost define a military neurosis as an unconscious bodily rebellion against service. The secondary gain was very strong—much stronger than the desire-to-get-well.

Whenever the severity of a patient's symptom complex was such that he simply could not adjust and remain healthy in the service, telling him he would be discharged worked wonders. In this case he could be informed that "when you get well enough you will go home." Now the terrific motivational pressure of wanting to go home has been removed from its secondary gain value and hitched to the desire-to-get-well side. Often it was so strong as to give symptomatic relief without insight. The soldier "got well" and left for home, the predisposing factors still coiled within him and ready to cause trouble under some future releasing stress.

Not nearly so good, and yet to some extent effective, was the telling of a patient that regardless of how he felt, the decision had been made that he was able to return to duty, and that would be his disposition on leaving the hospital. This meant giving him the motivation that if he had to do duty, why not be as well as possible? In the Special Treatment Company, where the cases described in this book were handled, it was found much better to make a decision as to disposition as early as possible in the period of treatment and so inform the patient. Uncertainty in itself is a most upsetting factor.

If a man had to return to duty, he was shown that at most he would have only a few more months of service in the Army, but he had to live with his body the rest of his life. He had to see that his health was more important, that it wasn't worth trading his life's happiness and health just to escape duty. That was adding all the power possible to his desire-to-get-well motivation. It was often necessary to explain to him just what this secondary-gain factor could do to his body. He would usually oppose that explanation with every resistance, conscious and unconscious, that his Ego could put forth. It is very hard to understand what we don't want to understand.

After VE Day, and especially after VJ Day, when nearly all patients were slated to go home at the completion of their hospitalization, an almost miraculous change came over the hospital population. Miles away from Hiroshima, that atomic bomb explosion jarred thousands of neuroses. Gone was the hostility and bitterness; gone was the antagonism towards the doctors and other professional workers; gone was most of the resentment and unwillingness to receive treatment. Instead, one got the picture of a bunch of happy, healthy boys who weren't even sick. While prior to this time it was expected that patients would exaggerate the severity of their symptoms, afterwards, really sick soldiers would claim that they were perfectly well and ready to go home now.

Of the cases to be described in this book, some improved because of the gaining of insight, others through pure motivational changes, most through a combination of the two. When insight has been secured but the pattern of motivational forces is untouched, the secondary gain factors can continue to maintain the symptom structure. On the other hand, when a "cure" has been secured through motivation alone, the dynamics lie as a predisposing force capable of causing the illness to return in the future. That's why an attack was generally made from both sides with the aim of securing more permanent results.

Sometimes the desire to go home could be utilized to "punish" the neurosis. Take the case of the patient whose dynamics are very tough, deeply imbedded, and hard to uncover, and whose mental ability is limited so that even though they are uncovered he cannot comprehend them. We then try to increase the strength of the motivational stream of wanting to go home. The therapist would inform the patient that *he could not go home until he improved* regardless of how long he had to remain in the hospital. If this technique had to be used as a final resort it became a "sweating-out" process or endurance contest in which the stubborn neurotic complex was pitted against the patient's desire to go home, with the man's life-long health as the stakes. Usually the desire to go home won out, and slowly but gradually the neurosis gave way, dissolving the symptoms.

Drive for Social Approval

But the desire to go home is not the only motive inside our patient. He is a whole bundle of individual drives. If we can discover them and harness their energy toward pulling those symptoms down, we will have been doing good therapy. One of the most important is the drive for social approval. All of us want to do those things which will make other people like and approve of us. More scientific researches are attempted and books written to gain the approval of others than for purely unselfish reasons. This is a very strong force in our patient's body which we can hitch to our getting-well cart. In some persons it is more highly developed, but everybody has some of it. If we can bring to his attention how much his wife, parents, children, or girl friend will approve if he gets well, we've added more power to our side. Unfortunately, people make a great fuss over the "wounded veteran." Sometimes carrying a cane or using a crutch becomes a mark of approval. The next time you want to give a veteran a great deal of attention and sympathy for his paralyzed leg, think twice. If he is an orthopedic casualty with demonstrated organic damage, reassurance that you like him is all to the good. But if his disability is the result of an hysterical reaction, the more attention and sympathy you give him the less likely he is to recover. Your approval of him gets aligned with the secondary gain which is keeping him sick. Then his body has "learned" a new and very bad lesson. He has found out that being a disabled veteran brings public approval and satisfactions that he could not get as a well man, and even if that isn't recognized consciously, and it probably isn't, it will be noted unconsciously and become part of the motivational structure.

There are many variations of this drive for social approval. We would like to be part of a group, to identify with it, and be accepted as a "regular fellow." If the soldier patient is with a number of men who have either recovered or are getting well, he will identify with them and will also improve. But if he is in with a group whose symptoms are chronic, his too will tend to become fixed.

Among the patients living in barracks it was interesting to note the similarities of behavior within each outfit. Where the motivation was favorable for getting well, this attitude extended more or less to all members of the group. When new patients were admitted for treatment who had been previously with companies where there was much complaining and hostility, their own attitudes soon evidenced a marked change. They quickly found out that "cussing the Docs" and the treatments was not *the* acceptable behavior in the new outfit, and that they in their attitudes were simply out of tune with the gang. Accordingly, they adjusted and changed. Often, a few weeks later, no more loyal and enthusiastic members of the group could be found. This almost always coincided with a marked change for the better in their illness. This motive of group approval was further utilized through *group-therapy sessions* (Cotton, Shulack, Kaplan and Watkins, 1945) in which the patients had opportunity to air their gripes and to receive certain superficial insights about their condition in a group discussion led by a professional therapist. A new patient placed in a group which was enthusiastic and positively oriented towards getting well couldn't help catching the spirit himself regardless of how disillusioned and embittered he had been to begin with. Attitudes, like diseases, are contagious.

One of the treatment techniques in the handling of severely ill soldiers was to give them "buddies" on first coming into the company —buddies whose symptoms had been much like their own, but who now were largely recovered. The new patient immediately found friends with whom he could identify and whose attitudes were in a constructive direction. The therapist always noticed how much the resistance was lowered at the next treatment session and how much easier it was to establish rapport.

In this way the group was usually composed of patients who had made rapid strides in getting well. New ones were added gradually and absorbed. On one occasion, when nearly all the "old boys" were discharged, and an entirely new group accepted at once, there was not this carry over. It took some time to melt away the strong and mutually reinforced antagonistic attitudes of an unassimilated group.

The same technique was most effective in breaking the resistance to hypnotic treatments. Patients who first refused them changed their minds and requested to be hypnotized after other almost-well patients had mentioned how the "sleep treatments" (as the soldiers called them) "couldn't hurt you and did you a lot of good." Others who had previously had certain unconscious resistances, and who were either not hypnotizable or were so only to a limited degree, became able to enter a deep trance whereby rapid, intensive treatment could be given.

Utilizing Other Motives

Another drive on which the therapist might draw was the desire to please parents or wife. This was sometimes double-edged, since many of the cases proved to be ambivalent toward family members. Some of the patients, while consciously professing great affection for parents, because of repressed hostility were unconsciously setting up symptoms which would effectively block parental ambitions.

Drives for affection and for sexual satisfaction were strong, but again there was the possibility that a particular symptom had been set up unconsciously to prevent sexual intercourse with the wife. So motives of this type could be used effectively by the therapist only when he understood much of the patient's dynamic structure.

The desire to accomplish or complete something was a most effective drive and could be drawn upon in such activities as painting or making gifts in a crafts show. Some soldiers would work patiently for hours building a model ship or plane, proudly displaying it during a group therapy session. The making of bracelets and shell jewelry proved very popular with others. If the patient, however, undertook a project and then failed or did not complete it, he not only lost the benefit of this motivation but he regressed and lost further confidence in himself. Patients were encouraged to undertake only projects they could complete.

During the treatment sessions the therapist usually explored early childhood objectives in life. What kind of person did the patient want to be? What were his goals? Did he want to go further in school and, if so, what kind of course did he want to take? For what kind of career was he aiming prior to his entrance into service? When these motives were understood, the therapist then had to devise ways by which they could be hooked to his desire-to-get-well. One of the fundamental axioms is that the stronger the motives used, and the more of them that can be harnessed, the sooner the patient will get well.

And so we find that discovering a man's wants is quite important. To cure George we must determine what are the motivational forces in his body, both the constructive ones and the destructive ones. Then our job is to harness all the strong and good ones we can onto the desire-to-get-well factor and detach all others from the secondary gain. These are fundamental psychological tactics in the battle for health.

Developing Individual Insight

Now let us briefly consider the second term in our therapeutic formula, that of *insight*. Symptoms are language. A neurotic symptom has a definite meaning behind it if we are only astute enough to read. That is what we mean by the word *dynamics* or *psychodynamics: the inner significance of certain conflicting forces manifested in the form of an external symptom.* There was not only a general reason why our patient broke down in combat and became ill. There was also a specific reason why his symptom took the form of a paralyzed back instead of a paralyzed arm, or a stomach pain instead of a stutter. We could give him, through group instruction and therapy, a general insight into reasons why people break down into neuroses, but only individual study and attention resulted in an understanding of why his symptoms developed as they did. The symptom, being the external manifestation of an internal conflict, is like the coded symbol for a hidden meaning. The therapist is the decoding expert. Whether the symptom be a stutter, a paralysis, an amnesia, a phobia, vomiting, or a "nervous" pain in the stomach, head, back, or any part of the body, it still is language. Each symptom is a symbol and has its own individual meaning, but until the dynamics are uncovered we are unable to read that meaning. By resolving these dynamics we free the individual from his conflicts, and the symptoms disappear.[1]

Often we had to be content with so altering motivational factors as to pull the symptoms down and leave the dynamics still repressed. We hoped that the stress on the individual would never again be great enough to release the symptom structure. Such is frequently the case. Very few of the veterans who went home "cured" of psychoneurosis really acquired much insight into their dynamics. Most recovered because of motivational changes, but down inside them the potentialities for a repeat are still coiled. However, the chances that they will ever again be placed in a situation as stressing as combat are also slight. In the motivational cure the predisposing dynamics were not touched, but the stress was relieved and will probably not again be strong enough to reinitiate the neurosis.

---

[1] A distinction is usually made between symptoms in the hysterical or obsessive-compulsive neuroses which are presumed to have specific *dynamics* or inner meanings behind them and the *psychosomatic symptoms* which are considered to represent a more generalized visceral response to emotional stress without specific inner psychological significance. Whether this distinction is a valid one is subject to controversy. However, we shall be more concerned here with the first type, in which definite *dynamics* are indicated.

Generally the time available for therapeutic treatment was not sufficient to uncover all the dynamics. Only a complete analysis could do that, but each patient might have been given some insight. This relieved part of the "predisposition factor" in the formula so that it would require more stress than formerly to unleash again the neurotic symptoms. Even if he only knew that his illness was a way of shutting out his wife because there were certain aspects of sexual intercourse with her that were not satisfactory to him, he had received some insurance against recurrence of the symptoms. Many cases had to be left with only symptomatic or motivational cures. The therapists were never entirely happy when this occurred. The patient was usually quite delighted that he had been "cured," but the therapist knew the dangers of recurrence that still remained, so the attempt was made to give each at least some insight into the nature of neurotic illnesses even if time was not available to uncover individual dynamics. This could be accomplished largely in group therapy sessions.

There are three steps in the acquiring of insight:

1. Understanding the general reasons for a neurosis and how it can be caused
2. Accepting the fact of having a neurosis
3. Understanding and accepting one's own dynamics

Each of these three steps became an educational job, a battle against the many resistances thrown up by the neurosis to prevent its resolution. Much progress usually was noted if the first two steps could be achieved. That often gave enough insight so that motivational pressures could accomplish the rest in pushing down the symptom structure.

The first hurdle was the easiest. If he understands the explanations given, he will have achieved the initial step in his therapy. But no real progress will have been made unless he is ready to take the second jump and accept the fact that he has this type of illness. This step is difficult because people have often used the words psychoneurosis, neurosis, "psycho" or neurotic in a slurring or deprecatory manner. Being thus diagnosed is regarded as an insult. One tends to feel that he is being accused of feeble-mindedness, lack of will power, malingering, or just plain cussedness. He believes that someone is pointing an accusing finger at him by calling him neurotic. His ego is being attacked, and it means that he is some lower species of mankind.

In helping the patient over this hurdle he must be reassured that fine, intelligent, and capable people often suffer from neurosis; that the pages of history are covered with the achievements of great men and women who were afflicted with incapacitating neurotic symptoms. He must be led to the idea that he is not to blame for this difficulty, that it is not his fault, or that he could have avoided it by exerting his "will power." He should learn to realize and accept the fact that his neurotic complexes are the product of predisposition and stress; that often this predisposition represents unfortunate and traumatic childhood experiences which he could not help. Neurosis is not a matter of blame. No person is perniciously and viciously responsible for the fact that nervous maladjustment has developed in him disabling symptoms. He has to be shown that frankly admitting a neurotic disorder does not represent any challenge to his pride. There is nothing in such an illness which should bring about the disapproval of others any more than having tuberculosis, appendicitis, malaria, or diabetes. The world will be a much better place in which to live when people get over the idea that an organic illness is honorable, but that a functional disorder is to be discussed in hushed terms and never admitted to one's family or friends. Both must be treated objectively as illnesses.

Many a soldier had become embittered because an unthinking physician had told him, "It's all in your head" or "It's in your imagination." This statement certainly did not make the patient well. It turned him against medical assistance and made him especially distrustful of psychiatric attention, the only treatment that could really help him.

Therapy becomes effective only when it actually induces the patient to change some of his attitudes about himself, his illness, and the world. Whether we are changing the energy dispositions and forces through motivation or through the giving of insight, we are making certain fundamental alterations in the body just as surely as if we were intervening in bodily processes by medical or surgical treatment. That is why insight *cures.* But to *heal,* it must be a genuine, thorough insight—not a detached, intellectual understanding, nor a superficial, lip-service acceptance. It must represent a rich, deep, inner-emotional experience involving every fiber of the individual's being, re-educating his entire energy-pattern system. It has to be an emotionally corrective experience. This is what is meant by the statement that *insight cures.* And it is this type of *insight* to which we refer when the term is used in the following chapters.

A few final words on the techniques by which the therapist initiates insight within the patient. Usually he can view the dynamics before the patient sees them. It then becomes his aim to lead the patient toward an understanding of the same things. It will be much easier for the therapist to see dynamics because he is not trying to maintain this neurosis in himself. Accordingly, he will not have all the resistances which are established to prevent insight. But in getting his view of the dynamics across to the patient, all his educational skill, tact, and diplomacy will be called upon. Attempting to force too much insight too suddenly may be disastrous. The patient cannot accept. Either he rejects because his resistances have not been pierced or, if they are, and he cannot assimilate the new insight, he develops an anxiety state. In some of the cases to be described in Part III it will be noted how considerable anxiety was initiated as the heart of a conflict was approached. It is for the therapist to determine just how much can be understood at any one session. He will have to decide what can be done and what should best be left untouched. He will not open up a conflict, demolish the neurotic defenses the patient has set up to control anxiety, and then leave him floundering at that point without resolving the difficulty and freeing him. Attempts to give too much insight too rapidly can sometimes even cause suicide.

Since in the Army all therapy is necessarily of a limited type the therapist should map out for himself as soon as possible how far he can go and where he should stop. There are certain inner recesses of each person which it is better to leave untouched. No therapist should attempt to play God and try to mold the perfect human; he must try only to help the patient adjust reasonably well to normal living without severe pains or unhappiness and with some insurance against the recurrence of neurotic distress. That, and no more, is his goal.

FUNDAMENTAL CONCEPTS IN THE TREATMENT

1. The diagnostic formula	Predisposition plus stress equals neurosis
2. The therapeutic formula	Motivation plus insight equals cure
3. Four factors in a neurosis	a. Symptoms
	b. Dynamics
	c. Secondary gain
	d. Desire to get well
4. Treatment	a. Motivate to get well
	b. Develop insight

PART II

HYPNOTHERAPY

CHAPTER 5

HYPNOSIS, PAST AND PRESENT

Mesmerism

The time is 1778, and the place Paris. We are standing in a large hall. The windows are covered, and it is dark and quiet. In the middle of this room is a wooden tub about a foot high and fifteen to twenty feet in diameter. The tub has a wooden cover, but there are holes in this cover, and from these holes pointed rods protrude. Standing and seated around the tub are a number of quiet persons. Walking among these persons is a man clothed in a brilliant silk robe passing his hands over the patients and touching them with an iron rod.

One senses that something very extraordinary is happening here. And indeed there is, because here, for the first time, the world is witnessing a systematic use of hypnosis for medical therapy. At this time, however, it is not known as hypnosis, but as animal magnetism.

The man in the bright silk robe was Dr. Franz Anton Mesmer, a Viennese physician. It was his belief that the human body was like a magnet, and that disease was caused by improper distribution of magnetism. Mesmer maintained that certain persons threw off an almost invisible gas or fluid which he called *animal magnetism,* but he held that this quality could be transferred to inanimate objects and thus became part of them. Persons who were diseased could have the magnetic forces of their bodies readjusted by contact with some magnetic source. It was his contention that he was able to transfer this magnetic fluid to the large tub and that the patients could then be healed by contact with the rods protruding therefrom. So hypnosis made its first appearance before the scientific and medical world clothed in mysticism and based on a fallacious theory (Hull, 1933).

Mesmer's period of active therapy was short-lived. In 1784 the French government appointed a committee to investigate the truth of his therapeutic claims. Included in this group was Benjamin Franklin. After a number of experiments this commission concluded that there was no such thing as animal magnetism and published its report. Shortly afterward Mesmer left Paris and returned to Germany. The

43

findings of this committee exploded the false theory on which Mesmer's work was based. However, they did not explain the therapeutic success he had secured, and they discouraged reputable scientific study in a field which was and still remains much neglected. The practice of hypnotism, for that is what it was, was continued by followers of Mesmer and became known as *Mesmerism*.

During the next fifty years, most of the major phenomena of hypnosis were discovered, such as the trance, induced hallucinations, anesthesias, amnesias, etc. By 1825 the world knew that these phenomena were capable of performing rather startling transformations within individuals. It still did not know what they were, nor how they operated (as, indeed, it does not know yet).

Braid, Liébeault, Bernheim, Charcot, Breuer, Freud

No new, significant contributions appeared until about 1843. At that time an English physician by the name of James Braid (1899) [1] carried on a series of experiments from which he concluded, as had the French Commission, that there was no such thing as a magnetic fluid. But, instead of rejecting the phenomenon of hypnosis, he recognized its therapeutic importance and developed an improved method of inducing trance. This involved the fixation of the eyes upon a small object. Braid also first used the word *hypnotism* and performed a number of painless surgical operations under trance conditions.

At about the same time a group of men in France were developing a similar view which culminated in the work of Liébeault (1892), a physician who practiced at Nancy. He seems to have made wide use of direct suggestion for the alleviation of various types of illnesses. Liébeault's work was not adequately recognized until the middle 1880's. At that time he became associated with Bernheim, a professor in the medical school at Nancy. Bernheim (1895) was converted to the value of hypnotic treatment by observing the "cure" of a sciatic patient. These two men, rejecting the theory of animal magnetism, placed considerable stress upon the psychological aspect of hypnosis and were the first to describe it as a form of *suggestion*.

Charcot (1890), a prominent neurologist in Paris, also performed extensive experiments with hypnosis and once again tried by controlled studies to prove the existence of an animal magnetic force. The controversy which developed between the Paris and Nancy

---

[1] Dates following names identify entries in the Bibliography.

schools is classic. It culminated in the triumph of the Liébeault-Bernheim group, who were able to demonstrate conclusively that hypnotic phenomena were not due to magnetism, but were psychological in nature. During the 1890's, through the work of several men, including Janet (1925), a student of Charcot, the use of direct suggestion under hypnotic trance became a full-fledged medical technique. Simultaneously other scholars, notably Breuer and Freud (1912), discovered the possibilities of "exploding" psychological complexes through abreaction, or the reliving under trance of traumatic experiences.

Abandonment of Hypnosis by Freud

During the early 1900's the practice of medical hypnosis, because of an unfortunate set of circumstances, ran into a blind alley which brought about its abandonment for nearly thirty years. First, it was discovered that the therapeutic attempts to eliminate symptoms by direct suggestion under trance, or through the abreaction of traumatic experiences, were frequently ineffective. This discouragement was further increased by the overenthusiastic application of the technique to all types of disorders. The many inevitable failures tended to turn medical men against it.

The second major reason for its decline was the failure of its followers to develop an effective, dynamic psychopathology. The men who practiced hypnosis were doing so blindly. They did not know what they were doing, nor why it achieved results. It remained for Freud and the psychoanalysts to establish a theoretical conception of neurotic disorders and develop an accompanying therapy.

This might have reawakened an interest in the field had it not been for the unfortunate, premature rejection of hypnosis by Breuer and Freud. Freud found that the abreactive and direct suggestive methods practiced at that time could not successfully overcome deep, unconscious resistances. Furthermore, because of popular misconceptions and prejudices the practitioner of hypnosis was in some danger of accusations of malpractice. For these reasons Freud abandoned its practice and devoted himself to the development of the dynamic theory of psychopathology known as *psychoanalysis,* and the therapeutic methods of free association, dream analysis, and analysis of transference. It is not our province, at this point, to go into a further description of psychoanalytic theory, except to note that Freud taught (see Freud, 1935) that "psychoanalysis . . . only began with my rejection of the hypnotic technique." Because of the tremendous prestige of Freud, the master and founder of psychoanalysis, his followers accepted this as a final instruction to avoid the use of hypnosis. As a result, the analysts lost very early a valuable therapeutic tool, while the practice of hypnosis was left largely to those psychologists and physicians who were not sympathetic to the psychoanalytic viewpoint.

Most of the objections of Freud and his followers that under hypnotic trance the natural Ego resistances are laid aside (and hence cannot be worked through and resolved), and that hypnosis reaches only very superficial layers of the unconscious, have not been corroborated (Wolberg, 1945, 1948). And now, some thirty years later, a new interest in the technique is evolving.

During the past three decades the clinical and therapeutic use of the method has been extremely limited. Charlatans and showmen have used hypnosis for stage demonstrations to entertain the public. Naturally, this aroused a fear in physicians that they would be considered unethical if they also used it in their treatment. Most of the development during this period was due to the research psychologists (Hull, 1933). The therapy described in this book is based upon both psychoanalytic studies and experimental findings of the psychological or nonanalytic group.

Theories of Hypnosis

Perhaps the most significant question that can be asked is, "What is hypnosis?" Frankly, at the present time, the answer must be, "We don't know." There are many theories, no one of which appears to be adequate. Merely calling it *suggestion* only tacks on another label. It certainly does not describe what happens within the body.

It has been visualized as a form of *dissociation,* or a splitting of segments from the personality structure. Janet (1907) espoused this theory. While it is true that a hypnotized person can act very much like an individual who is dissociated, hypnosis appears to include much more. *Dissociation* is still only a term used to describe a form of behavior about whose basic nature we know practically nothing.

Salter (1944) has tried to explain it on the basis of a conditioned reflex, and indeed, word-stimuli frequently trip off in the hypnotized patient a set of action patterns much like a conditioned response. Yet the concept of the conditioned reflex appears to be quite inadequate to explain the process. The gap between psychology and neurology, still a wide gulf, leaves us with no true knowledge as to what happens physiologically within the brain when any idea or psychological process occurs. Physiological explanations of hypnosis have usually been pure conjecture, while the psychological ones have clothed themselves largely in a verbiage which is more descriptive than explanatory.

However, it is possible to describe the types of behavior which can and cannot be elicited under hypnosis. First, we do find that persons whose sensory-motor reactions are suggestible tend to be more hypnotizable. For example, we may expect an individual to be hypnotizable who, while his eyes are closed, sways a great deal and is very unsteady when suggestions of falling are given. Likewise, if he responds to the suggested idea of heat or cold on the body he tends to be more hypnotizable. We know, further, that the prestige of the hypnotist is important and that the confidence or faith which the patient has in the hypnotist is a crucial factor. Hypnotizability has not been effectively correlated with any other trait. It seems to bear little or no relation at all to intelligence (Hull, 1933). Possibly it, like many other psychological traits, is normally distributed among the population. Adequate proof on this point is still to be secured. Probably a few persons are highly hypnotizable, a few others are completely nonhypnotizable, and most lie somewhere in between.

Trance Phenomena

In the next chapter, methods for inducing the trance state are described in detail. However, they all involve the limitation of distracting stimuli or, as we might say, the restricting of the patient's environmental field and the inducing of relaxation through the repetition of monotonous suggestions. The patient entering an hypnotic trance will first merely relax, then close his eyes. Next, he will follow such simple suggestions as "You are now unable to open your eyes," or "Your hand is so heavy you cannot raise it." In a deeper stage of trance he can be given more active suggestions, such as "Your hand is rising in the air," or "Your eyes are opening, but you will remain in a sleep." During this stage of trance it is quite possible to require the subject to perform foolish and ludicrous actions. It is elementary suggestion phenomena of this type which, as exhibited by show people for entertainment on the stage, have disgusted the professional person and the intelligent layman and turned them against its more practical use in the therapeutic field.

Still more important is the actual restriction of the senses through direct suggestion, as for example, the anesthetization of a part of the body, rendering it unable to feel pain. This is usually astonishing to the layman, yet it is actually an elementary phenomenon.

Since hypnosis apparently reaches deeper and more unconscious layers of personality structure, subjects under trance have been found to possess *hypermnesia,* or superior memory. They can describe in detail events that happened to them at a very early age or recite selections which they had committed to memory years ago and had since forgotten. While hypermnesia still requires scientific validation by objective experiment, those who work in the field generally accept its existence. The evidence for it is common and overwhelming. A complicating feature, however, is the fact that the patient will sometimes "remember" a fantasied or imagined experience instead of a real one. It is not always easy to distinguish between a true and an imagined memory.

The patient may also be *regressed* under reasonably deep trance to an early age level. He not only remembers what happened then, but he acts in every way like an individual of that age (Spiegel, Shor, and Fishman, 1945). For example, when regressed to the age of seven he will read, write, and play games like a seven-year-old. There is at present controversy as to whether this is a form of "play-acting" (Young, 1940) or a true reversion to an early type of behavior (Wolberg, 1945). The writer is inclined to believe that nothing is ever forgotten by a person, and that later-acquired ideas and behavior patterns are merely superimposed upon earlier ones. These in a sense, have pushed the earlier systems down into the unconscious part of the personality structure. Ample precedent for this view exists in the psychological findings on the retroactive inhibition of learned material by similar-type material memorized afterwards (Swenson, 1941). The writer feels that under hypnotic regression more recently learned patterns are inhibited or blocked off—dissociated if you wish—thus permitting the earlier patterns again to become operative. Lindner (1944) has reported the successful regression of a patient to the first year of life.

One most interesting hypnotic phenomenon is that of *posthypnotic suggestion.* If a subject, while under trance, is given instructions and told he will follow them when he awakens, he does so and is generally unaware of the reasons why he acted accordingly. In fact, anything that can be suggested under trance can be suggested posthypnotically, provided trance is deep enough. Hypermnesia, amnesia, anesthesia of any part of the body, visual or auditory hallucinations, compulsions, obsessions, and the initiating or removing of pain can also be suggested posthypnotically, as can alterations in fundamental attitudes. These behavior patterns will be discussed at greater length in Chapter 7.

Apparently, the deeper the hypnotic trance, the more profound and the more permanent are the alterations in behavior patterns achieved through direct suggestion. The description of advanced phenomena will be left to later chapters, but enough has been said already to indicate that personality adjustments—some superficial and some deeper in nature, some temporary and some more permanent—can be brought about in the energy-pattern system of a hypnotized patient. It is exactly this type of adjustment which is our aim in motivating or developing insight in the person afflicted with a functional disorder. This should point to the important role which hypnosis is prepared to play in an effective psychotherapy.

Misconceptions About Hypnosis

There are certain misconceptions and prejudices about the field which might be clarified here. Some of these are widespread and serve as an effective barrier to the more extensive use of hypnosis. One is the fear by the uninformed that a patient may not emerge from trance—that the therapist will have difficulty in "bringing him out." This danger is probably nonexistent. During seven years prior to the completion of this book the writer has had occasion to hypnotize several hundred subjects. Never has it required more than ten seconds to bring any of them out of even the deepest trance.

Perhaps more valid popular fears are that hypnosis may be used by an unscrupulous person to bring about criminal behavior in a subject, that a person may be hypnotized against his will, or that he may be made to disclose, under trance, material that would be self-incriminating. Until recently the scientific view has been that persons cannot be forced to commit criminal acts under hypnotic trance; that they will refuse to do anything which violates their basic concepts of right and wrong. Often quoted is the case involving a young woman who was hypnotized before a group of professional men and told to remove her clothes (Janet, 1925). Instead, she instantly emerged from trance and slapped the hypnotist. Furthermore, it is commonly held, both in lay and scientific circles, that the individual cannot be forced to enter a trance against his will. Fairly conclusive experiments by Wells (1941) and Rowland (1939) have demonstrated that persons under trance conditions can indeed be induced to carry out dangerous and criminal actions through the suggestion of criminal compulsions to them. The writer concurs in this view-

point, which is also held by Estabrooks (1944). The case of the
young woman reported by Janet is invalid. It represented only a
clumsy, tactless, direct assault against her natural motivations. It
subjected her system to a sudden psychological shock resulting in
her being jarred out of trance. Likewise, the initiating of anxiety
and the failure of psychotherapy is nearly always the consequence
when the therapist directs a frontal attack against natural resistances
and inner drives.

In certain informal studies (Watkins, 1947b) the writer was able
to bring about criminal-like behavior in deeply hypnotized subjects
through the distortion of reality by suggested hallucinations and
delusions. These avoided a direct conflict with the right and wrong
concepts held by the subject. Suggestions were aligned with already
existing motivational structures. For example, an army private, not
neurotic, but normal, with a stable personality and good recommenda-
tions as a soldier, was induced under deep trance to make a homicidal
attack with the intention of strangling a high-ranking officer. (Even
striking a superior officer is a court-martial offense in the Army.)
The subject was told that the officer was a Japanese soldier trying
to kill him, and that he must kill the Jap first. His ferocious leap at
the officer, something he would have been terrified to do when out of
trance, required the interception of three husky assistants to prevent
severe harm to the officer.

In another case the same experiment was tried using two officer
friends. The suggestion was given one of them that the other was
a Jap soldier and that he must "kill or be killed." The subject not
only made a powerful attack on his friend, but also whipped out and
rapidly opened a large jack-knife which neither the writer nor his
assistants knew the subject possessed. Only rapid interception by
one of the assistants trained in Judo prevented a serious stabbing
from taking place. It will be noted that in both cases the subject was
not told he was going to kill an army officer, or another friend, but
that he was protecting his life against the attack of an enemy soldier.
However, reality was so distorted and hallucinated as to cause him
to take murderous and antisocial action. Nevertheless, both of these
subjects would have been convicted of murder if they had been permitted to complete their actions and the court had believed the traditional scientific view that criminal behavior cannot be induced under
hypnosis. The extent to which a suggested compulsion alone without
hallucinations could initiate hostile behavior has not yet been tested.

The point of view that individuals actually can be induced to
engage in criminal and immoral behavior under hypnotic trance is

apparently growing as evidenced by a recent legal case. A recent Associated Press dispatch [2] reports the sentencing of a hypnotist to five to fifteen years in prison upon conviction of a breach of the "felony morals act" on a young woman. At the trial a state psychiatrist testified that "some persons when hypnotized could be induced to commit immoral and even criminal acts."

It may be argued that immoral or criminal behavior can be elicited under hypnosis only if impulses to perform these acts are already present. This may indeed be the true situation. However, this makes the responsibility of society to control hypnotists no less. The psychoanalytic point of view holds that in the unconscious part of personality known as the Id there exist in everyone primitive instinctual drives of a hostile and erotic nature. These are controlled in the normal person by the development of the Super-Ego. The Super-Ego, governed by the duty principle, forces the Ego to adjust and reconcile the pleasure-seeking Id drives to the realities of ethical and social demands. In deep psychoanalysis immoral and criminal impulses are commonly found in every person analyzed. There are sound biological and anthropological reasons for hypothesizing their universality. Hence, it would not be illogical to assume that if under hypnosis Super-Ego controls might be temporarily blocked, anesthetized, or even softened, these more primitive impulses might be made operative and initiate actual antisocial behavior.

As to the second contention, namely that individuals cannot be hypnotized against their will, the writer has upon several occasions successfully hypnotized subjects known to be highly suggestible who had been offered sizable sums of money to keep from entering trance. The subject was seated at a table. A ten-dollar bill was then placed in front of him. He was next told that the money would be his provided he would not go to sleep and could keep from entering trance. In several cases a deep trance was induced in less than thirty seconds while the patient was staring at the ten-dollar bill and ineffectually trying to keep his eyes open. Cases of this type, however, are the exception and certainly do not apply to most persons, where voluntary cooperation is almost always essential.

As to the third point—that individuals can be induced under hypnotic trance to divulge information which would be self-incriminating—that also is true. Seldom can material which has been voluntarily suppressed be withheld once the patient has actually been placed in a trance. The writer conducted a number of experiments

[2] Datelined Martinez, California, April 1, 1948.

in which monetary bribes were offered subjects to withhold pieces of information (1947b). When placed in trance they "spilled" every time, either verbally or in writing. Examples of this included the securing of material which the subject, an enlisted WAC in a Military Intelligence department, had been ordered by her commanding officer not to reveal. In another case the experiment was discontinued when it became obvious that the subject, a research worker in a government arsenal, was revealing vital and secret war information. This she began to do in front of a professional group of approximately 200 persons. Her disclosure of this information, if she had been permitted to continue, would have subjected her to a general court martial.

The writer, therefore, concludes that:

1. Hypnotic suggestion, when used indirectly and subtly, can cause *some* subjects to perform antisocial and criminal acts which they would not normally do.
2. At least a few persons can be hypnotized against their will.
3. Secret or self-incriminating knowledge may be disclosed by a subject under hypnotic trance.

Restrictions on the Use of Hypnosis

It is apparent from this that hypnosis is indeed a dangerous tool in the hands of a criminal or unethical hypnotist. So, also, are knives, guns, and narcotic drugs. Yet society does not abolish them for this reason. It merely places restrictions about the sale and use of weapons and requires that the prescription of narcotic drugs be limited to those who are professionally and ethically prepared to assume the necessary social responsibility. Society must do likewise with hypnosis.

The most valid objection to the lay use of hypnosis lies in the fact that under trance a person's inner, unconscious Ego—his soft, under-personality structure—is laid bare. He thus becomes much more easily molded for better or for worse. The actual steps in inducing hypnotic trance are rather widely known, and the description in Chapter 6 of the methods used by the writer adds little new in this area. The induction of trance and gaining of access to a patient's unconscious is comparatively simple and can probably be learned by anyone.[3] Likewise, it is not difficult for a layman to read in a surgical

---

3 At Welch Convalescent Hospital the writer conducted a one-month class in hypnotherapy (1947c). There were a dozen students, psychiatrists and psychologists. The methods

book how to use a scalpel. However, society still does not permit a man, unless he is surgically trained and thoroughly versed in human physiology and anatomy, to cut into the soft inner tissues of the human body and operate. The same should be true regarding hypnosis. The psychological harm a blunderer may do in unnecessarily initiating phobias, stirring up conflicts, increasing anxiety, or inducing harmful compulsions, further underlines the constant warning given in this treatise to the layman—*leave the practice of hypnosis and hypnotherapy to the professionally trained clinician.*

At the present time there is a new interest in hypnotherapy and hypnoanalysis. General physicians, psychiatrists, and psychologists are becoming increasingly aware of its potentialities. This brings up the question as to who *should* hypnotize and practice hypnotherapy. It is much easier to say who should not than who should. We might suggest that the practice of hypnosis could be limited to the psychiatrist, to the clinical psychologist, and to the psychologically trained or psychiatrically oriented physician. It is a specialized technique requiring a good knowledge of psychology, psychopathology, and psychodynamics—the anatomy and physiology of mental behavior. He who does not have considerable training in these essentials, whether he be a psychologist or physician, had better refer cases needing hypnotherapy to the specialist, just as the general practitioner will not ordinarily perform a lobotomy but will refer to the skilled surgeon.

A Reading List

Professional people may wish to delve further into the field of hypnosis. For a scientific account of its development and objective research studies the reader is referred to Bramwell (1930) and Hull (1933). Jenness (1944) presents a less comprehensive but more up-to-date summary than Hull. Young (1931, 1941) has also published critical reviews of the literature. An authoritative account of modern hypnoanalytic procedures has been given by Wolberg (1945, 1948), while an excellent treatise on this subject has also been released by Brennan and Gill (1947). LeCron and Bordeaux (1947) have published a comprehensive and practical reference which is divided between a discussion of theories and facts about hypnosis and brief hypnotherapeutic procedures in the treatment of various

---

of teaching included lecture, discussion, demonstration, and supervised practice with actual subjects. Instructional time totaled twenty hours. All the students were successful in learning how to induce trance and initiate the various hypnotic phenomena as described in Chapters 6, 7, and 8 of this book.

emotional conditions. An interesting account of hypnosis, designed more for the lay reader, has been published by Estabrooks (1944). Those therapists interested in detailed reports of various cases and techniques are referred to the excellent set of papers by Erickson (1935, 1937a, 1937b, 1938, 1939a, 1939b, 1939c, 1939d, 1939e, 1943a, 1943b, 1943c, 1944a, 1944b, 1945) and by Erickson and Kubie (1938, 1939, 1940, 1941). Other interesting recent developments have been reported by Fisher (1943), Kubie (1943), Kubie and Margolin (1942, 1944), Simmel (1944), Wells (1944), and many others whom space does not permit us to mention.

CHAPTER 6

INDUCING TRANCE STATES

Many professional therapists have hesitated to use hypnosis. Frequently, this is because they do not know how to induce the trance state or are afraid of failure if they attempt to do so. This beginning hurdle is a difficult one, especially since the therapist who has a fear that he will not succeed usually transmits this uncertainty to the patient. That factor alone can cause him to fail.

This chapter is designed for the benefit of those *professional therapists* who wish to learn how to use hypnosis and who need instruction in what is actually said and done to induce the hypnotic state.

Approaches to Hypnosis

There are two fundamental approaches to hypnosis. The first is the overpowering or dominating one, in which the hypnotist virtually orders the subject into trance. It is a highly emotional approach and is most commonly used by entertainers on the amusement stage. When effective it is very rapid, the subject frequently entering a deep trance in a few seconds. For purposes of therapy, however, it has many grave limitations. It is based on fear, while the chief values derived in the uncovering of conflicts under hypnotic trance lie in the positive transference relationship between therapist and patient. Only mutual confidence and rapport can bring this about. Therefore, this method of inducing trance destroys the fundamental basis of the patient-therapist relationship.

Accordingly, the therapist prefers a persuading technique, one in which trance is induced through voluntary acquiescence. The patient is persuaded to enter an hypnotic condition through his complete trust in the therapist. Perhaps the psychoanalyst would describe the first method as the *father* approach and the second as the *mother* technique. It is customary for our fathers to dominate us directly. Our mothers generally control us by more persuasive methods. It seems quite possible that the father approach would have serious repercussions for a patient who is suffering from an Oedipus complex. He might identify the therapist with his hated father and reject him accordingly.   So let us concentrate on the more persuasive methods of inducing an hypnotic state.[1]

Each therapist will develop his own variations of the methods given here, but several approaches will be presented in detail, including word for word just what the therapist does and says when inducing the hypnotic condition.

Postural-Swaying Method

The first one to be described might be called the *Postural-Swaying Method*. With some persons it is most rapid. An individual who either does not respond at all or requires many minutes to go into trance by a reclining method may enter a trance in a few minutes by this method. There is also the advantage that it can begin merely as a test of suggestibility. If this test proceeds satisfactorily it can be turned into an actual method of inducing trance.

The therapist speaks to the patient as follows: "Now Jones, I'd like to have you stand here with your heels and your toes together and your body erect, shoulders back. That's right. Breathe comfortably and easily with your hands at your sides. Now close your eyes. Just imagine that your feet are hinged to the floor and your body is like a stick pointing upward in the air, free to move back and forth. You will probably find after awhile, you will become unsteady. Don't worry, if you should fall, I'll catch you." (This last remark is given in a rather matter-of-fact way, almost as a side comment. If previous suggestibility tests have been given, and the therapist is quite certain the patient will enter trance, he may modify this statement by saying, "Don't worry, I will catch you *when* you fall.")

The therapist then continues: "Now while you are standing there, breathe very calmly and easily. Just imagine that your body is floating up into space. Don't try to do anything, and don't try *not* to do anything. Just stand there and let yourself drift." The therapist is then silent for a time, perhaps fifteen seconds up to a minute. If the patient is suggestible he will sway back and forth slightly.

The therapist should place himself at the side of the patient where he can line the back of the patient's head or the tip of his nose against a mark on the opposite wall so that a slight backward or forward swaying movement can be easily detected and measured. It is even convenient to have a card against the wall on which black vertical lines

---

[1] The dominating approach might be effective when working with male homosexuals or females having an Electra (father-fixation) complex.

have been ruled about an inch apart, thus making it easier to determine the amount of sway. Usually the therapist will soon detect the rhythm of the swaying, since it is almost impossible for anybody to stand perfectly still. There will always be some swaying, although it may be slight in the more unsuggestible patients. One will generally find that the more suggestible the patient, the greater will be the amplitude of the swaying arc.

The therapist next begins to reinforce this swaying by timing his remarks to coincide with it. As soon as the patient has reached the extreme forward part of the arc and begins to sway backward the therapist says, "Now you are drifting backward." Frequently this will cause the patient immediately to catch himself and to reverse the direction, whereupon the therapist instantly follows it with, "Now you are drifting over forward." As the swaying continues the therapist reinforces it with "Drifting forward, drifting backward and forward, backward, forward, backward," etc. The tone is low, soft, and firm. The therapist should be about one to two feet away from the patient's ear and should repeat the suggestions in a low, soft monotone from which all harshness has been deleted. It should have an almost pleading quality, monotonous like the drone of a bee. There should be no change of pitch, and the patter should be continued steadily. Occasionally it may be varied from "drifting forward" to "Swaying forward, swaying backward, swaying over backward, now swaying forward," or "Leaning forward, backward, forward, backward," etc.—on and on in a monotonous, repetitious voice.

As the therapist observes the amplitude of the swaying arc increasing, he may make his voice somewhat less pleading, less soft, and more dominant and controlling, even injecting some emotional pitch into the "forward, backward, forward, backward."

When the amplitude of the swaying arc has become quite substantial—six or more inches—it is probable that some light degree of trance has been induced. Suggestibility should then be checked by beginning a command of "forward, backward" a little before the patient has reached the maximum sway of the arc. If the patient is suggestible, and there is a degree of hypnotic trance, he will interrupt the natural sway in order to follow the therapist's suggestion. The past remarks of the therapist have so closely followed the patient's swaying behavior that the patient begins to think to himself, "What this man says is true, I am swaying backward. Then I do sway forward." Consequently, the therapist's prestige is increased, and the patient begins to follow the suggestions instead of leading them.

From this point on the therapist can generally assume the more dominating role and direct rather than follow the swaying of the patient.

To induce deeper trance the voice tone is now made much firmer, and the swaying suggestions are given somewhat more rapidly. *"Swaying forward, swaying backward, forward, backward,"* the volume of the voice growing stronger and stronger. Finally, attempt is made to induce the patient to fall over backward into a deep trance. The emphasis on the "backward" is increased, and on the "forward" diminished, and the verb is changed from "drifting" or "swaying" to "falling, *falling backward,* falling forward, *falling backward,* falling forward, *falling over backward,* falling, falling, *falling, falling"* rather rapidly and in a higher-pitched and more emotional tone. If a deep trance has been induced, the patient will increase the amplitude of his sway until he can no longer stand erect. He will then fall over backward in a deep trance state where he may be caught by the therapist and eased into a waiting chair.

If the patient is in a light trance only he may start to fall backward, but catch himself by placing one of his feet back, or attempt to sway sideways or steady himself voluntarily in some manner. This indicates to the therapist that a deep trance has not yet been induced, and he can then do one of two things: he may either continue the monotonous repetition of "falling forward, falling backward," etc., to induce a deeper degree of trance; or he may reassure the patient that he will not fall by placing a hand lightly behind his shoulder. This allays fears which might arise and interrupt the hypnotic process. After the patient realizes that he will not be permitted to fall and hurt himself, he tends to lose the signs of anxiety which may have begun to appear. He may then allow himself to fall back against the therapist's arm, whereupon the therapist continues the suggestions, "Falling over backward, falling backward, falling back into a deep sleep, back into a deep sleep, deep sleep, deep sleep," and then eases the patient gradually over into a chair. This, preferably an arm chair, should have been placed behind the patient. He can also be gradually lowered back upon a couch which has been located conveniently near.

If the patient is either completely limp or in a stiff catatonic state when he is placed back on the chair or cot, it is evidence that a fairly deep degree of trance has been induced. If, however, he is able to help himself either by taking steps backward or by putting his hands on the armchair and guiding himself into it, then only a light ·or hypnoidal trance has been induced.

With the patient seated or lying down, and a light trance induced, a deeper level may be reached by continuing the suggestions or by the use of a metronome, which will be described later. Whether or not the patient is ready for therapy at this point will depend upon the depth or intensity of work to be done at that particular session. This can be determined only after the therapist has had considerable experience in hypnotizing patients.

Lindner (1944) defers actual treatment until a subject has been able to acquire thorough facility in attaining deep trance and exhibiting the advanced phenomena. This writer prefers to initiate treatment at once and undertake deeper hypnotherapy as increased rapport makes these lower levels accessible. Moreover, it appears as if interviewing under light trance, even hypnoidal states, is quite fruitful. Free associations and dream recapitulations are much richer even under a light narcosis.

The postural-swaying method has a great advantage in that it appears quite harmless to the patient. The therapist merely needs to tell him at the beginning that he wishes to "check reflexes," observe his "nervous reaction," give him a "reflex test," or determine his ability to relax while on his feet. Furthermore, this method of trance induction is not the one popularly established in the public mind. There is often less anxiety and apprehension than when the patient is seated or told to recline on a cot while the therapist makes passes with the hands in front of his eyes. The patient merely thinks that he is taking some type of "nervous test." He doesn't feel he is being placed "in the power" of the therapist. The most important element in this as in other "persuading" methods is the elimination of fear by a soothing, firm, reassuring voice. Once the voice begins it should continue in a steady patter without interruption and with an even tenor of pitch and speed.

A good rule to be followed in all methods of trance induction is to *avoid challenges until you are certain you can meet them.* Do not tell the patient that he will be unable to open his eyes until it becomes evident that he cannot do so. This will require shrewd observation of his reactions and a correct judgment of his condition. Each time a challenge is made in which the therapist is successful (that is, the patient cannot meet the challenge) the therapist will have made significant progress and can then continue into the induction of a deeper degree of trance. However, if a challenge is issued which fails, the therapist loses prestige and further immediate attempts to induce hypnosis are likely to result in failure.

Eye-Fixation Method

Another common method is that of *Eye Fixation* on some bright object. This can be done with the patient either seated or lying down on a couch. Some patients will respond quickly when seated. Others expect to lie down, because they are to receive a "relaxation or sleep treatment." The fixation object may be a shiny pen, pencil, bright light, or even one or two of the therapist's fingers. But, it should be held fairly close, three to eight inches away from the eyes, and in such a position that the patient must strain his eyes upward. If the object is that close, a high degree of convergence will be forced. The eyes of the patient tend to cross and point upward. This, of course, is extremely tiring to the eye muscles. The therapist thereby gains as his ally the strong natural desire to relieve this fatigue by closing the eyes. Here, as in the postural swaying method, the therapist builds upon and reinforces by suggestion any small natural muscular tensions and movements which appear.

Let us suppose that the patient has been told to lie down on the cot, and the eye-fixation object has been placed in position.[2] The therapist might then talk to the patient as follows : "Now, just stretch your arms and legs out. That's it; relax all over. Breathe easily and calmly, slow, in, out. That's good. Get the feeling of lying down to sleep without a single care in the world. Imagine that you are float-ing in a boat [3] on a warm, sunny afternoon, easy, calm, and relaxed, all through yourself. Just let the tension go, all through your legs, through your neck muscles, through your arms, your hands, your eyes and your head. Float away; don't try to *make* yourself go to sleep; don't try to *keep* from going to sleep; just let yourself drift very calmly." Suggestions of this type might be repeated over and over again. It is essential that a calm, steady flow of patter of this type be continued; that the voice be low, firm, resolute, solid-pitched, without harshness in it, and with a soft, persuading, pleading type

---

[2] The writer frequently uses a 10-watt blue electric light bulb. This has been found effective, patients reporting that as they entered trance they felt as if they were sinking into a blue cloud. The entire field of vision became a soft, blue light. Blue was subjectively chosen because it is a cool, restful color. Green might evoke certain eerie or fear-provoking associations in the minds of some patients. When this light was affixed to the wall with an adjustable bracket the therapist was relieved of the fatigue of holding a bright object over the eyes of the reclining patient. This left his hands free to take notes.

[3] In describing to the patient the scene of lying in a boat the therapist should use his imagination as much as possible and give it free rein. The more vivid he makes the adjectives, the better the picture he conjures into the patient's mind, the more likely it is that the patient will react with an hypnotic sleep.

of timbre. It can be almost a sotto voce, slightly-above-a-whisper volume. The therapist then continues : [4]

> You will probably find after a while that you feel sort of drowsy and rather sleepy, just imagine how it would be if your eyelids were very, very heavy, you would feel as if a thousand-pound weight were tied on each eyelid, trying to pull it down, and it would seem as if the eyes kept wanting to come down, as if it would feel so very, very good if they could just naturally close and you could go into a calm, easy, restful type of sleep, and the eyelids keep getting heavier and heavier and heavier and pulling slowly downward, until it does not feel as if they could possibly stay awake, and you feel sleepier and drowsier, and a comfortable glow comes over your entire body, all the nervous tensions that you have had today seem to float away, you feel as if your body was just drifting, and you were floating off into a nice comfortable, dark,[5] warm space, drifting, drifting, drifting, you get more and more drowsy, more and more sleepy, see how well you can relax, how easy and comfortable it feels, how much more you would like to go into a very, very deep sleep, and now you feel that your eyes are slowly closing, slowly closing, slowly closing, slowly closing, now you feel as if you are going off into a deep sleep, deep sleep, sleep, sleep, deeper sleep, the eyes are closing, closing, closing, almost tightly closed, almost tightly closed, almost tightly closed, tightly closed, tightly closed, *tightly closed.*

At this point the therapist speaks the last "tightly closed" in a rather firm, solid, resolute, voice, with a louder pitch, displaying confidence in what he is saying. At the same time he places the index finger of his hand rather firmly just above the bridge of the patient's nose and between his eyebrows. This tends to reinforce the verbal suggestions of eye-closure with tactile emphasis. Suggestions should be given through all possible sensory channels—touch, sound, and sight. The more senses utilized, the more effective the suggestions will be.

This last "tightly closed," spoken in a firm, confident, strong voice with the simultaneous pressure of the finger above the nose bridge, is actually the first challenge issued by the therapist. He does not

---

[4] Much of the following verbal report of the trance-inducing suggestions is given without the use of punctuating periods or complete sentences. The sentences are merely tied together by commas. This is done because a period implies a break in the monotone and a drop in voice pitch which is not best while giving the suggestions. The sentences are actually run together. Practice them that way.

[5] One patient woke up at this point. He explained that he had a fear of the dark, and the idea mobilized his resistance to the hypnotic process. Trance was then rapidly induced by using such visual imagery as: "You are floating up into the light, into the sun, and the deeper you go into a sleep the more comfortable and bright everything will be." When possible know your patient's fears and avoid associating to them.

give it until the patient's eyes have almost completely closed. In determining when to try this first challenge he is guided by the breathing of the patient and by other signs of relaxation. Usually, the eyes will first take on a staring appearance. They may blur with tears. The eyelids may wink or flutter. As trance comes on it is likely that they will slowly close, and the eyeballs will roll upward. Only practice and experience will prepare the therapist to know the right moment to change the suggestion of "tightly closed" to a challenge by manner and volume of voice. Always keep the suggestions close to the reality of the patient's behavior. Do not try to anticipate or lead too far ahead.

Notice the reassurance constantly given that the patient will feel better as he goes into the sleep—more comfortable.

With anxiety patients, one will often notice a tendency for tension to increase, indicating repressed hostility. The patient apparently is unconsciously reacting in a negative manner. Reassurance can sometimes be given merely by putting the hand on the shoulder or by stroking the arm or the muscles of the neck to induce greater relaxation and build up rapport.

If after several minutes of suggestion of this type, five at least, the patient's eyes do not close, it is wise to tell him to close his eyes—a simple direction as if it were naturally part of the treatment. ("Just close your eyes now.")

The therapist should be quick to observe any tiny reactions of the eyes and to capitalize on them. Thus, if the eyes blink, which they often do, the therapist immediately remarks, "Your eyes are so tired, they keep blinking as if they want to close, they can hardly stay awake, they don't want to stay awake, they want to close." This is injected into the steady patter without a break and is precisely timed. If the patient's eyes have closed through suggestion and have not opened when the therapist has said "closed" in the final, firm, solid voice with pressure of the finger above the nose bridge, he is then ready to test the depth of trance further by giving an additional challenge as follows: "Now you will find that your eyes are so tightly closed that they will not want to come open. In fact, they will feel so tightly closed that it would seem as if the harder you tried to open them, the tighter they would stay together—the harder you try to open them, the tighter they stay together—the harder you *try* to open them the tighter they stick together, tightly stuck together, so very tightly stuck together that they would not come apart no matter how hard you try. They will not come apart no matter how hard you try. They will remain tightly closed. Try to pull them apart."

Read that last group of suggestions over again and notice how they gradually build up into a challenge. If the patient makes a half-hearted effort to open his eyes, wrinkling his brows, let him do it not more than once or twice and then immediately announce in a firm voice, "See, your eyes are tightly closed. Now you will be able to go into an even deeper sleep." In other words, do not continue having him try to meet this challenge, but let him fail once or twice and then immediately take it for granted that he cannot succeed and divert his attention from any further attempts.[6]

Inducing Deeper Trance

He is now ready for the next step in entering a still deeper trance. The writer has found the following an effective device to accomplish this.

I have placed the point of my finger on your forehead. Radiating out from the point will be a dull, numb, glowing sensation. It spreads in all directions—through your scalp, down into your face, your nose, your lips, the chin and into the neck. It sweeps on like an all-engulfing wave. As it comes over you it makes you want to go down into a deeper sleep. It makes your body feel as if it were not part of you any longer, but sinking out into space. And the numb, cool, glowing feeling gets ever stronger, ever stronger, making you feel increasingly happy and comfortable. Now it sweeps down into your shoulders and courses out into the arms, down through the elbows, the wrists through the hands and out into the fingers making the tips glow with the comfortable numb feeling. Then it sweeps back up the arms and irresistibly down into the chest, the stomach. It makes your body get heavier and heavier. Now down the thighs, and the knees, into the lower leg, the calves, the ankles, down into the feet, spreading back into the heels and fanning out into the toes. Then with ever-increasing force it begins to roll back up your legs sending you down, down, down into a comfortable, dull, numb, heavy, glowing sleep, etc.

The "wave" is then just as vividly described rolling back up the body. The more picturesque the description, the more effective the suggestions. This device will usually bring about a deeper trance. It can be employed several times with various tests of trance depth interspersed.

---

6 In his more recent handling of civilian cases the writer is lessening the use of "challenges" to indicate trance depth. The patients treated in Company F were known to be hypnotizable. This is not the case with the average civilian patient who presents himself to a clinician for treatment. Greater caution must therefore be used since premature "challenges" may only serve to mobilize increased resistance in the lightly hypnotizable.

After each depth of trance has been successfully reached and proved by tests the suggestion might be given, "You can [7] now go into a deeper sleep, deep sleep, deep sleep. You are relaxing all over, down into the deepest and darkest sleep you have ever been in." As previously mentioned, the word "dark" may be used except with patients in whom a phobia toward the dark is suspected. However, repetition of the phrase, "Down into the deepest and darkest sleep" is usually very effective.

At this point a challenge might be given which involves a larger group of muscles than those in the eye. If this test is successful, it is certainly indicative of a deeper degree of trance than that exhibited by eye closure and catalepsy. Take the patient's two hands and clasp them together, the fingers interlaced. Then tell him to imagine, "The blood and power are coming down into your arms, through your arms, through your wrists, down into your fingers," and as you say this stroke the arms and wrists down into the hands and continue: "Just imagine that the hands are getting tighter and tighter together, until the fingers are gripping each other with fingers of steel, tighter, tighter, *tighter*," giving these last commands in a resolute, firm, and commanding manner. "Make the fingers grip each other so tightly that no matter how hard I try, I cannot pull them apart." At this point the therapist takes a couple of the fingers and appears to make an effort to pull the fingers apart, failing in the attempt, of course. He then continues (notice how this works up to the challenge) :

"You see, the fingers are so tightly gripped together that I cannot pull them apart no matter how hard I try. No matter how hard we would try, those fingers get tighter and tighter together, and it seems as if the harder we try to pull them apart, the tighter they grip each other. No matter how hard we try, they will not come apart. No matter how hard you try, they will not come apart. No matter how hard *you* try, they will not come apart." Notice how the suggestions have run the gamut from *"I can't* pull them apart" to *"We can't* pull them apart" to "You *can't* pull them apart" to *"You* can't pull them apart." If the fingers seem to be gripping each other firmly, and it appears certain the patient cannot separate them, then the therapist issues a direct challenge such as, "You see, no matter how hard you try they will not come apart, because the harder you try to pull them apart, the tighter they will stick together. Try to pull them apart— see, they will not come apart."

---

[7] Notice use of the term "can" in a permissive sense. This does not challenge.

The challenge should again be interrupted while the patient is still trying and before he succeeds in pulling them apart. This can be done in the following way: "All right, you see, they will not come apart; now you can relax and can go into a still deeper sleep." The patient's failure to meet the challenge is made to appear as an actual achievement on his part. The therapist then takes the patient's clenched hands and gently draws them apart.

Testing for Depth of Trance

If the patient has not been able to meet the challenge of opening his eyes or unclasping his hands, you should now be able to induce a catatonic state in his arm or a paralysis and anesthesia by direct suggestion as follows: The therapist lifts the arm up into the air, and then while stroking it, says to the patient, "Your arm is becoming stiff and rigid, straight like a board, stiffer, and stiffer. It cannot move up. It cannot move down. It is losing all movement and all feeling. It's losing all sense of touch. It doesn't hurt. It has no feeling or pain. It's all numb, completely through. No matter how hard you try you cannot move it up or down, and it will not have any sense of feeling whatsoever." [8] The arm will usually become quite stiff and rigid, extending out into the air. If the therapist slowly removes his own supporting hands the arm will stick straight out, unbending, by itself. Anesthesia can be checked by pinching it or yanking out a few hairs on the arm, observing carefully the patient's eyelids at that moment to see if there is any fluttering or wincing. Of course, pricking with a sterilized needle will also indicate whether there is any sense of pain. It is wise after the patient has emerged from trance to question him concerning his reaction to these tests. If he had reached a stage of deep trance he will not even remember what was done. If he had achieved a medium trance he can recall it, but will state that he could not have changed or controlled it—that he felt impelled to follow the therapist's instructions. A patient who has experienced only a light trance will usually say that he could feel the arm pinched, but that it was somewhat numb. Careful records should be kept about the degree and intensity of the patient's reactions in each trance session. These can prove very effective in guiding the therapist during future meetings.

After the test the patient's arm is stroked, and he is told, "Your arm is relaxing. The feeling and movement are coming back into it,

---

[8] A firm, commanding voice full of confidence should now be employed.

and it is going down normally." A test involving hand levitation, which indicates a deeper trance, can now be tried.

The patient is told, "Your hand is slowly rising up into the air. It is floating as if it were a cork bobbing up to the surface of the water, as if it were pulled by invisible chains. You do not have to pull it up, and you *cannot* keep it down. The higher it rises into the air, the deeper you will go to sleep. And the deeper you sleep, the deeper you will *want* to sleep. The hand will slowly float up into the air, until it touches you on the face, and when it touches you on the face, that will be a sign to you that you are in the very deepest possible sleep." [9] Suggestions of this type are continued and reinforced, sometimes by a slight pull on the shirt sleeve if necessary, until the patient's hand does float up and touch his face. The hand-levitation test given in this way is usually indicative of a fairly deep degree of trance. Patients are often amnesic to it after emerging from sleep.

An interesting variation in the suggestions given to induce hand levitation when the patient is obviously negativistic is as follows: "I am going to put pressure on your hand by pushing mine down on it. You will notice shortly that the more strongly I press down the lighter it will tend to get. It will tend to respond by rising up and pushing back against my hand, and the longer I push against it, the stronger will be its tendency to rise. Soon the forces floating your hand upward will be greater than I can meet in trying to hold your hand down." When the upward pressure of the patient's hand begins to get very strong the therapist gradually lifts his. Whereupon the patient's hand will rise up into the air and continue to force the therapist's palm higher.

Use of Metronome in Inducing Trance

Two fundamental methods for inducing hypnotic trance, postural swaying and eye fixation, have been discussed. Another technique, which is very simple and often quite effective both as a basic method of inducing trance and as a supplementary device to deepen it, is the use of a metronome. The metronome should be placed near the cot, but where it cannot be observed by the patient. It should be set at a very slow rate. The writer uses about fifty beats to the minute and muffles the tone by putting it in a closed cabinet because some patients claimed that the loud tick was more disturbing than soothing.

After the usual suggestions of relaxation are given to the patient he is told, "Now I am going to turn on a slow ticking sound. This

[9] This test is described by Dr. M. H. Erickson (1945a).

will help you to go to sleep. Listen very carefully to it and to nothing else. It goes like this." The metronome is turned on. Then the therapist continues, "Just imagine each tick saying to you, 'deep—sleep, —deep—sleep,' and the deeper you go into sleep the deeper you will want to go. How comfortable you will feel all over. Just keep on listening to this ticking sound which says over and over again, 'deep—sleep, —deep—sleep.' " The therapist may even continue speaking the words "deep—sleep" for a little while, timing them to coincide with the ticking.

Another variation of this technique is to suggest to the patient that as he listens to the ticking he will imagine himself slowly going down a ladder or stairway. "Each tick is saying 'step—down, —step—down,' or 'deep—sleep, —step—down,' " etc. He may be told, "As you go down this ladder you will feel that you are going down into a deeper and deeper sleep." The writer commonly uses the eye-fixation method to induce eye closure and eye catalepsy. After tests for these have been successful he turns on the metronome with the suggestion that it is saying "deep—sleep" or "step—down" and leaves the patient for a period of ten minutes to a half hour. It has been found that this is effective in inducing a deeper degree of trance. It also saves the strength and energy of the therapist. Repeated suggestions of sleep continued in a monotonous tone of voice for an hour, or even for twenty minutes, are very fatiguing. Occasionally the patient will be told, "Now I am going to leave you here, listening to this ticking sound which will help you go into a deeper sleep. I am going away for a little while. When I come back you will be in the very deepest possible sleep." Sometimes the suggestion of hand levitation previously given is also made at this time, such as, "When you get into the very deepest sleep, the deepest you can possibly reach, your hand will slowly rise up in the air until it touches you on the forehead and stays there. This will be a sign to you that you are in the deepest possible sleep." If this suggestion has been effectively planted the therapist merely needs to come back to the treatment room at occasional intervals to observe whether the patient's hand has risen and is touching his forehead. This serves as an indicator that sedation under the metronome has been sufficiently continued to induce a deep trance. Some therapists have used a variation of this metronome method in which they amplify the sound of the patient's own breathing and play it back into a head set which he wears (Kubie and Margolin, 1942). The essential part is the routine, monotonous sound, and the restriction of the patient's attention from distracting stimuli.

Other Techniques

The writer has found a modification of the *descending-a-ladder* technique to be very effective in deepening a light trance state. It goes as follows:

> I want you to imagine you are standing at the top of a stairway. As you look down, the stairs get darker and darker and seem to fade away into space where you can't see. On this stairway is a thick, rich, soft, velvety carpet. This carpet has such a soft plush finish that you sink into it as you gently walk down the stairs. And everything is purple, a deep vivid purple, a purple which gets darker and darker the farther down the stairs you go. Now you are walking slowly down those stairs, down into a sleep, the deepest and most comfortable sleep you have ever been in. I shall walk beside you and count steps. Each count is one step down, one—two—three—four—. Down, down, down, step down, deeper, deeper, five—six, etc.

The therapist would often count up to a hundred this way, drawling the words out very slowly in a droning voice: "For—ty twoooo, for—ty threeeee, for—ty fourrrrr," etc. Every thirty or forty counts he would once more reinforce the picture of the soft carpeted steps and the deep purple hue. After a hundred counts a test of deeper trance depth might be administered, or a shift might be made to the suggestions of the "numb glow" spreading down the body. Some patients were quite unable to visualize "a numb glowing wave spreading down the body," or "the dark purple stairs." When visual imagery was weak, it was better to use the postural-swaying method, ease the patient over on a cot, and give ten to thirty minutes of metronome sedation.

Another technique is the *Waking Method*. The therapist should be quite sure of his patient before attempting this. It usually will not be tried the first time. If he is certain the patient is highly hypnotizable, the therapist proceeds as follows: "Now just close your eyes." (In this method the patient is usually seated or reclining.) "Imagine that the muscles in your eyelids are getting tighter and tighter and that a great deal of power is pulling the eyelids down, making them feel as if they were tightly stuck to the lower lids. They keep getting tighter and tighter and *tighter*." While the therapist is saying this, he observes the patient's eyes carefully to see if the lids are really pressing more tightly together. In the highly suggestible subject this will be so. If it does not occur, the patient is probably not suggestible enough to use the waking method of trance induction. After a minute or two with this type of suggestion the usual challenge that the patient cannot open his eyes is made in a confident manner as described in the eye-fixation method. If this is successful, the patient is then told to clasp his hands and the suggestions of increasing tension in the grip, followed by the challenge that he cannot pull his hands apart, are given. Deeper trance is induced by suggesting arm catalepsy, paralysis, etc. The only difference between this and other methods is that the word *sleep* is not used. The patient is taken directly from the waking condition to the trance state as control is secured over progressively larger muscle groups.

Ordinary sleep can be turned into hypnotic trance. In this technique, the therapist attempts to gain control of the sleeping patient by using a soft, whispering monotone which is not loud enough to awaken him. Thus, he might say, "You are now in a very, very deep sleep. You feel comfortable all over. You will stay in this deep sleep, but you will be able to hear me very clearly while in your sleep. To prove to yourself that you are in this deep sleep, but can hear me, your hand will slowly rise into the air," etc. It may take some time before the attention of the sleeping patient can be secured.

The hand-levitation suggestions can be expanded as follows: "Your hand is getting lighter and lighter. The fingers are beginning to leave the cot. They are beginning to float up into the air. They are being pulled up by invisible chains. You do not have to bring them up yourself, and you *cannot* keep them down. They want the hand to pull up more and more, up, up, up, up higher. Now your hand is beginning to lift. Now you can feel it coming slowly up into the air," etc.

Self-hypnosis is also possible (Salter, 1941). It is probably not to be recommended. The patient might try to experiment with himself when not in the presence of the therapist and get into difficulty. However, this method might be illustrated by the case of an actual patient who was known to be highly hypnotizable. He came for a treatment session one morning and asked, "Say, Doc, could I put myself to sleep?" He was told, "Why, certainly. Just lie down and relax as usual. Start looking up at that small spot on the ceiling. Now begin to count very slowly to yourself up to fifty, and as you do, feel that you are going into a deep sleep. By the time you reach fifty you will be sound asleep." The patient stared at the ceiling. In approximately thirty seconds his eyes closed. At the end of a minute the usual tests for trance-depth were administered and indicated a medium trance. After the initial instructions had been given, no words were spoken until the tests were made.

Tests of Hypnotic Susceptibility

Friedlander and Sarbin (1938) have developed a number of possible scales which might be used to estimate depth of trance. Among those which have been most widely used is the Susceptibility Test devised by Davis and Husband (1931), a suggestibility scale which assigns numerical values to various degrees of trance depth. Hypnotic phenomena that can be induced at the respective score levels are listed. This is convenient to the therapist, as he can assign a numerical score in reporting on the depth of trance in any session. This tells others what phenomena the patient was capable of exhibiting and what ones were beyond him at that particular session. This scale is useful in testing for trance depth. The Davis Scale is here reproduced, plus several additions (*) which are based on the writer's experience:

THE DAVIS AND HUSBAND HYPNOTIC SUSCEPTIBILITY TEST

Depth	Score	Objective Symptom
Insusceptible	0	
Hypnoidal	1	
	2	Relaxation
	3	Fluttering of lids
	4	Closing of eyes
	5	Complete physical relaxation
Light trance	6	Catalepsy of eyes
	7	Limb catalepsies
	*8	Hypermnesia, slight
	10	Rigid catalepsies
	11	Anesthesia (glove)
Medium trance	13	Partial amnesia
	15	Posthypnotic anesthesia
	*16	Hypermnesia, marked
	17	Personality changes
	18	Simple posthypnotic suggestions
	*19	Regression
	20	Kinesthetic delusions; complete amnesia
Deep trance	21	Ability to open eyes without affecting trance
	23	Bizarre posthypnotic suggestions
	25	Complete somnambulism
	26	Positive visual hallucinations, posthypnotic
	27	Positive auditory hallucinations, posthypnotic
	28	Systematized posthypnotic amnesias
	29	Negative auditory hallucinations
	30	Negative visual hallucinations, hyperesthesias
	*32	Negative visual hallucinations, posthypnotic

In the trance sessions described in the cases in this book trance depth was sometimes indicated by the above scores and other times merely as *Light, Medium,* or *Deep.*

Le Cron and Bordeaux (1947) have published a revision and expansion of the above scale based on their extensive experience. Scales of this type are badly in need of objective experimental validation. ·

Although the two basic methods of postural swaying and eye fixation, either seated or reclining, will be found adequate in most cases, no definite rules can be given. A patient may respond to one method of trance induction and not to another. Some hypnotists begin the suggestions of sleep by having the patient close his eyes at the start instead of fixating them on an object.

Most hypnotists like to give some type of suggestibility tests before trying to induce trance. They fear the loss of confidence by their patient if they fail, and they do not want to attempt hypnotic work unless they are assured of success in advance. Most of the suggestibility tests described in the literature involve definite challenges which will bring about a "loss of face" to the therapist who administers them to a resistant or nonhypnotizable patient. Here is a useful one which is both highly indicative of hypnotizability and does not involve a "challenge." The patient is seated (or he can stand) and told to extend both arms out in front of him, palms extended and downward, with the hands close together, but not touching. He is next instructed to close his eyes and then told to imagine that "A large bucket has been placed on top of your left hand. (The therapist strokes or lightly touches the hand.) Now, imagine that somebody is pouring water into the bucket, and it is becoming heavier, and heavier, and heavier." There are a few moments of silence. The therapist watches the patient's hands carefully to see if there is a noticeable tendency for the left hand to sink downward. After the test has been discontinued the patient may be asked whether he felt any difference in the sensations of fatigue in his left and right arm. A check on this test is to tell him, "Now the bucket is being taken off of your left hand and being placed on top of the right hand, and somebody again is pouring water into it, making it heavier and heavier." If now the right hand shows marked sinking below its previous level on line with the left hand, the patient is usually quite hypnotizable.

The failure to respond to this test, however, does not mean non-hypnotizability, although it generally implies that the induction of trance will not be easy.

Sarbin and Madow (1942) have reported a study indicating that the Rorschach test may be used to predict hypnotizability to some extent. They offer the ratio of whole to major detail responses as a significant index. When W is greater than 40 per cent D, the subject was found to be highly hypnotizable.

A survey of cases of neuroses drawn from the writer's civilian practice for which both Rorschachs and tests of hypnotizability were available shows only a slight correlation, as the following table indicates:

	Hypnotizable	Nonhypnotizable
W > 40% D	4	2
W < 40% D	9	14

In another study Brenman and Reichard (1943) found that hypnotizable subjects tended toward more "labile affectivity in Rorschach scores" than subjects resistant to hypnosis.

In general the Rorschach has not yet been found to have definite predictive value in the determination of hypnotizability.

Approach to Patients

The methods of inducing trance outlined in this chapter by no means exhaust the possible methods. Each hypnotist will develop many variations of approach for himself. A number of other techniques for trance induction are rather thoroughly described by Le Cron and Bordeaux (1947) and Wolberg (1948). Each therapist can adapt his own variations to the basic techniques given here. A method that works well with one patient may not succeed with another. It is usually a good idea to find out which technique is best for each patient and to so record it. The more time that can be spent in actual therapy under trance, and the less time spent in inducing trance, the better.

The beginning professional therapist will find difficulty when he first starts to hypnotize his patients. He is afraid that he will not be successful. This fear in itself often prevents him from being successful because it is unconsciously transmitted to the patient. The attitude toward the patient must be one of kindly firmness, in which the therapist does not irritate by bragging or making strong claims. Avoid mobilizing resistances. The patient must have confidence that the therapist knows what he is going to do and is able to do it. Observing other hypnotists will help the beginner. After he has practiced one of the fundamental approaches enough to know that he can keep up the necessary steady patter in the uninterrupted, slow, well-modulated voice, the novice should select as his first subject one who is known to be highly hypnotizable. It is important that he be successful in his first attempts to hypnotize. If he fails, he may develop such a fear of trying that he cannot hypnotize anybody. That is why it is best to learn hypnosis under the direction of a skilled hypnotist. In the class developed at Welch Hospital (Watkins, 1947c), this success in the initial attempt was found to be most important.

The amount of time required to induce a deep trance depends on several factors: the patient and his personality structure, the freedom from distractions, the personality of the therapist, the strength of the patient-therapist transference, the technical skill of the therapist, and many others. Some patients may reach a deep trance at the first session in a matter of seconds, although few persons are naturally this highly hypnotizable. Some persons may be completely unhypnotizable regardless of the time spent in attempting to induce trance, but probably most individuals can be hypnotized to some extent if the therapist is skillful and patient enough. Erickson, who is one of the most experienced and careful workers in the field, points out that the average new subject cannot usually be hypnotized until after several hours of patient, nonroutinized effort have been spent. At Welch Hospital the writer found it possible to induce a moderate degree of trance within one thirty-minute session in about half of the cases examined, but it is quite possible that a selective factor was operating here, those patients referred to Company F being more hypnotizable than the average.

Shortly before the closing of Welch Hospital, experiments were being conducted which indicated that time and energy could be saved by recording sleep suggestions, as described in this chapter, and playing the recordings to the patient. This saved the therapist's breath and energy for the therapy which followed the monotonous work of inducing an initial trance state. Hypnotizing in groups may also be done as a time saver.

In gaining the patient's confidence, especially if he is one of the first hypnotized by the therapist, it may be necessary to make the patient feel that he is quite experienced with hypnosis. The patient will sometimes ask, "Can you hypnotize me?" The answer, of course, should be, "Yes." This can then be qualified to point out that not all persons are able to enter trance at all times under all conditions—that while the therapist has hypnotized people, and can probably hypnotize the patient, there may not be 100 per cent success the first time. This gives the therapist a loophole in case he is unsuccessful. This matter should be handled tactfully, but firmly.

Use of the postural-swaying method is recommended for beginners because the patient does not need to be told that he is going to be hypnotized. His resistances are not mustered. He does not feel that he has to defeat the therapist. If it is not successful, the therapist does not feel that he has failed to deliver something he has promised. He has only told the patient that he is administering a "reflex test," or "studying his nervous reactions." The word "hypnosis" does not even need to be mentioned.

No attempt should be made to hypnotize the hostile, resisting patient until a higher degree of understanding and rapport has been secured. The therapist must establish a mutual confidence. It is possible, occasionally, for a resisting subject to be placed in a trance without his cooperation (Watkins, 1947b), but this is rare. There will usually be enough unconscious resistances to the treatment to cause the therapist a great deal of difficulty. If conscious resistance is also added, inducing trance becomes almost impossible.

Factors that are important include the prestige of the operator. A mild build-up is all to the best advantage. Some other person, a fellow patient or another doctor, can tell the new patient, "Oh, yes, he can put you to sleep. He has put me and a lot of others to sleep." And reassurance from another patient that "The sleep treatments won't hurt you at all; they do you a lot of good" may break down most of a patient's initial resistance. It was often found effective to give the patient an orientation for hypnosis, a few suggestibility tests, and then to leave him with other patients who were undergoing hypnotherapy, and for whom results had been achieved. A successful demonstration of hypnosis is also quite effective in increasing the hypnotizability of a patient. A specific example of this is described in another paper (Watkins, 1947a).

Unresponsive subjects can be made more so by light dosages of sodium amytal orally (3 gr.) administered about a half hour before the induction of trance is attempted. Of course this should be under the prescription of a physician if the therapist is a nonmedical clinician.

Inducing trance is an art. No two hypnotists will use identical methods, but they will follow the same general principles. These include:

1. Establishing rapport with the patient and building up prestige in his eyes

2. Securing a high degree of attention so that external stimuli are excluded

3. Using a monotonous group of suggestions by voice, metronome, or other comparable auditory and visual stimuli

4. Utilizing challenges when they can be successful and avoiding them when the patient can meet them

5. Maintaining at all times a confident manner

The recent treatise on hypnotism by Le Cron and Bordeaux (1947) describes a number of very useful devices for inducing trance in resistant subjects.

Again, the caution must be given here that hypnosis is not something to be tinkered with by the layman. If you are not a professional psychiatrist or psychologist who knows what he is doing, do not try to hypnotize people. Hypnosis can be a powerful influence to help people get well, but anything which is strong enough to help them is also strong enough to hurt them. In the hands of the amateur, hypnosis may cause a great deal of psychological distress. Never encourage its use for entertainment purposes. It should be kept where it belongs, in the professional treatment office or clinic, the advanced classroom, or the research laboratory, and practiced only by the professionally trained person.

CHAPTER 7

HYPNOTHERAPEUTIC TECHNIQUE

Role of Hypnosis in Psychotherapy

In the last chapter several methods of inducing trance states have been described. While Wetterstrand (1902) and others have treated with prolonged trance, the greatest therapeutic value of hypnosis does not lie in the state itself, but in the psychotherapy which can be accomplished under it. Hypnosis, like a surgical scalpel, is a tool. It must be wielded with skill if it is to be of value therapeutically.

It should be emphasized here that hypnosis does not replace other types of psychotherapy. Rather, it is an additional aid, making other psychotherapies more effective by enabling the therapist to work with deeper levels of personality structure. One has the feeling that a patient under hypnotic trance is more plastic, more subject to change and to molding influences. Analogies are frequently misleading, but a convenient one might be used here to illustrate this point. When practicing psychotherapy on a conscious individual, the therapist feels he is slowly molding and changing personality like a sculptor chipping marble. It is a difficult, painstaking process. If the sculptor could immerse his block of marble in a solution which would make it soft and jellylike, he could then more quickly and rapidly mold the figure in the desired direction. After the block was removed from the solution it would solidify again in marble form. The psychotherapist by placing the patient in an hypnotic trance appears to be working with a personality structure which is softer and more moldable than one in the conscious state. Through the use of suggestion, motivation, and insight under trance, changes in behavior can be effected which would be very difficult to accomplish in the conscious state.

It is not true that hypnosis eliminates resistance—that patients can be easily turned into their opposites or made into criminals. Nor is it true, as some psychoanalysts have written, that the Ego abdicates when under trance (A. Freud, 1937). The hypnotized patient is not mere putty in the hands of the therapist. He exhibits a definite personality structure. He has his likes and dislikes. He demonstrates attitudes, and his points of resistance are such that he can, when necessary, say "no" to the therapist very definitely and firmly. However, one gathers the impression when working with a patient under trance that his entire mental life is more subject to study, his behavior and personality softer and more moldable.

As previously mentioned, early results with hypnosis were disappointing largely because of the clumsy techniques used. Simple direct-suggestive attack against symptoms was often the only method employed—and this rather crudely. As will be evident throughout the cases to be described, this method alone seldom produces permanent results.

Direct Suggestion

The simplest and most commonly used technique of hypnosis is that of direct suggestion. Here the attempt is made directly to manipulate symptoms under trance. We should distinguish between the suggestion during trance and the posthypnotic suggestion. In the first, movement might be restored to an hysterically paralyzed limb, but the immobility returns before the patient is awakened. In the second, special instructions, suggestions, and commands are given to the patient, and he is told that he will carry these out after he awakens from the trance. The attempt then is to make the effect permanent. Carelessness in the use of posthypnotic suggestions may leave the patient burdened with new and unnecessary compulsions or obsessions. This is one of the strongest reasons why the layman, untrained in psychopathology, should not experiment with hypnosis.

Two general rules might be given about the use of suggestion. First, the deeper the trance, the more effective the suggestions will be, and the more likely it is that they will be carried out. Second, it will require a deeper degree of trance to make suggestions stick posthypnotically than to have them achieved only under trance. Many persons think that anything can be suggested—that the patient can be forced by direct suggestion to achieve the impossible and to perform actions contradictory to his entire nature. While it is true that a person can be *bent* under hypnotic trance to reveal suppressed information or to perform deeds which he would not normally do in the conscious state, there are definite limits beyond which he cannot be taken. The skilled therapist at all times takes account of the resistances of the patient and makes his suggestions such that they are reinforced rather than opposed by natural motives. Herein lies his skill in applying psychology. In the early work with hypnosis the patient was merely told under trance that he would perform this or that action and was expected to carry out the instructions. Much more skillful is the use of logic, persuasion, reasoning, and aligning suggested actions with natural drives already within the patient. Remember, the hypnotized patient is a person, a very definite person with likes, dislikes, attitudes, and an integrated personality structure. True, this structure is softer under trance than in the conscious state, but the patient must be dealt with as a person, not as a mere automaton or slave. The suggestion should be given in line with a person's natural drives and in the most logical and persuasive manner.

One of the most common suggestions is that of alleviating a symptom, for example: "As I put my hand on your forehead the pressure will make the pain diminish in your head. Your head is beginning to feel much better, much more comfortable. The pain is leaving it; the headache is going away. I shall now count slowly up to 25, and as I do the head will begin to feel better. By the time I reach 25 your headache will be completely gone. One, two, three, . . .," etc. On reaching "twenty-five" the therapist says, "Now your headache is completely gone. You feel much better. When I wake you up you will feel cheerful and comfortable, and will not have any trace of a headache." Notice how this suggestion is built up. It will be more effective and permanent when given this way than if the patient is merely told, "When I wake you up your headache will be gone."

Suggestions need to be learned by the patient. We know that repetition is one of the fundamental principles of learning. Therefore, a suggestion should be given repeatedly, using different words, stating it over and over, placing it in a meaningful context, rationalizing it so that it makes sense. Notice that the patient was told that pressure of the therapist's hand on the forehead would alleviate the pain. This makes more sense to the hypnotized patient than if he is merely commanded to lose his headache. In the same manner, direct suggestive attacks can be made against insomnia, nausea, anorexia, or almost any symptom.

Actually the patient is *taught* a suggestion. All of the psychological principles of learning, such as repetition, recency, satisfaction, pleasure-pain principle, the principle of "belongingness," and other well-known educational laws should be applied. Stories, instructions, suggestions, and commands should be made pleasant and interesting. Description should be given in meaningful and vivid terms. Language which is at the patient's level of understanding should be employed. Everything that is known about the arts of persuasion, education, salesmanship, and effective public speaking should be applied by the therapist in altering the personality structure of a hypnotized patient through direct suggestion.

Direct suggestion should not be considered as a method of curing an illness. Its chief place in hypnotherapy lies in the opportunity it offers the therapist to alleviate symptoms temporarily until a deeper study of personality difficulties can be made, and to aid in the more effective application of advanced techniques. It is a device useful for *manipulating rather than eliminating symptoms.* True, some cases in which the maladjustment is fairly superficial seem to be cured by simple direct-suggestive attack against the symptoms. Several cases of this type are described in this book, but these are probably the exception rather than the rule, and the permanency of the "cure" is open to speculation.

One of the great values in being able to alleviate pain, if only temporarily, is the increase in prestige which the therapist will enjoy and the consequently greater rapport with his patients. This helps all his psychotherapy to be more effective. The patient places great confidence in the therapist when he knows that his "doctor" has the ability to remove pain (or to induce it). At the end of each trance session it was quite common for the therapist to suggest euphoria. This generally left the patient positively oriented toward continuing treatment.

A very interesting technique is the use of direct suggestion under trance to set the stage for a quick reinduction of trance. Thus, the patient may be told as follows: "When you wake up, you will feel very good. I shall count up to five, and your eyes will open wide awake on the count of five, but any time I hand you a yellow pencil, you will instantly go back into a deep sleep." Notice that this gives the therapist almost instantaneous control. He has set posthypnotically a mechanism within the patient which permits him to induce trance in a matter of seconds. How this can be most effectively used will be demonstrated later.

Another powerful use of direct suggestion is to alter attitudes. Again the persuasive and logical attack is more effective than the direct command. For example: "During the next week you will begin to feel much less hostile toward the company commander. Notice some of the good traits that he has. You will not be so critical of him as you realize that his apparent strictness is only a part of his sincere desire to take good care of his men. You will not feel that he is personally trying to attack you or hurt you. You can then be more friendly toward him." Here the attempt is made through suggestion to effect a change in an attitude of rejection toward some given individual. This is given not through command, but through persuasion. No attempt is made to reverse the attitude immediately, but rather the change is made to appear gradual and logical. Frontal assaults against deeply entrenched attitudes usually result in rejection, not only of the desired attitude, but frequently of the therapist also. They may cause anxiety or disinclination to continue hypnotherapy sessions. The good automobile salesman never makes the mistake of contradicting a prospect and trying to command him to reverse his opinion. Yet many therapists do exactly that when using hypnosis. They attempt instantly and without preparation to reverse their patients' feelings and attitudes. Later they report that "Hypnosis was not effective," or "The effects are very temporary and wear off." Hypnosis is no substitute for tact.

Other uses of direct suggestion to alter attitudes might be as follows: "You will begin to enjoy your stay here at the hospital" or "You will realize that the facilities and equipment are to help you and are available to you. You will see that this is much different from many parts of the Army under which your freedom has been more restricted. You will come to appreciate more the efforts of the doctors, social workers, and company officers to help you. Your hostility to the Army will gradually melt as you begin to feel that something constructive is being done to help you here," etc. Through suggestive methods of this type attitudes for or against any person or group can be changed. If the suggestions are skillfully given, every evidence indicates that this change is not merely temporary but involves fundamental alterations in the personality structure. Attitudes toward life, attitudes about rationalizing, compensating, daydreaming, prejudices, even desires toward alcohol and sex can often be *adjusted* through the skillful use of suggestion and persuasive methods.

It may be desirable to set up certain compulsions, such as, "Each morning at ten o'clock for the next week you will have an overwhelming desire to come in and receive your treatment." This might be used with patients who notoriously lack a time sense, or who for other reasons of resistance are tardy or absent from their appointments.

Another effective use of suggestion is to prepare the person for insight just prior to the revelation to him of some fact which might be disturbing. In other words, a *readiness* is suggested to him. The patient is placed in a trance and informed, "When you wake up you will be told something new and interesting about yourself. You will understand it and appreciate it. You will make it thoroughly part of you. You will not feel anxiety. It will not upset you or make you ill. You are very strong now; you are strong enough to accept a new insight." The patient is then brought out of the trance, and the critical point is discussed with him. This usually results in more genuine acceptance and less resistance. Afterwards, the patient can be placed back in trance and told, "You have just had a new point about you explained. You can understand it clearly now and accept it. You will believe it from now on. It will be part of you." To be certain that this is true, the patient might be questioned periodically under trance and asked to explain the points that have been discussed with him.

Thus suggestion can be used to lower resistance and to increase acceptance of a new disturbing insight. Sometimes it is desirable to explain a point to the patient under trance. At other times material of a pertinent nature uncovered in trance can be revealed as follows: "When you wake up you will remember distinctly everything we talked about while you were asleep." [1]

Direct suggestion can be a very useful tool in the hands of the careful psychotherapist, especially if he realizes its limitations. He must not use it crudely, clumsily, or stupidly, attempting to reverse at once the whole previous trend of a person's behavior.

It is a good idea to have a complete record of each treatment session. Sometimes a suggestion will be made inadvertently which will carry over and set up some undesirable compulsion or obsession in the patient. The skilled therapist, before he awakens the patient, considers carefully everything he has said and cleans out or removes any undesirable suggestions. However, in a long session some of these may slip by. Precise notes on what was said and done enable the therapist to rectify the error at the next session. The writer recalls one such occasion. While using the dissociated hand technique (to be described later) he induced the hallucination in the patient that his hand was not connected to his wrist. After a long hypnotic session the patient was brought out of trance, and this hallucination was not specifically removed. The patient was most perplexed and disturbed because he had the sensation that his hand was disconnected and

---

[1] The writer's most recent practice favors a more nondirective or "permissive" approach. Instead of informing the patient under trance that he *will* remember traumatic and repressed matters when he wakes up, the therapist now prefers to *ask* him while still under trance whether he *would like* to recall these after he awakens. He is told that if they would cause too much anxiety he doesn't have to remember them until he feels strong enough to do so, at which point he can. Often he will "choose" to remember part of the uncovered traumata and will recall the rest later in the therapy by himself as recovered Ego strength permits him to face the new insights.

floating in air.   It was necessary immediately to reinduce trance and to remove this hallucination.   There have been reports of persons who have been unnecessarily burdened with compulsive ideas by amateur hypnotists.   The hypnotherapist must realize that he is dealing with a softer personality structure and be careful not to leave undesirable dents in it.

Direct suggestive attack against symptoms is an elementary hypnotic technique, and we have stressed here the importance of insight for permanent "cures."   Yet it must not be forgotten that the older hypnotists, Braid, Liébeault, Bernheim, Janet, and others, have reported hundreds of direct-suggestion cures apparently permanent in nature.   Bramwell (1930) gives an extended account of these.   It is a psychotherapeutic weapon which, if skillfully wielded, must not be underestimated.

Uncovering Techniques

You will recall that in the first section of this book the therapeutic formula was given as: *Motivation plus insight equals cure.*   Direct suggestion under trance is essentially an attack on the motivation factor in this formula.   It represents a specialized kind of motivation. Achievement of insight has been designated as our second major goal. And it is in the opportunities for uncovering unconscious conflicts that hypnosis offers its greatest assistance.   The modern tendency is to use the hypnotic tool as an uncovering device, a psychological X ray of the underlying strata of personality rather than as a method for symptom manipulation.   It is very interesting to secure a case history from a patient by conscious interview and then to re-interview the subject under trance.   The case history secured under hypnosis is usually much richer with emotional content and detail.   Through it one obtains not only facts about various events in the man's life, but also his feelings, attitudes, prejudices, and interests at the time. Sometimes statements secured from the patient under trance will contradict those made in the conscious state.   This is readily understandable when we remember that completely contradictory ideas can exist side by side in the unconscious mind.   Discrepancies of this type may mean that the true facts have been concealed or repressed through inner conflict.   Or the statements made in the conscious state may be true, and those reported in trance may be fantasies.   Because it is not generally possible to verify trance statements and because under trance the patient may conjure up these dream-fantasies, some have argued, "Hypnosis is not reliable."   To the analyst, the patient's fantasies may be as important as facts in treatment. Furthermore, discrepancies between stories in the conscious and trance states may most significantly indicate conflict areas.

Interviewing under trance is used to secure both suppressed and repressed material. By *suppressed* is meant that which is voluntarily concealed from the interviewer, such as incidents which the patient feels are too embarrassing to reveal. Repressed material, of course, includes that which is below the threshold of consciousness and of which the patient is not aware.

The securing of suppressed material is comparatively easy once the trance state has been induced. The possibilities of hypnosis in the questioning of enemy prisoners or interviewing of suspected criminals seems promising. The discussion of delicate material under hypnotic trance is frequently desirable when conditions make it difficult for the patient to speak of the trouble in the conscious state. For example, the writer once treated a young woman whose difficulty included a homosexual maladjustment. The homosexual side of the problem was never mentioned consciously by the patient. The treatment for this angle of her problem, continuing for several months, was carried on entirely in the trance state. Her other maladjustments, of an educational nature, were discussed when she was awake. The therapist in this way was informed at all times of both aspects of the problem and the progress of the treatment. Yet the patient was never embarrassed by having to discuss it in the conscious state. The treatment in this case was apparently successful, since she ceased the homosexual practices and did not develop compensatory symptoms. The patient apparently never did realize consciously that she had discussed the sexual side of her problems with the therapist.

Uncovering *repressed* material is much more difficult. In Chapter 8 methods of reaching the deeper layers of repressed material are described. Ordinary direct interviewing under trance probably uncovers only suppressed and some lightly repressed ideas.

The same traits which make a person a good interviewer in the conscious state will make him a good interviewer of a person under trance. All his interviewing skill will be called upon. Tact and delicacy should be used. Contrary to some opinions, suggesting an answer to the patient will not necessarily cause him to respond by saying "yes." In fact, if the suggested answer is not correct, the patient will often reply with a vigorous denial and set forth his reasons —again evidence that hypnosis is not mere suggestion alone. Everything that has been written about good interviewing technique applies in interviewing a patient under trance. Resistance points, when located, should be handled skillfully and tactfully. Generally, there will be a closer bond of rapport between therapist and patient under the trance condition than in the conscious state. The patient's discussion can be expected to be richer, more meaningful, and less inhibited. Interviewing under trance should be considered merely as an extension of normal interviewing.

Hypermnesia Under Hypnosis

One of the most interesting hypnotic phenomena is that of *hypermnesia* or superior memory. A hypnotized patient can remember many things about his life which he could not recall otherwise. One subject was able to recite the valedictory address he delivered on his eighth-grade graduation some sixteen years earlier. In the conscious state he could not even remember the title, but under trance he recited the fifteen-minute speech word for word without a single hesitation. It is this quality which makes the interview under trance much richer and more meaningful for uncovering conflict-laden material. Fortunately, it is not necessary to initiate a deep trance before hypermnesic results can be secured. Superior memory is evident under a light trance or even hypnoidal state.

Closely allied to hypermnesia is the phenomenon of *regression*. Under trance a person may be regressed, that is, taken back to previous levels of behavior and thought. Thus, when carried back to the age of seven, he will not only remember in detail his thoughts, actions, and school friends in the first grade, but will describe the pictures on the wall or the teacher, will read as he did in the first grade and will write his name the way he did with his first childish scrawl. In every apparent way he has once more *become* a first grader, aged seven. After adequately deep trance has been induced, instructions such as the following may be used to carry the patient back to the earlier age level of functioning: "Now you are going to forget all about where you are and how old you are. You are going back and becoming younger and younger. You are becoming nineteen years old, eighteen years old, seventeen—, sixteen—, . . . 9, —8, —7, —7, —7. You are a little boy seven years old. You do not remember anything that has happened since that time. You are seven years old. You are sitting at your desk in the first grade of school. You are looking at the teacher. She is smiling at you. What is her name?" The patient will usually respond by naming the teacher. Adequacy of regression can then be checked by asking him who sits in front of him, who sits in front of that person, and so on until he has named enough pupils in the first grade room to satisfy the therapist that regression is established. He can also be asked his age and be requested to sign his name. If regression is satisfactory, he will give his age as seven and write his name like a small child. (See Figure 5.)

Figure 5. Samples of Handwriting of a Subject Regressed to Various Ages Under Hypnotic Trance

Several cases occurred in which regression was incomplete at first. The patient in describing what happened in the first grade would use the past tense instead of the present tense. Then, after considerable questioning, the regression would apparently become more adequate, and the patient begin to enter and participate thoroughly at the first-grade level. He would then use the present tense in describing his actions.

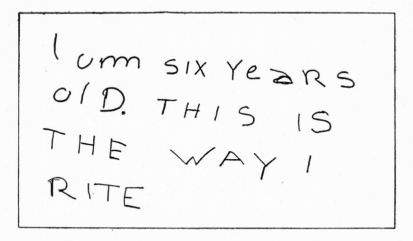

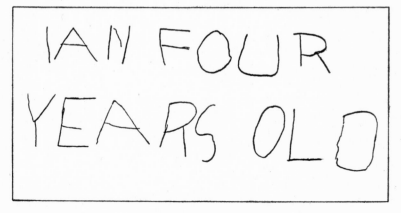

Figure 5. (*Continued*)

Regressed to Age Four: Subject could not spell but "drew" the single letters as words were spelled to her.

Note again how, in regressing the person, he is not merely commanded to be seven years old. First, amnesia for his present age is suggested. Second, he is carried back through the years. Third, he is told his age and in what grade he is at school. Fourth, he is placed in a specific setting in the schoolroom. This is made more realistic by having the teacher smile at him. It cannot be too greatly emphasized that diplomatic and even dramatic skill is necessary for effective work in hypnosis. The writer feels that many of the failures reported by some disappointed users of hypnosis were largely the result of their superficial reliance on the direct-command technique and their belief that the hypnotized patient does not need to be treated as a person.

Horizontal exploration of personality structure at various ages becomes an extension of the interviewing-under-trance technique. The patient is first regressed to the age of seven, four, twelve, eighteen, or other desired level, and regression is tested. When its adequacy seems established, interviewing skill is used to bring out the attitudes, feelings, parental relationships, sibling rivalries, loves, hates, and fears held by the subject at that particular age.[2]

From the scientific viewpoint regression and hypermnesia are still controversial. Some research studies appear to prove their existence (Spiegel, Shor, and Fishman, 1945). Other experimenters do not find that true regression occurs under trance (Young, 1940). Even though their existence is yet to be established firmly by experimental methods, those who have worked therapeutically with patients will tend to accept the reality of these phenomena. As therapists, go ahead and use them. You can achieve results.

Often the effectiveness of interviewing at regressed age levels will increase if the therapist actually plays a dramatic role. For example, he might regress the patient back to the age of five and then say, "I am the person whom you love best. Who am I?" Or, "I am a person whom you fear a great deal," or "I am one you hate." Again the therapist might say, "You are in the living room of your home. Your mother is just coming in the door. She is now going to speak to you, and you will answer her. 'Good morning, son, what are you doing?'" The patient will then respond to the therapist as if he were the mother. He may disclose experiences and feelings which at the age of five he would not tell to anybody but his mother. In his manner of conversation he will reveal the kind of affection he had toward his mother—or the hostility which may have been present. The therapist may rapidly change roles, becoming brother, sister, friend, associate, employer, sweetheart, or wife. For example, he can explore attitudes toward the marital partner at different years during the married life while a maladjustment was developing. Needless to say, he should not identify himself in these dramatic roles unless the patient is in such a deep trance that he will be amnesic to it all on

---

[2] The school of nondirective therapists should investigate the possibilities of using their techniques with hypnotic trance.

awakening—or can be made so by direct suggestion. Otherwise, the patient may become distrustful and suspicious of the therapist. Horizontal exploration of the personality becomes an intensive interview at a selected age level. The therapist uses all his interviewing skill and identifies himself with any person to whom the patient would be most likely to have revealed significant information at that age.

Not only is horizontal exploration valuable, but also *vertical exploration.* This includes tracing the origin and development of specific fears, hates, affections, sex experiences, religious thoughts, attitudes, etc. The ability to cross time lines rapidly is often a great asset. A specific example of vertical exploration occurred in a case of reactive depression treated by the author. While re-enacting a traumatic experience which occurred on the Anzio beachhead, the patient said that his fear of crowds of people and his shyness had been somehow precipitated by being buried alive by a shell explosion. The reason for this connection was not understood until after a period of "vertical exploration" in which his attitudes toward people were systematically uncovered through the preceding years. During this he recovered a memory of his first day at school. The elder boys "ganged up" on him in the cloakroom, threw him to the floor, and piled coats on top of him. He was saved from this incident by the intervention of the teacher. This brought a fear of groups of people and associated smothering with them. The fear was gradually outgrown but was reinvoked when he was smothered by the shell explosion.

Often it will be desirable to trace an attitude toward a relative at ages four, seven, nine, twelve, fifteen, eighteen, etc. Under a deep trance it is very easy to jump to the desired age levels. For example, if the patient has mentioned hostility feelings directed toward his father while he was regressed to the age of six, the further development of this might be explored as follows: "Now you are forgetting all about being six. You are growing older and older. You are seven years old, eight years old, nine years old, ten years old. Now you are ten years old. You are a much bigger boy. What is your name? How old are you?" etc. When the patient has successfully answered these last two questions or others designed to establish adequacy of regression, he is then asked, "Is there anybody whom you hate or dislike?" If he does not now identify his father as a disliked person, he might be next questioned more directly such as, "Do you dislike or hate your father?" If at the age of ten he still answers "No," one would infer either that certain significant changes in the father-son relationship had occurred between the ages of six and ten or that the hostility had become more deeply repressed by the age of ten and would require intensive depth-techniques such as analytic or projective methods before it could be uncovered.

It was found desirable to explore horizontally first at various significant age levels. From the data uncovered, important trends would be extracted for intensive vertical exploration to determine origin and development.

The most significant ages for horizontal exploration were found generally to be the preschool years three to five; the first year of school—ages six to seven; the early adolescent period—ages twelve to fourteen; the age at which the patient became independent of parental authority; and the age at which romance and marriage occurred.

Quite often resistances are uncovered during trance-interviewing as well as in the conscious state. These are evidenced by signs of anxiety, tension, fidgeting, tremors, moving about, wrinkling of brow, refusal to speak, desire to change the subject, etc. The person who is accustomed to notice and observe these fine points while interviewing will also see the same factors arising in the hypnotized patient. Of course, these are frequently of great significance because they point to areas of unconscious conflict. Indicators of this type must be carefully noted by the therapist for further and deeper study. The symbolic significance of postural changes occurring during psychoanalytic sessions has been emphasized by Deutsch (1947).

Apparently no one has yet tried analytic or hypnoanalytic sessions with the Keeler Polygraph (lie-detector).[3] The therapist relies on his observational skill to detect blocking, tenseness, signs of anxiety, and other external indicators of internal conflict. In this machine age, clues to significant repressions might be gained if analytic probing were combined with an instrument of this type which records changes in internal visceral behavior as a result of emotionally charged associations.

Many neurotic conditions can be effectively treated by the methods described in this chapter. However, even the most skillful of interviewing techniques under trance or regressed trance may not uncover deeply repressed material. More advanced and delicate "depth" procedures must be employed. So we will continue in the next chapter with a description of some of these more complex techniques.

---

[3] Inbau (1942) has described the uses of this instrument.

Outline of Elementary Hypnotherapeutic Techniques

1. Direct suggestion employed to alter:
   a. Symptoms
   b. Attitudes

2. Uncovering techniques:
   a. Interviewing under trance
   b. Hypermnesia and regression
      (1) Horizontal exploration
      (2) Vertical exploration

CHAPTER 8

ADVANCED HYPNOTHERAPEUTIC TECHNIQUE

In earlier chapters the relation of the Super-Ego to repressed, conflict-laden material has been discussed. The Super-Ego was described as a judging and censoring force within the person. Ideas or meanings which would cause too much anxiety to be faced directly must be repressed into the unconscious.

Of course, we already know that the material which would be most significant in an individual's maladjustment is probably also most unacceptable to him in the conscious state, hence most surely repressed. This material, of which he is unaware, may be an actual incident in his life about which he has become amnesic. On the other hand, the difficulty may lie in an inner significance or meaning which he will not face. In Chapter 7 it was mentioned that the simpler interviewing techniques under trance were useful in obtaining suppressed material and rather lightly repressed material, but that complex methods were necessary to uncover more deeply repressed ideas.

Getting these ideas out past "the censor" reminds one of the old Greek story of Ulysses and the Cyclops. You will recall that Ulysses and his men blinded the one-eyed Cyclops while he was sleeping, but that the Cyclops kept the men penned up in a cave. Ulysses and his men were able to escape only when each was tied to the underbelly of one of the huge goats which the Cyclops kept in the cave at night. The Cyclops, feeling the top of the goats' backs as they went out to pasture in the morning, permitted them to leave the cave. The men escaped through disguise or camouflage. In like manner ideas of a traumatic nature are encouraged to escape into the conscious mind by being camouflaged or disguised. Methods of eluding the censor by disguising these ideas are needed so that the Super-Ego will permit them to come into the conscious state.

Dissociated Handwriting

One manner in which this may be done is through the use of *dissociated handwriting* (Erickson and Kubie, 1938, 1940). Perhaps it can be best illustrated by giving the actual suggestions made to the patient in employing this device. He is first placed in a deep trance, adequacy of depth being thoroughly tested. The patient is then told, "A numbness is coming over your right hand. It is losing all feeling, all movement, and all sensation. You cannot feel it at all." The hand is lightly rubbed. This is continued until complete paralysis and anesthesia have been induced. The patient is then given the hallucination that the hand is no longer connected to the wrist: "Your hand is now floating away from the wrist. It is no longer a part of your body. It is standing by itself out in space. You will stay in your sleep, but you will open your eyes and observe that the hand is floating in space and that it is not part of you. See, it is not connected to your wrist any longer." Slowly the patient opens his eyes and "observes" the hallucination that the hand is not connected to his wrist. The eyes of the patient are then closed, and he is told. "The hand is no longer part of you; you do not have any control over it whatsoever. It is completely outside of you. It is a little person who is all-seeing and all-knowing. It can look down deep inside and see all about you. If there is something that you cannot remember, the hand will be able to remember and write out the answer. If there is something which is too painful for you to talk about, the hand will write it. If I should ask you a question, and you do not give me the right answer or tell the truth, the hand will write out the correct answer. You have no control over it. It is completely independent and outside of you." [1] The hand is then given a pencil and placed on a pad of writing paper, while various questions are asked of the patient. Sometimes it requires further suggestions to stimulate the hand to begin, but once started it may write voluminously. The therapist may have some difficulty keeping it on the pad of paper and supplying fresh sheets. Often, when a direct question is asked, the patient may give one answer while the hand writes the direct opposite, or he may refuse to speak or may show a great deal of anxiety. The hand may then write a significant statement giving a clue to the cause of the anxiety.

The *hand-technique* was used most effectively in a number of the cases described in this book and was sometimes decisive in breaking into the heart of a conflict. The hand, being dissociated from the rest of the person, is put in the position where it is not responsible to "the censor"—at least, it is not as much responsible. However, even with a dissociated hand one still finds the resistances and the reluctance to touch on certain subjects. The same necessity for skill

---

[1] Notice the use of repetition. Repetition makes for better learning and increases the strength of suggestions.

in questioning or approaching and solving difficult points is required even though deeper levels of the personality have been tapped. Significant material will often emerge with the dissociated-hand technique which cannot be brought out by direct interviewing under trance. Of course, it is quite possible to combine regression with the dissociated hand. The hand can be regressed to any desired age level.

Attempts have also been made to dissociate the voice in the same way, placing the vocal organs outside the limits of restriction of "the censor" and thus relieving the person of responsibility for what he is saying. The writer's experiments in this line to date have had at best only limited success. In these he tried to dissociate the voice through inducing anesthesia of the lips, tongue, and vocal organs, and with suggestions that these organs were no longer a part of the body. Further studies in this direction might prove very interesting.

When writing with a dissociated hand, there is a tendency for the subject to "warm up" just as he does when he first begins to talk under trance. At the beginning of the session responses are short, made rather slowly, and with obvious effort as though there were considerable resistance. One can almost feel the ensuing process of being "thawed out." As the patient proceeds, more and more significant material emerges. The hand writes more easily, freely, and voluminously. Admissions of an important nature, which could not be secured at the beginning of the session, often are easily obtained later. That is why points of resistance must be carefully charted and reviewed later in the session—or at subsequent sessions.

There is an important precaution to observe. At the end of a session involving a dissociated hand, the hand should be returned to normal and reassociated with the individual before he is awakened from trance. Feeling and movement are returned by suggestion. Then the hallucination that the hand is disconnected from the wrist is removed, and the patient is told that his hand is now completely normal. Before being awakened he can also be told that he will remember everything the hand wrote, or certain selected parts of the material. Or, he can be instructed to remember nothing which the hand wrote. The hand may also be dissociated posthypnotically and the writing done independently by the hand while the patient is awake. It is also possible in the suggestible patient to initiate automatic handwriting without first inducing trance at all.

A variation of this technique is convenient as a time-saver. A "hand," writing on a sheet of white paper, is hallucinated and the patient instructed to observe what it writes. It is not known whether this is as effective as having the message reported by motor behavior in real handwriting.   However it has been so effective that the writer has recently been using this device more than the dissociated hand.

Automatic writing by the dissociated hand is most useful in breaking through a significant point of resistance. Material will sometimes come out through its medium which apparently cannot be elicited in any other way.   In the *permissive* approach, though, it is often wise to ask the patient whether he is ready to read that which the hand has written and not to insist that he do so if he is not yet strong enough.   He may be promised in advance that he will not have to read the writing unless he wishes to.

The therapist should practice and become skillful with as many different uncovering techniques as possible.   He can then combine and integrate them.   Like a good tactician he chooses the right weapon for a job and knows the values and limitations of each of his tools.

Projective Techniques

Psychologists have recently been doing considerable experimentation with projective techniques.[2]   By these are meant unstructured situations presented to a subject which give him a great deal of latitude so that he may interpret them in terms of his own personality—that is, he can structure them in line with his own inner mental concepts and attitudes.

The best known of these is the *Rorschach Ink-Blot Test* (Klopfer and Kelley, 1942; Beck, 1944, 1945).   Here the patient is shown cards on which are ink-blot forms and is asked to tell what he sees in the blots.   Inferences may be made about his personality structure by the manner in which he deals with the ink-blot material.

Likewise, a person often reveals many important facts about his emotional and ideational life if he is presented indirectly with stimulating situations when he is not on guard.   The answer to a direct question, even under trance, must pass "the censor."   If the patient is given a great deal of freedom in a situation in which he does not feel he is being judged, he may project out significant conflicts.   Thus the hypnotized patient might be told, "In front of you there is a large movie screen.   On the screen is unfolding a story, a real story about people.   You will see various characters there, and you can describe what is happening to them."   The patient is thereby encouraged to dream or fantasy.   Since we ourselves are usually the most important people in our own minds, almost inevitably one or

---

[2] For a survey of these methods see Bell (1948).

more of the characters on the screen in this dream can be identified with the patient himself. As he tells us what this character does, what happens to him, how he feels about people or how people react to him, he is often telling us a great deal about his own inner feelings.

Variations of this technique involve *looking into a crystal,* or looking at a blank card or sheet of paper and being told to visualize pictures on it. Sometimes the patient can be given more directly structured suggestions, such as, "There is a large scroll unfolding in front of your eyes. There are words on this scroll. You will be able to read them. They say many things that are very important to you." The patient might then be told, "You will be able to read this scroll aloud as it unfolds." Or, he might be instructed, "I will leave you for a little while, and you can read to yourself what it says on this scroll." When the therapist returns he may suggest either that the patient tell him what was on the scroll, or that the patient will be able to remember what was on the scroll when he awakens. The matter can then be discussed in the conscious state.

Generally, the more the situation is structured, the less significant will be the material which emerges. If the patient is told, "You will read material on this scroll which is of great importance in your problem," he will bring forth ideas which have been subject to considerable internal censorship. If it is merely suggested that an imaginary story is going to unfold, and he is not told that it will apply to him, he will give greater freedom to his imagination. With less control it may wander more widely afield from the immediate problem, but there will often be much less censorship in that which does emerge. The degree to which the projective situation is structured, directive or nondirective, is a matter of professional judgment. You must decide whether you want all wheat, but low quality (highly structured and controlled), or lots of worthless chaff with a sprinkling of high-quality kernels (relatively unstructured and nondirective).

As a projective screen the patient may be shown a blank card, a crystal, a wall, or similar surface while he is in trance but with his eyes open. Or, his eyes may be left closed and any of these hallucinated for him so that he may project images. Data do not yet seem to be available as to which method is the more desirable.

Illustrated in Chapter 18 is a method which proved very successful. It involved giving the patient a hero as a projective character. Usually a name was selected somewhat similar to that of the patient. Let us say the patient's name was *Wilson.* He would be told, "You are now floating out into a dream world and dreaming about a person, a young man by the name of *Williams* [Eluding "the censor," yet

providing elements for identification.] This young man has many
problems and troubles. You are going to be able to make up a story
about him. Of course, this is all imaginary, but you can tell what
is happening to this young man, Williams, how he is feeling, and
what are his real problems." The chances are strong that the patient
will identify Williams as himself and proceed to tell a significant story
about this dream character which is actually a deeper, more revealing,
and more intimate tale about his own difficulties as they are—or,
equally important, as he sees them in fantasy.

If the patient is induced to imagine a drama or story, the whole
situation can be dramatized, and the therapist can accept one of the
roles. He might then suggest that the patient play the part of the
young man by the name of Williams. The two dramatize a situation
in which inner conflicts of the imaginary person, Williams—who has
been identified with himself by the patient, Wilson—are enacted.
The method of *Psychodrama* has been developed by Dr. J. L. Moreno
(1946) especially for use with psychotic patients. It can be a
useful technique with neurotic patients who are under hypnotic
trance.

If the patient is told that he will *dream,* the dream may be made
to emerge at the present time, or later. He can be instructed to
describe it as it emerges or to remember it and discuss it at a later
time, perhaps the next day. He may be told only that he will remember the dream. Nothing is said about his disclosing it. Later,
he can be questioned about this dream either under trance or in the
conscious state. Sometimes it is desirable to suggest that he will have
a dream tonight when he goes to sleep and that he will remember it
in detail when he awakes in the morning.

Under trance a dream about any selected topic can be initiated
and consummated within a few minutes. For example, "You will
have a dream concerning your true feelings toward your brother."
If he has had a dream recently, he may be told that he will re-experi-
ence the same dream. Perhaps he has forgotten parts of it. Or,
perhaps the dream was incomplete, being interrupted at a crucial
point. This is commonly the case where battle dreams awaken the
patient. He may be told under trance that the next night he will
experience the same dream again, and this time he will complete it without awakening. The same previously discussed principle
regarding highly structured versus relatively unstructured projective
stimuli apply also in suggesting dreams.

Dreams are unconscious doubletalk. Like a symptom, they tell a
concealed story disguised through elaboration and symbolism. Under

trance patients can more easily associate to their dreams and interpret them. The methods of dream interpretation described by Freud (1938) and Stekel (1943) can be greatly facilitated when the patient is under hypnotic trance (Farber and Fisher, 1943; Kanzer, 1945). Sometimes the patient will directly interpret his dream symbols without the need of free association.

The resolution of neurotic dreams is one of the best tests of the progress of the treatment. With each therapeutic gain in insight the patient's dreams usually take a more benign turn and show the complete resolution of the conflict only when the point is reached at which treatment may be safely terminated. Either hypnotically induced dreams or the spontaneous variety will serve as indicators of progress, regression, or the course the therapy should next follow. After the treatment has been essentially finished, induced dreams can be used in conjunction with the projective techniques to locate the sources of remaining anxiety or other symptomatic residuals so as to permit a concentrated "clean-up" attack. Perhaps some point in the interpretation is not clearly understood and hence still partially rejected unconsciously. Hypnotically induced dreams and projections can tell the therapist and patient where this is and enable them to concentrate on this point. The writer has found the recalling and interpretation of dream fantasies, both induced and natural dreams, to be one of the most productive of the hypnoanalytic methods. He now uses these methods to a considerably greater extent.

A recent promising development in the field of projective psychological methods for uncovering unconscious conflicts is the *Thematic Apperception Test* (Murray, 1938, 1943; Tomkins, 1947; Stein, 1948). In this, the patient is presented with various pictures. He is asked to tell what is happening in the scene, what led up to it, and what is the outcome. In other words, he is asked to imagine a story or theme suggested by the picture. In the recent forms some twenty pictures are used. Since subjects will often identify with various characters in the pictures, called heroes, it is possible, by analyzing what happens to these heroes, to discover much about the inner unconscious content of the patient's emotional life. The actions, dealings, affects, and attitudes of the heroes are analyzed, as are the environmental forces which press down upon them. The relations of heroes, parents, siblings, friends, wives, and sweethearts are frequently significant. Whether the stories have happy or unhappy endings also tells much about the inner mental state. These test pictures are even more revealing when administered under hypnotic trance. Thus, a patient can be regressed to any age level, and the particular dynamic conflicts of that age studied. This is similar to the projective technique of movie reading or dream production previously mentioned, except that a more specifically structured stimulus is presented in the form of an actual picture.

All of the projective methods discussed so far have involved visual stimuli. The writer has recently experimented with the presentation of vague or unstructured auditory material for projective interpretation. The tautophone or verbal summator (Shakow and Rosenzweig, 1940) is a phonographic instrument which plays "jabber-talk" or jumbled speech. Subjects are asked to listen and tell what the voices are saying. In a variation of this device, a whispering record was made on the Dictaphone. One could hear a whispering voice, but no actual words could be distinguished. This whispering record was played to patients under trance, and they were asked to describe what the voice was saying—or a dissociated hand was instructed to write out the "whispered message."

The arts are expressive techniques whereby human feelings and emotions may be made manifest in the form of some medium: pictures, music, drama, dance, sculpture, or poetry. There is no reason why almost any of the arts could not be called upon as a projective technique for a patient under hypnotic trance. That type of art might be most effective in which the patient is most naturally talented. Many of the world's great poets and painters have indirectly described their inner conflicts in their creations. The writer has often observed examples of expressive and creative activity by subjects under deep hypnotic trance. This is definitely contradictory to the older concept of the hypnotized person as an automaton, subject to the hypnotist's "will."

The making of drawings, finger paintings, or sketches has been used as a projective technique, especially in the study of children (Elkisch, 1945). The possibilities for their use under hypnosis need much study. In one case a patient, using a dissociated hand, responded to questions about his fears, which he could not verbalize, by drawing the picture of a man with a queer, twisted, and misshapen figure. Later, it was found that this represented a childish fear of a character actor in motion pictures, the late Lon Chaney. He had acquired this fear as a young boy when he saw *The Hunchback of Notre Dame.*

Free association has always been a basic psychoanalytic technique. The patient is encouraged, while in a relaxed state, to discuss and describe the various thoughts that pass through his mind and make no effort to control them.   He must talk about all of them, regardless of how foolish or embarrassing they are. This is based upon the assumption that each association, no matter how ridiculous it seems, has definite psychological meaning. If this material is permitted to emerge without artificial restraint, it will point to significant inner conflicts. This technique of Free Association can also be performed under trance—and under regressed trance. The possibilities here need much more exploration. Psychoanalysts, who are already skilled in the use of this method in the conscious state, should investigate the opportunities for it under hypnosis.

Jung (1918), a disciple of Freud, developed a list of 100 words as association stimuli. The patient is given a word and asked to respond with the very first word that comes into his mind. Time of response is checked, and the actual association noted, as are evidences of anxiety. If a word brings about a significant association, this is discovered through the response, by the amount of time required to secure a response, or through signs of anxiety. Another list which has been more standardized is the Kent-Rosanoff (1910). It is interesting to administer a free-association word list and then to give it again to a patient under trance regressed to various age levels. Significant changes in the response pattern are often important indicators of conflict areas and also are useful in determining developmental changes which occurred during the intervening age period.

Free association is listed in this book as a projective technique. The writer sees it essentially as one of the many projective methods. In the *Rorschach* an unstructured ink-blot is used to arouse patient associations.   In the *Thematic Apperception Test* it is a picture which does the job.   In the *Jung Word-Association Test* a word is given the patient by the therapist to induce an association.   And in *Free Association* the patient in one idea presents himself with the stimulus which evokes the next response or association.   It is a self-structuring projective technique in which each response becomes the stimulus to pull out the next response, or association.   Free association under trance can be employed in the same way as the psychoanalyst uses it in the conscious state.   Some patients who are blocked and unproductive when fully conscious are able to associate easily under hypnotic trance.

One of the most interesting depth-techniques is the *dissociating or splitting of the personality structure* into two or more segments for separate study.   The patient can then throw himself into a psychodramatic production in which he takes more than one role.   The axis of splitting should be along the lines of the inferred conflict.[3] For example, the patient is told,

> We are now going to make up a story about a pair of twins by the name of Madden. One of these we will call George Madden, and the other one will be John Madden.[4] Let us imagine that George and John Madden are in the same outfit in battle. George Madden has always been a very well-meaning young man. He tries to do that which is right, but there is much evil in his brother, John Madden. John is always trying to urge George to get into trouble. He suggests many things for them to do which are against George's better nature. You can now make up a story, a dramatic play, about these two boys. Make it as vivid as possible. Tell the story first by taking the part of George and then by taking the part of John. Act it out as you think it should be.

This permits the patient to identify with George, the better character, which he has probably been trying to do consciously anyway, but also to play the part of John, who symbolizes those repressed forces or more primitive drives within him which have been operative only at an unconscious level. In dramatizing the story of George versus John the patient is actually re-enacting his own inner conflicts. Sometimes the therapist will initiate the beginning of this play and then interpose questions as an outside or third party. This technique can be combined with many others, such as regression, free association, and any of the projective techniques. It is also possible to use dissociated-hand methods in conjunction with multiple personalities, letting one hand write for the John personality and the other for the George personality. (Naturally, the right-handed person will exhibit poor muscular coordination when trying to write with his left hand. Most individuals, however, are able to make letters and words that are legible. See Figure 6, Chapter 22.)

An interesting minor technical device for securing a resistant association is to prepare the patient for an idea as follows: "I am going to count up to five. When I say the word 'five,' a very significant idea will instantly come into your mind, and you will tell me what it is. One, two, three, four, *five*." This can sometimes be used

---

[3] Some projective techniques are well adapted to indicate conflict areas. For example, the *Bellak TAT Blank* (1947) allows for analysis of each TAT story to show ambivalences of the following type: Super-Ego—Id, compliance—autonomy, passivity—counteraction, achievement—pleasure, etc.

[4] These two names might have been used if the patient's real name was something like George Miller. The similar name was chosen, of course, to encourage identification. Sometimes the presentation was made nondirective, the patient being asked to describe and name the multiple personalities as he wished.

to recover a lost name which the patient has been unable to recall even under trance (Watkins, 1947a). "I shall count up to three. At the count of three this man's name will suddenly appear in front of you, and you can read it. One, two, *three*." Or again, "I shall count slowly up to ten. When I reach ten you will know what it is that you fear." This sometimes brings about a significant recall which cannot be secured otherwise. It is especially fruitful in overcoming minor resistances. If this fails a still further extension of this method is as follows: "When I count up to five the name of that which you fear will come to your mind, but you will see it as a *jumbled word* in which the letters are all twisted." On the count of five the patient will then frequently give a nonsense word. Readjustment of the letters will sometimes turn it into a very significant term. This technique is especially effective combined with the dissociated hand, permitting the hand to write out the twisted word with the mixed letters. An intermediate stage between securing the actual word or jumbled form of it is to suggest that the number of letters in the word will emerge on the count of five, or some other number or letter —such as, "I will start saying the alphabet. A number will pop into your mind when I reach the letter K."

Psychological Testing

Psychological tests—intellectual tests, aptitude tests and *personality tests*—are all designed to furnish certain information about a person's aptitudes or maladjustments in his mental life. These tests can also be given effectively under trance, and, of course, under trance regressed to any desired age level. In an unpublished study [5] the writer once gave rather exhaustive batteries of diagnostic reading tests and photographed eye movements of a college student regressed to various age levels from six up through eighteen. The qualitative and quantitative development of her various reading skills could be traced in this manner. It was possible to determine what type of reading instruction she must have had at various grades and what her chief difficulties were at these age levels. The opportunities of using such clinical diagnostic tests as the Bender Gestalt, the Rorschach, the Wechsler-Bellevue, the Minnesota Multiphasic, and other psychological testing instruments under regressed trance appears promising.

---

[5] John G. Watkins, and Benjamin R. Showalter, "The Development of Reading Skills as Exhibited under Hypnotic Regression."

Psychological Meaning of Symbols

Finally, the *deeper interpretation of symbolic material* uncovered, in line with classical analytic theory, offers a vast area for advanced study. Freud has pointed out that often an individual's fantasies are as important as his more objective ideas; that conflicts frequently emerge clothed in symbolic form in the dream life of a person; that certain types of symbols commonly represent certain sexual or other concepts. There is, therefore, a wealth of possibilities for the skilled psychoanalyst to discover latent tendencies in patients through the symbolic interpretation of material that has been uncovered by any of the techniques thus far described.

Analysis of Transference Reactions

One of the fundamental therapeutic methods used by the psychoanalysts is the analysis of that close interpersonal relationship between the patient and therapist known as *transference*. In the course of a protracted treatment it has usually been found that the patient begins to manifest irrational attitudes toward the therapist. These may vary from profound hostility to gestures of extreme affection. These attitudes may manifest themselves in the patient's dreams, associations, and in his manner of behaving toward the therapist. Thus, during a stage of positive transference the patient may most enthusiastically praise the skill of the therapist, may relinquish some of his symptoms as a friendly gesture, or may report highly erotic dreams in which the therapist is the object of his affections. On the other hand, when the transference is negative, the patient may be late for his appointments or forget to come. He may most actively criticize the methods and personal characteristics of the therapist. Since the therapist has been consistently playing an objective role toward the patient, these attitudes obviously do not stem from reality but originate in some subjective strivings within the patient.

These reactions find their origin in the transference to the therapist of attitudes and feelings developed toward other close associates in the past. Unconsciously the patient appears to be regarding the therapist as mother, father, brother, sweetheart, etc. He is thus behaving toward the therapist as if the therapist were one of these persons. The changes in the transference may reflect a change of roles which the patient is projecting onto the therapist.

Transference reactions occur not only toward the therapist but toward many others within the patient's social environment. For example, his hostility toward a business associate may stem from his identification of that man with his domineering (and hence hated) father. Or he may assume a dependent, child-like role toward his wife because unconsciously he views her as a mother substitute. Probably a large number of our social reactions to each other are based on the transference of earlier attitude patterns rather than the reality of the situation.

In the therapeutic situation these irrational reactions become a powerful leverage as the clinician interprets them to the patient. The patient is forced to achieve insight into his immature behavior patterns because in the transference relationship he experiences them at first hand. The old motto, "Seeing is believing," takes cognizance of the fact that we learn most readily and appreciate most deeply that which we have intimately experienced. An insightful interpretation by the therapist carries much greater weight when backed up by a personal and immediately perceived emotional experience. Many analysts believe this proof through analysis of transference reactions to be the only real and thoroughgoing way in which basic attitudes can be altered. They feel that insight arrived at through other methods is likely to be superficial or "intellectual," and hence that it may not permanently affect basic personality.

While conceding the great value of analyzing transferences as a method of achieving therapeutic insight, we prefer to take the position here that the insight is our basic goal and that the analysis of transferences is only one of many methods whereby new behavior patterns may be learned. The study of learning as it takes place in transference reactions should be more closely investigated by our experimental psychologists along with the other principles and methods of learning. Likewise, our psychoanalysts might improve their methods considerably and shorten the time of analyses if they took greater advantage of the many significant findings by experimentalists in the psychology of learning. Learning, faulty and good, appears to be at the heart of neuroses and their treatment. Thus J. McV. Hunt summarizes (1948), "I cannot refrain from stating the proposition that therapy for a patient is learning and for a psychotherapist teaching. It is high time that the practitioners of this art should examine the science of the learning process."

Transference reactions occur under hypnosis as well as in the ordinary conscious state, and the same principles of manipulation and interpretation apply in these circumstances. Wolberg (1945) has written rather extensively on the integration of handling these reactions with other hypnotherapeutic procedures.

Transference reactions usually tend to manifest themselves only after an extended period of continuous treatment. Hence, their analysis as a therapeutic method is more feasible during the prolonged treatment of a well-entrenched, chronic neurosis than under war conditions in the Army.

Since there has already been some psychiatric screening before men are inducted into military service, the military neurosis is more likely to be related to the element of stress than predisposition. On the other hand, the civilian neurosis which has developed in the absense of severe stress probably is rooted in the severe predisposition of immature adjustments and early traumatic experiences. Therefore, from the standpoint of both etiology and time available for treatment, the method of analyzing transference reactions is less well adapted to the handling of the military neurosis.

For these reasons the analysis of transference did not become a major method of treating the cases described in this book. Where insight rather than a motivational cure was achieved, the emotionally corrective experience was generally reached by other learning methods than analysis of transference.

Abreaction

The term *abreaction* should be discussed at this point. By this we mean the emotional reliving or re-enacting of traumatic experiences. This actually involves a great expenditure of energy and a release of anxiety. It has been done quite effectively in narcosynthesis, where the patient under the influence of sodium amytal or sodium pentothal releases pent-up battle anxieties (Grinker and Spiegel, 1944). During these dramatic sessions the patient may cry, weep, stride about, pound on the walls, or shout. He relives a whole dramatic or guilt-laden experience. This can be done under hypnotic trance as well as under the influence of the barbiturate drugs (Alpert, Carbone, and Brooks, 1946). It is of value, both in anxiety reactions and in hysterical reactions, where the anxiety has been systematized and structured. Simmel (1944) in describing his hypnotherapy during the first World War mentions that he often used a dummy which could be identified as the enemy, the personal enemy of the patient. On this the patient was encouraged to secure his revenge. Under the high emotion of an abreactive trance he would tear the dummy to shreds. He would then be told that he had now destroyed his enemy and did not any longer need to feel rage and hostility. He was thus relieved of guilt over apparent cowardice. At the same time, there was a loss of pent-up anxieties. This appears to be a valuable extension of the abreactive technique in that it enables the patient not only to talk out his anxiety, but also to act it out and thus bring about more total bodily participation.

During abreaction there is an emotional catharsis or release. It is much like "getting it off your chest." Abreactions will frequently arise during use of the psychodramatic method while the patient is under trance. They should be exploited to the full by the therapist when they occur. Under abreaction the nature of hidden aggressive impulses can be studied to determine objects at which they are directed.

It is often possible through an abreaction to permit the patient to project out deep-seated, repressed hostilities toward father, mother, wife, brother, sister, or friend. Not only is a certain amount of relief afforded, but also the therapist gains a great deal of valuable information about the inner motivational structure. Abreaction can, of course, be initiated at any regressed age level.

Abreactive sessions will be most valuable if the therapist will prod by dramatic and emotional suggestions the most thorough participation of the entire patient psychologically and physiologically (Watkins, 1949). Afterwards, it is essential that the release of the inhibited guilt, rage, or fear impulses be followed by intellectual and emotional reintegration and insight. Through such a re-enactment of the conflict the opportunity is offered the therapist to bring the original frustrating situation to a more satisfactory and realistic solution. An emotionally corrective experience is undergone which "completes" the unfinished strivings, which are the repetitive core of the neurosis, and relieves the need to continue its symptomatic manifestations. The neurosis is basically an interrupted or uncompleted reaction trying compulsively (but futilely) to complete itself. This striving to complete unfinished business has been stressed by the Gestaltists (Koffka, 1935) as a basic motivation. They have termed this the *principle of closure*. Experimentally it has received verification in the work of Zeigarnik (1927) and Ovsiankina (1928), whose findings have been summarized and integrated by Lewin (1935). The psychoanalysts also have emphasized this compulsive striving to complete the unfinished reaction as the *repetitive core* of the neurosis (Kubie, 1943). Therefore our "closing" of the system through hypnotic abreaction, just as in completing it by analysis of transference reactions, does resolve neurotic conflict. The procedure is based on sound theory and is backed by substantial experimental and clinical findings.

Freud, among others, found that some neuroses did not respond to the abreactive method. While we certainly cannot expect any single procedure to be effective in all cases, it is quite possible that many of the reported failures of abreaction to cure (both hypnotic and narcosynthetic abreactions) have been due largely to inadequate attention to the two fundamental points of total participation and subsequent reintegration. Merely sticking pentothal into a man's arm is not enough.

The In-and-Out Method

In Chapter 7 an example was given of the use of direct suggestion to prepare a patient to accept an insight. A variation of this, called the *In-and-Out Method,* can be used in the therapeutic interview. The patient is linked to some object by posthypnotic suggestion so that trance can be reinduced in a matter of seconds. He can then be placed in a deep trance in a moment, prepared for a revealing statement, and brought out of trance at the count of five or some other established signal. The statement is next discussed with him. He is shown the trance-inducing object; whereupon he immediately becomes hypnotized again. His degree of understanding and acceptance is checked by questioning under trance. The statement is further explained and elaborated to him under trance. He is prepared for the next one, awakened, etc. An entire session may develop into an *in-and-out* interview used for uncovering new material or integrating already discovered points. The writer has held sessions in which the trance state was induced twelve to fifteen times within a single hour. This technique of weaving back and forth between conscious and hypnotic states helps the patient to reintegrate concepts at both levels. It is in this reintegration that significant insight is formed, that permanent changes in the personality structure are achieved. It is in this welding or bridging of the unconscious to the conscious that the therapist can change the entire Gestalt or pattern and thus achieve a more permanent and lasting cure.

Teaching Under Trance

Acquiring insight is a process of personality education. As mentioned earlier, the good therapist must be a good teacher. The ability of the patient to grasp new concepts and use them to break through resistances and change his neurotic mechanisms or relinquish his infantile drives is directly related to the didactic skill of the treating clinician. The therapist's ability to couch his interpretations in meaningful terms to the patient and to reduce the patient's intellectual defenses by evoking full-fledged emotionally corrective experiences is a characteristic of the effective therapist secondary only to his perceptual skill in deducing dynamic relationships.

The patient is taught the meaning of a point in the conscious state. He is taught it in trance, and the two are welded together. This teaching or integrative process may often go back to different age levels. The teaching is then under regressed trance. Harmful attitudes that were acquired through the stupidity or maliciousness of friends and parents can be retaught, reintegrated, and given a more beneficial meaning through explanation and elaboration under regressed trance.

It is even possible to *alter memories* (Erickson and Kubie, 1941). Thus, a particularly unfortunate occurrence which has happened to the patient at an early age can be re-enacted (abreacted) and reinterpreted to remove some of the awesome and fearful features. Checks made months afterward show that at least in some cases this altered memory has become a permanent part of the patient's life. He "remembers" it in the reinterpreted or *adjusted* form. This technique was used with good results on several occasions, but it does not seem to have a therapeutic effect as dependable as resolution of the conflict through emotionalized insight.

Memories which have been altered at the regressed age of four can be checked by advancing the person to any later age, such as seven, nine, fourteen, or seventeen to see that the altered memory, rather than the original one, is *recalled*. While this method needs much further scientific experimentation, it promises new possibilities in readjustment of early unfortunate experiences.

In suggesting insights the therapist may often prefer to do so slowly. For example, "During the next few weeks you will gradually come to realize that down deep inside, you have always had a great amount of hostility toward your brother. This new understanding will emerge a little at a time. You will work on this problem during the next two weeks and approach an understanding of it."

We must remember at all times that under trance we have a person with individual attitudes and resistances. Changes in the fundamental personality structure are not simply and easily secured by mere direct command. He who resorts constantly to direct suggestion will find many failures. Even with all our hypnotic weapons we must patiently and gradually initiate changes in the personality involving acceptance and understanding of new insights.

Planning Therapy in the Individual Case

In the various treatment sessions described in the case studies to follow there were definite individual plans of attack. This tactical scheme was very flexible. Before each session the plan was prepared after reviewing previous notes. The therapist outlined what he hoped to accomplish and the methods he proposed to utilize. He usually followed these unless something happened in the course of the session which required a change of plan. Sometimes there were "hot sessions" in which the therapist received a "break." He did not hesitate to take advantage of these and alter the plan, if necessary.

Occasionally notes were recorded by an assistant so as to free the therapist to meet the questioning and interviewing demands of the occasion. In some sessions the relations between the therapist and patient were of such a delicate nature that no third party could be permitted in the room while trance was being induced because the rapport would be impaired. In these cases either the recording assistant was invited into the room after trance had been secured or after the hallucination had been induced that there was nobody else in the room except the therapist and patient. At other significant sessions the therapist took notes while conducting the interview. This was not always satisfactory as material would often come at a faster rate than he could record and still meet the evaluating and questioning demands of the situation. He would in this case have to rely upon memory. The desirability of hidden microphones and recording devices is obvious.

There was a rather common strategical plan of attack in the various hypnotherapeutic sessions. In the first hour suggestibility tests were given. This was followed by an orientation into the nature of hypnotherapy. Next, trance was induced and tests were made to determine what depths could be reached. These were followed by suggestions tending to increase rapport and to enhance the prestige of the therapist in the eyes of the patient. Following this, the attempt was made to see how far the symptoms could be manipulated under trance. Precautions were generally taken not to remove all the symptoms if the underlying dynamics were not understood. Sometimes, part of the symptoms would be removed, leaving a few incapacitating ones until more of the inner motivational system could be disclosed. In the next stages of the treatment simple interviewing and regressive methods were tried. Finally, if still necessary, the various depth techniques involving dissociated hand and projective methods were employed.

The general rule of procedure was to start with the more superficial manifestations and later attack the deeper conflicts. The simplest methods which could accomplish the job were preferred. Operations were kept within the predetermined areas of the problem. If a man could be relieved of his severe headaches without the necessity of digging into an entrenched Oedipus complex, this was done. The job in an Army hospital is minor, not major psychological surgery.

It should be evident from Chapters 7 and 8 that the therapeutic importance of hypnosis does not lie in the trance itself. Its significance is much greater than the attempts to eliminate symptoms by direct suggestion, however valuable this method may be at times. Its greatest advantage lies in the increased opportunities it offers the psychotherapist to employ a wide variety of uncovering and integrating techniques.

Outline of Advanced Hypnotherapeutic Techniques

1. Dissociated handwriting
   a. Under trance
   b. Posthypnotic
   c. Automatic writing without trance

2. Projective techniques
   a. Projective psychological tests
      (1) Rorschach Ink-Blot Test
      (2) Thematic Apperception Test
      (3) Jung Word-Association Test
   b. Psychodrama
   c. Crystal gazing (card gazing, movies, scroll unrolling, etc.)
   d. Dream and fantasy production
      (1) Dream interpretation under trance
   e. Art forms
   f. Free Association
   g. Dissociated personalities

3. Psychoanalytic interpretation of symbolic material

4. Analysis of therapist-patient transference

5. Abreactive techniques

6. Teaching and re-integrating under trance

7. Altering memory-structure

8. In-and-Out method

PART III

INDIVIDUAL CASE STUDIES

CHAPTER 9

FOREWORD TO THE CASE STUDIES

Exposition of Techniques

Many excellent descriptions of the treatment of cases by various techniques have been written. Good casebooks are available in non-directive therapy, psychoanalytic therapy, hypnoanalytic therapy, etc. However, the writer in his search to improve his own therapeutic skill has often read these with a feeling that what would have been most valuable to him was omitted. For example, one writer may state, "This was then interpreted to the patient." Perhaps other readers have had the same reaction as this writer in wondering just what the therapist said in making the interpretation. What words did he use? How did he use his voice? What was his general manner? Why did he choose to make the interpretation at this point? Why did he make it in this particular way? Afterwards, did he feel that this was the best way to have handled the point? If not, in what way did he think his technique could have been improved? In other words there has often been a lack in case reporting of word-for-word recording and of critical evaluation and exposition of the therapy in reporting it as it happened. This does not give the reader opportunity to profit from the mistakes of others. It does not afford him a chance to learn therapeutic skills and tactics successfully employed by other clinicians. The emphasis has usually been on the pathology and dynamics of the case. True, this gives the reader a good understanding of emotional conflicts, but it does not help him in developing his technical skills in the actual handling of the patient.

A casebook may be equally valuable when it reports errors in judgment and therapeutic strategy. We cannot always be right in our treatment of a case, but we can faithfully report what we did and the results as best we can evaluate them. If we have failed, at least we can help others not to repeat our mistakes.

It is with this general attitude in mind that the following case chapters were written in order to share with the professional reader as intimately as possible the experiences, the successes and failures, which were our lot in the Special Treatment Company (Company F,

Third Battalion) of the Neuropsychiatric Treatment Branch of Welch Convalescent Hospital.

The course of the treatment in each case is presented with an emphasis on the techniques employed. Progress reports and transcriptions of therapeutic sessions are interspersed with critical comments on the methodology employed and explanations of the reasons for using various tactics.

Method of Recording

During the therapeutic sessions extensive notes were taken. Immediately at the end of each hour a complete report of the session was recorded on Dictaphone cylinders as nearly as possible, word for word, exactly as it had occurred. The reports of the interviews as described in the case chapters were taken from the transcriptions of these records. It is to be regretted that automatic recording devices were not available in order that our written record here would not contain even the slightest deviation from what actually transpired within each therapeutic hour. However, within the limits of our recording method every effort has been made to preserve fidelity of report. Names and identifying circumstances have been altered to protect the anonymity of patients, but the essential features in the background, development, and treatment of each case have been accurately described. To report completely everything that was said in every therapeutic session for these cases would require many times the number of pages that it is possible to use in this book. Hence, word-for-word reports are given of the most crucial sessions and the significant parts of sessions. Procedures used and patient reactions which did not appear to be of great importance are briefly summarized instead of being described verbatim.

Follow-up Data

Follow-up inquiries have been made, and where it was possible to secure later data on the health and adjustment of the patient subsequent to discharge from the service these findings have been included. Unfortunately, repeated efforts to contact and trace many of the patients have been unsuccessful.

It is hoped that the case reports as they are recorded here will be of substantial assistance to professional clinicians who wish to learn more of a therapeutic technique through the mutual sharing of experiences.

CHAPTER 10

APHONIA

The telephone bell jangled. Over it came a voice saying, "Lieutenant, this is Major C. We have a patient down here with an aphonia—can't speak above a whisper. He's had amytal and pentothal narcosis with no apparent effect, and he'll have to be discharged. However, we wondered whether his hysterical condition might respond to hypnotherapy, and we are sending him up to you to see what you think. He can be transferred to Company F if this is desirable. When can you see the man?"

The therapist replied, "I have an open hour at two o'clock this afternoon, Major, and—just one other point—have you definitely decided that this man is no longer suitable for military service, so he can be reassured that the treatment in this company will not interfere with his returning home?"

"Yes, this man is of no further value to the service. He has had functional stomach trouble for the past five years, including nausea, vomiting, burning, and cramping. He has also had chronic, severe headaches most of his life. He'll have to be given a CDD, but perhaps you can help him some, at least with the aphonia symptom, which is his most disabling characteristic."

At two o'clock that afternoon, the therapist was seated by his desk when a timid knock sounded on the door.

"Come in."

The knock was repeated. "Come in!"

Slowly, the door opened, and a rather sallow-faced, slim-looking boy, somewhat hunched over, shuffled into the room. The soldier seated himself beside the therapist's desk, nervously fingering his cap and gazing around the room.

"You're Walter Ball, I believe," began the therapist.

The patient merely nodded his head and continued to stare in a frightened fashion toward the door through which he had just entered.

There was another moment of silence, finally broken by the therapist with, "Walter, tell me about how you feel. What bothers you most?"

Then the patient responded in a whisper that was barely audible, "I can't talk."

"How long has this been going on?" (The therapist knew very well how long it had been since this symptom began, but most neurotics like to talk about their symptoms, and it is a good way of establishing rapport, since the patient feels that his "doctor" is interested in him.)

As the patient began to realize that he was not being accused of malingering, and that his symptom was accepted, he warmed up somewhat and related the following facts about himself, many of which were also available in the social history in his chart. He was twenty-five years old and had spent a year and a half in military service. Although he had been overseas some four months, he was not in combat. He had been sent to the Panama Canal, but was returned to the States in three months after having been hospitalized for "stomach trouble." He had been born in a rather poor family, and his father was engaged in farming in a Southern state. He himself had worked on the farm and done other miscellaneous common labor jobs, had been married four years, and had two children. He claimed that he was once interested in athletics, but now had no interest in such activities. Three months earlier, while engaged in rather monotonous duties in the States, he developed first a hoarseness and then finally a whisper, and had to be hospitalized again. Since his wife had been ill, he had received a convalescent furlough and gone home for a few weeks, but upon return to the hospital there was no improvement in his condition. He voiced a great deal of bitterness and hostility toward the Army and toward Army officers who, he felt, had mistreated him.

Orientation of Patient for Hypnotherapy

It was obvious that the extreme hostility toward the Army and toward Army officers would make it difficult to hypnotize the patient, so he was given the usual orientation discussion first. This was designed to answer questions, to establish a more friendly relation between the therapist and the patient, and to allay anxieties. It went somewhat as follows:

"Walter, you've been sent up to Company F because your doctor felt that you needed special help and treatment to get you to feeling better. In this company, we have a number of fellows who have certain nervous difficulties like you do. Many of them have felt the same as you do about the Army. The first thing I want to say is that *we are not going to promise to cure you.* Nobody here is going to slap you on the back and tell you that we'll fix you up at once. You know and I know that when a fellow is sick like this it's not easy to get over. But while I'm *not* going to promise to cure you, I *can* tell you that most of the fellows who come up here to Company F do get to feeling a lot better, and some of them become almost well."

Notice that we have in this patient a strong, unconscious desire not to get well because "not getting well" means a medical discharge, while getting well might mean return to duty. This motive, as we mentioned before, can be either conscious or unconscious. Let us give Walter the benefit of the doubt and assume that he is, at least, not completely aware of it. Nevertheless, in the orientation this factor must be handled. By our telling the patient that we would not promise to cure him, the neurosis itself received a certain encouragement. Note the almost wary actions of the patient on first entering the office. It is as if the unconscious were saying to him, "Look out! Better be careful. This doctor may cure you, and if he does, they'll send you back to duty." But when the patient is told that "we do not promise to cure you," the neurosis is pacified. Walter relaxed in his chair, and it was immediately noted how much his anxieties had subsided. Although consciously a patient wants to get well, also unconsciously he doesn't, because his symptoms are serving a certain purpose. For Walter, they are good for a medical discharge from service. The orientation continued:

"Now, I want you to know, Walter, that the decision has already been made to close your chart for a medical discharge. This will be done as soon as you get better. We don't feel that your condition is such as to warrant your being returned to duty, but we can't send a man home who has lost his voice and can hardly speak, so you will be closed to go home as soon as you get better, and the quicker you get better, the sooner you will be out of here." Notice how the motivation power is now switched from the secondary-gain side to the desire-to-get-well side of our neurotic mechanism. Prior to this, getting well meant return to duty. Now, getting well means going home sooner.

But, at this point, we notice in Walter a certain defensive reaction, a very slight freezing; and we suspect that, unconsciously, a part of him is saying, "Look out for this guy, Walter; he's trying to trick you. They're just promising you this so that you will regain your voice. They can send you back to duty then." So, we continue the orientation as follows:

"Perhaps you're like a lot of the other boys here, Walter. They've been transferred from one Army post to another, from one hospital to another; they feel pretty much kicked around. Many of them say that promises have been made to them that haven't been kept." (One can almost see the unconscious nodding of agreement in Walter.) "I understand how you feel. I've been in the Army two years myself and know a little of what it's like." (The therapist here attempts to get the patient to identify with him.) "We've found here that more than anything else the fellows like to know what the score is. So, while we can't promise you we're going to cure you, we *can* promise you that you'll know what's going on and that you won't be told one thing is going to happen to you while something else does. When I say your chart is going to be closed, it will be closed. You can count on it. Does that make sense?"

The manner in which the patient reacts, rather than his actual words at this point, indicates to the therapist whether or not he really accepts what has just been said. One notices a very definite thawing in Walter's manner. He begins to smile. His speech, even though in a whisper, comes much more freely and with less hesitation and blocking. He is relaxed in his chair, and the tensions have largely disappeared. He begins to take an interest in what is being said because, *now,* what is being said is important; it has something to do with his going home, and going home and escaping from military service are the most strong, vital drives in his whole body. Regardless of the true symbolism back of his symptoms, this is a powerful secondary gain tending to maintain them.

Let's summarize what we should have accomplished so far in the orientation. First, we have, psychologically speaking, played both ends against the middle. The neurosis has been reassured by the fact that, "we don't promise to cure you." This has enabled it to relax its vigilance and to feel that it is fairly safely entrenched. On the other hand, we have pointed out to the patient that "most fellows get to feeling much better here." This makes him consciously believe that transfer to a special treatment company to receive therapy is desirable. Second, by indicating an understanding of his hostility toward the Army and Army officers (possible father figures) and by getting a certain amount of identification of the patient with the therapist, we have broken down a great deal of the resistance which otherwise might completely prevent any effective treatment. By not promising to cure him, there has been added a certain ring of sincerity and authenticity to all the other remarks, because, consciously, Walter doesn't think he's going to be cured, and unconsciously he hopes he isn't. We have also reversed the motivational springs, so that maintaining his symptoms means continued stay in the Army and in the hospital, while loss of symptoms means return to home. We next decide to try to break down resistance to the hypnotic treatment, and the orientation is continued:

"Walter, I want you to notice my arm." The therapist holds it out very rigid with all muscles tight and in a high state of tonus. "Why doesn't it go up or down?" Walter looks a little surprised, shrugs his shoulders, and replies,

"Why, because the muscles are holding it out there."

The therapist continues, "That's right. Notice these top muscles, though, are trying to pull it up, and the muscles on the other side are trying to pull it down. They're working against each other, aren't they? What do you suppose would happen if I were to keep my arm that way for a long period of time?" Walter appears to be mildly interested.

"I suppose it would get awfully tired, or sore, or hurt, or something."

"That's right. That's because the muscles are pulling against each other. They're in conflict, so to speak, and that's exactly what happens to a man's body when forces inside of him get into conflict with each other. What do you think would happen to a man's body if there were forces inside of him pulling one way, and other forces pulling another way?"

"I suppose it would make him sick or something."

"Of course it makes him sick. It can give him headaches, tie up his stomach so that it won't hold on to food but throws it up, make his heart beat irregularly, paralyze a leg or an arm, or it can even prevent him from speaking clearly." Walter raised his eyebrows rather quizzically and uttered the equivalent of a whispered "Hm-m."

The therapist next asked, "What must be done if my arm stays like this?" holding the arm rigidly out once more.

Walter said, "One of the muscles has got to be relaxed, so they don't conflict with each other, and the arm can be pulled up or down."

"That's exactly right, and that's what has to be done when the conflict is inside a man's whole body. It has to be resolved so that he doesn't pull two ways against himself at the same time."

Walter butted in, "Yeah, but I haven't got any conflict like that. There's nothing worrying me."

The therapist replied, "Yes. I imagine it doesn't seem as if you do worry, but did it ever occur to you that maybe a man could worry about things that he didn't know about?"

"How's that?" put in Walter.

"Just for example, who used to sit right behind you in the first grade of school?"

"Now, come on, Doc—you know that I don't remember that."

"Well, it's true that you can't remember it right now, but actually you haven't completely forgotten it. It's down inside you. It's what we call 'unconscious.' All the things that happened to you years and years ago, and some of the inner meanings they had, are unconscious inside of you. It's like the lower part of an iceberg, which you can't see. It's under water, but that doesn't mean it isn't there. And, in the same way, perhaps, these forces, these worries or nervous difficulties that you have, could still be inside you, and yet you wouldn't know about them." [1]

---

[1] In the explanations, simple, homely language free from technical terminology was used. This is an important point in the individual treatment of nonintellectuals. Too much professionally administered psychotherapy goes over the head of the average or less gifted patient. *Insight must be based on understanding—the patient's understanding, not the doctor's.*

The manner of making interpretations is of the greatest significance. Perhaps much of the resistance which arises in the course of working through deeper material is mobilized by offering interpretations in terms which are entirely unacceptable to the patient. This therapist has found it best to try to put one's self in the mental and emotional position of the patient and anticipate how one would react to various methods of presentation.

For example, let us suppose that one is treating a woman with considerable aggressiveness who through dream symbols indicates her latent homoerotic impulses and desires for masculine identification. To tell her that she has "penis envy" is a stupid procedure. Obviously she must reject the concept and mobilize her resistance against the idea in terms of her conventionalized training. Even though she ultimately accepts the correctness of this interpretation, much more time must pass before this unpalatable intellectual morsel can be emotionally assimilated. How much better it would be to proceed somewhat as follows: "Have you noticed how often in your life you have felt competitive toward men, how you have acted as though you looked upon men as beings who must be conquered or beaten? Perhaps you have even wished at times to be a man so that you might enjoy the advantages offered men in this culture. Do you think this may have caused you to reject the position and role of the woman—perhaps caused you to be more aggressive?

"Our dreams sometimes reveal motives within us through symbols which depend upon the most obvious associations to our repressed impulses. For example, from the earliest days we are taught the difference between boys and girls, between masculine and feminine, and we think of the difference in the shape of their genital organs as illustrating this distinction. The boy's possession of a penis and the girl's possession of a vaginal opening are, of course, the most noticeable differences between masculine and feminine. In fact, at the birth of a baby it is only by observing the shape of the genital organs that we can distinguish whether the child is a boy or girl.

"So in our dreams we often take some object shaped like the genitals to portray the idea of masculinity or femininity. Now in your dream last night you said that you saw yourself as wielding a big club to strike down or kill a number of men. Don't you think that in dreaming of your having this big club you may really mean that you wished to possess stronger traits of masculinity than the men whom you meet, and that therefore you could subdue them—that is, beat them at their own game? The big club, shaped as it is like a male genital, becomes the symbol of the masculine power which you wish you had in competing with the male sex."

An interpretation couched in such terms helps the patient to grasp the essential element of understanding her strivings toward masculinity without insulting her by the direct shock of calling it "penis envy." It is in the tactful skill with which he makes his interpretations that the therapist reduces resistance and speeds the therapeutic insight.

Walter chewed a while on that one. "That sounds sort of reasonable, Doc, but still, if I don't know what they are, there's nothing
that can be done about 'em. If you can't see 'em, you can't do anything about 'em." This last was uttered with almost an air of
triumph, as if the neurosis were gloating, "Well, I have you blocked
off there, anyway."

"That's right, Walter." (No contradiction. Controversial points
are treated by agreeing in general.) "They are very hard to get at,
but still we do have some ways of approaching them. For example,
do you ever dream at night when you go to sleep?"

"Sure, I dream some of the craziest stuff. Why, I remember, the
other night. . . . Say, what's this got to do with my whispering?
You aren't going to tell me that it's all in my head too, are you?"

The therapist cursed under his breath. Patients who had been
previously told that it was "all in your head" were notoriously resistant. This statement, made by some earlier aide or clinician, did
more to alienate the men and cause them to reject psychiatric treatment than almost anything else.

"No, Walter, I'm not going to tell you it's just in your head because it isn't just in your head. You and I both know that. But
also, it isn't just in your tongue and in your throat or your lips. It's
all through you; it's in your whole body where these forces are located. True, these forces are nervous, and have to do with your
nervous system. And it *is* true that your brain, which is the biggest
part of your nervous system, is in your head, but it's also little nervous
impulses that make your heart beat, make your stomach digest its
food, and they aren't in your head. These nervous forces, which we
said are unconscious, are everywhere in your whole body, and we
aren't going to be able to help you unless we can treat *all* of you."

The momentary flare-up of resistance subsided, and so the therapist continued :

"Now let's get back to that sleep. As you already said" (the
therapist here is probably amplifying the patient's statement a little
more than he originally intended) "there are things down in you
which normally you don't think about or know about, but which
come out when you are asleep, in the form of dreams. Well, we
know that lots of times it's possible, under a kind of natural sleep,
to get down and find out a little bit about these forces, the ones in
conflict with each other, which tie up your body so as to give it the
headaches, stomach pains—and which keep you from speaking
clearly."

Walter broke in, "What's sleep got to do with it?"

"Well," continued the therapist, "Let's go back to this arm again," holding his arm out stiff. "It's rather tight and tense now, isn't it? What's the opposite of tenseness in those muscles?"

"Why, relaxation," Walter grudgingly admitted.

"Of course," agreed the therapist, as he continued the attack, "We've got to try to help your whole body to relax. We must teach it how to relax, so these forces inside don't keep pulling it first one way and then another, and we can do it through relaxation or through putting it into a natural sleep. When you are under a natural sleep, we may be able to find out what are these nervous forces inside that are tying up your body. We want to relax them, so that they let go and quit fighting each other. Then you'll begin to feel a lot better. Maybe you'll talk clearly too."

Suspicion again arose as Walter inquired, rather anxiously, "You're not going to give me drugs or stick me with needles, are you? They stuck me with needles once before. It put me to sleep, and I felt awful funny and woozy, but it didn't do a bit of good."

"No," responded the therapist. "We're not going to stick any drugs into you or use any needles. I can promise you that." Walter sighed contentedly. "But we're going to *help* you to relax into a real, natural sleep. No drugs, nothing artificial. It's very natural, and you can do it by yourself. Nobody's going to try to force you to go to sleep. I'm just going to try to *help* you do it." (Note the permissive character of this attack. Already, the use of suggestion has begun; suggestion in the form that Walter will be helped, not forced, to go to sleep.)

"Well, when do I go to sleep? When are we going to get started? Do I go to sleep in the daytime?" The patient now seems ready for suggestibility tests, so he is told.

"I think first we had better study your nervous reactions. I want to see if you are going to be able to relax on your feet." And, before the patient can meditate on that one, he is immediately distracted with, "Do you mind standing over here and putting your toes and your heels together along this line?" A direct request for action has now been initiated, which does not leave time for a mulling over of what has been said, what commitments have been made, or a re-mustering of resistances. Walter stands up and places his feet, heels and toes together at the designated spot. The postural swaying test is begun as it was described in Chapter 6.

Walter did not seem to follow the normal reactions. Two minutes went by, three minutes, four minutes, five minutes. The therapist was continuing the monotonous suggestions of ". . . falling over

forward . . . falling forward . . . falling backward . . . backward
. . . forward . . . backward . . . " There seemed to be much unconscious resistance still on Walter's part to resist swaying in the
manner indicated.

At the end of six minutes, the therapist had decided that Walter
was not going to respond positively to the test and probably was not
very easily hypnotizable. Here is shown the common error easily
committed when the therapist prematurely gives up hope, because the
session was just about to be discontinued with the remark that, "All
right, you can open your eyes now and sit down," when Walter
began to sway in a rather dizzy-like fashion. His knees buckled, and
he collapsed in a semi-stuporous condition on top of a cot near by,
there being just enough voluntary control left to him to see that he
fell on the cot and not on the floor. There he lay quietly with his
eyes closed. There was obvious resistance, because suggestions of
hand levitation were not followed. It was apparent that only a light
or hypnoidal trance had been initiated, so direct suggestions had to
be avoided. Challenges, commonly used for indicators of trance
depth, were more likely further to mobilize resistance. So the therapist then tried this course:

"Just relax while you're lying there, Walter, and don't worry. I
know that you can hear what I say, and I also know that you're not
sound enough asleep but that we can talk. See if you can remember
anything which bothers you or worries you about which we might
talk."

Walter whispered a few remarks which were rather inconsequential in nature, but not even one single, significant lead appeared,
so a more superficial and direct attack against the speech symptom
was made, as follows:

While Walter had just previously been whispering it was noted
that, when sounding the letter "e" there would be an occasional
change from a whispered "e" to a sounded "ee." It would be short
and momentary, almost as though a very high-pitched string were
being plucked for an instant, but it was a definite, resonating sound,
so Walter was urged to concentrate on it.

"Say 'Eee.'"

Walter said, "Eee."

"Again."

"E."

"Now louder."

"E."

"Now hold it a long time."

"E-e-e-e," and in a wavering, thin voice, Walter emitted a full-fledged sound that was definitely not a whisper.

"Now, let's try saying 'speak.' "

Walter said, "Speak."

"Now, hold it."

"Spe-e-eak. Spe-e-eak."

"Now, let's try saying 'A-a-ay.' "

After three attempts, Walter said "A-a-ay."

"Now, let's say 'Oo-oo.' "

Again, after a few attempts, Walter said, "Oo-oo."

Each new sound seemed to require practice, but gradually emerged, and Walter was slowly retaught the sounds of the English language as if he were receiving a phonic lesson in the first grade. Motivation to speak was reinforced by practice as follows:

"Now say 'O-o-oh.' "

"Oh."

"Now say 'home.' "

"Home."

"Now say, 'Going home.' "

"Going home."

"Now say, 'I am going home.' "

"I am going home."

The implications here are obvious.

Next, Walter was told, "You will still stay in your sleep, but you will be able very slowly to open your eyes." The patient opened his eyes, but it was obvious that he still remained in a moderate trance condition. A piece of newspaper was placed in front of him, and he was asked,

"Now, let's see if you can read this?" Slowly, haltingly, Walter began to read, part of the time in a whisper, part of the time with audible sounds. First one column was read, then the next, then the next, then the next. As he continued his voice began to gain more firmness, more resonance. Less frequently did it return to the whisper and more often did it sound forth with a full-fledged vocal tone, until finally, after some twenty minutes of reading under trance, Walter talked and read in a completely normal voice. Walter was then asked, "Do you understand now that you are able to use your voice again?"

He nodded "yes."

"Will you be able to remember all that has happened and understand it when I wake you?" Notice that here a direct posthypnotic suggestion was put in question form, rather than in the form of an order. Again Walter nodded agreement.

"Then, if you're sure of this," the therapist continued, "I shall count slowly up to ten. As I do, you will gradually wake up, and you will be able to remember distinctly everything you could do while you were asleep. You will be able to speak as clearly and distinctly as you did just now. You will always be able to speak as clearly and distinctly as this." The count was given; Walter looked up and smiled.

"Go on and read me some more of your newspaper, Walter," said the therapist. Walter picked it up again and began reading in a completely normal voice. He seemed pleased. There was no great evidence of anxiety, but a look of astonishment.

"Are you speaking now as well as you did before you had your difficulty?"

"Yes, it seems that way, Sir," responded the patient.

So the therapist concluded the session with, "Well, we have made some progress. You do have control of your voice again, but we don't know all the reasons why it became the way it was. We will have a few more meetings to see if we can find out why, so we will be sure that it won't happen again. Then your chart will be closed so that you can go home, as you were told."

All this was accomplished in one meeting. It was the therapist's purpose to continue with more probing sessions and see if the dynamics underlying the symptom could be uncovered. However, unfortunately, outside matters intervened. Because of a family illness, Walter had to go home on an emergency furlough. Upon his return, administrative changes and discharge policy did not make it possible for the therapist again to see Walter before he was returned to civilian life.

Let us see what was actually done. From the lay point of view, a "cure" had been achieved in one session. From the psychiatric point of view, only a superficial change had been brought about in the patient. This had been achieved largely by suggestion and by a rearrangement of motivational forces within him, pulling the symptoms down without the extraction of the "dynamic springs." The total treatment time was a one-hour session.

If Walter does not get under too much stress and makes a reasonably good adjustment to the demands of civilian life, the probability is that he will not lose his voice again. This case illustrates the direct suggestion and motivational attack. As therapists, we cannot be satisfied with it, even though the patient and his family were quite happy at its outcome. It is possible that the underlying conflicts were comparatively superficial and not too deep-lying, in which case the direct suggestive therapy may have been quite adequate. At least we see that words can bring about motivational changes and that these can heal, in the sense of causing the disappearance of symptoms. Many are the patients, both civilian and military, who receive much less individual treatment than Walter. Perhaps this symptom, having served its basic purpose, will no longer be needed by Walter and hence will never reappear. We hope so.

Chronology of the Case

The patient was hospitalized with the aphonia after thirteen months of service on May 1, 1945. Three months of this was spent overseas, but none of it was under combat conditions. He was admitted to Welch Hospital July 30, and the crucial session occurred on August 10. He was not actually transferred to the Special Treatment Company but referred for the single session. He was discharged about the last of October to civilian life.

CHAPTER 11

AMNESIA

Richard Billings was a family man; at least, he was about to become one. Although he was an only child, he had a loving father and mother, and a wife who was on the point of presenting him with an heir. But Richard didn't know all this; in fact, Richard didn't know anything that had happened to him prior to a shell concussion received in battle five months ago, and he didn't recognize anybody he had known before that time. Richard found that his father, who visited the hospital, was a total stranger to him. He knew his own name only because others had told him what it was. Richard walked around like a man stunned. His eyes blankly looking forward, he would sit for hours on his cot, speaking to no one and ignoring everything that happened about him. When questioned, he would reply in a lackadaisical manner with a haunting hesitation, much as if he were groping for words or ideas. He paid little attention to staff members or other patients.

On entrance to the convalescent hospital he was referred to the Psychological Testing unit, where the Wechsler-Bellevue Intelligence Scale was administered. The psychologist in charge returned him to his company with the report that "The patient's behavior is completely listless, apathetic, and affectless. He is well oriented in the present, claims to have no recollection of the past and does not care what happens to him in the future. No estimate of his mental capacity can be made at this time."

A few days later the attempt was made to give him a Rorschach examination. This time the psychologist's report was as follows: "An attempt was made to administer the Rorschach to this patient, yielding results too meager to be meaningful. Four responses and six rejections were received. One was pure color; the others were form responses. Six of the ten cards were rejected. No meaningful evaluation can be made."

Some of the professional staff felt that Richard was malingering, that he was only trying to get out of the Army; but the consensus of opinion was that this was a true hysterical reaction, and two of the most experienced psychiatrists so diagnosed it. Richard walked about in his dissociated manner as much when he was alone, or apparently unobserved, as when he was in the doctor's office.

The writer was asked by the Battalion Commander to attempt by hypnosis to break through the amnesia of this nineteen-year-old soldier. After forty-five minutes of sleep suggestions, a very light hypnoidal trance was induced, involving only eye closure; but repeated attempts to bring about memory of past incidents failed, the patient insisting under the light trance that he could still remember nothing.

Failures of Barbiturate Narcosis

At this time, the attempt was made to combine hypnosis with sodium amytal. In the record which came with the man from another hospital, pentothal narcosis had been tried with some slight success. Under narcosynthesis he had reconstructed the part of his battle experiences immediately preceding the onset of amnesia. However, these were forgotten as soon as he emerged from the narcosis, and repeated attempts to bring them back again had failed. Accordingly, the therapist tried to induce a hypnotic trance while the patient's physician was simultaneously administering sodium amytal intravenously. The narcosis gradually became heavier and heavier. The patient finally passed into a very deep sleep; yet a true hypnosis could not be secured, nor could any memory for past material be elicited.

At this time, the patient's father came to the hospital. Although the patient could not recognize him, Richard was released to his father's custody and taken home on a convalescent furlough. It was arranged that, upon return from this furlough, if he was still amnesic, he would be transferred to the Special Treatment Company.

When Richard returned, he still had no memory of the past; in fact, he claimed that while at home he did not recognize his wife, his mother, nor any of his friends, and that it was very embarrassing to have people whom he could not recognize come up and speak to him. He appeared to accept his identity and some of the events of his past life because, as he stated, "People told me about them," but there was no true memory for these incidents. He was asked whether he knew about the coming birth of his child before he went overseas and was hospitalized. He said that his wife knew, and that she had told him before he went overseas, but he did not remember this—only that he had been informed that this had happened when he was home on furlough.

Attempts were now made again to induce hypnotic trance. After about five minutes of eye-closure suggestions, his eyes closed and then suddenly opened. The verbal suggestions were repeated. After a few minutes, the eyes again closed, and he was placed under metronome sedation for fifteen minutes. At the end of this time he awakened. The effort to induce trance was unsuccessful.

He was next given the Jung Verbal Association Test (1918). The patient made ready associations to common nouns, but he was unable to think of anything when abstract words were given him. He would merely study them for a period of time and then, in a blank, despairing manner reply, "I guess I just don't think of anything." Nothing of great significance was disclosed by the association test. However, it helped to increase the rapport between the therapist and the patient.

Some interesting responses on the test which might be indicative of his area of maladjustment were as follows:

Test Word	Response
Woman	(Long pause) "Nothing comes—don't know."
Pride	(Pause) "Don't know about that—within you."
Despise	"Don't know. Won't come.—hate."
Wicked	"Don't know."
Child	"Home—with my wife."
Speak	"I don't know."
Name	(Long pause) "Anybody."
Naughty	"Family."
Brother	"Don't know."
Love	"Mad."
Happy	"Don't know."
Evil	"Mine. —Act."
Door	"Mother."

After administration of the Jung test, a second attempt was made to induce trance, this time by the postural swaying technique. After a few minutes, Richard entered a light trance and was seated in a chair, but at that moment, a noise outside the room reawakened him. A little later, a third try was made. This time he increased his postural swaying until he fell over backwards. As he fell, he again awakened.

Prior to his furlough, the patient had asked a great deal about going home and said, "Maybe, if I went home, my memory would return." This had been one of the factors leading to suspicion on the part of some of the professional staff that here was a case of malingering. However, after he had gone home on furlough and still had not regained his memory, the patient's argument became rather invalid, and he recognized it as such. Accordingly, some other motivation was needed to help in overcoming the resistances, to make him hypnotizable, and to relieve the amnesia symptom. Since repeated previous attempts to break through the amnesia had failed, it was felt that rather drastic motivation must be used. The job required a block-buster and not merely small arms fire. Imagine the effect of the following on a neurotic patient who has broken down under the stress of military service, especially combat; and who has escaped from it all by a thoroughgoing amnesia:

"Richard, you went home on furlough, and you still were not able to regain your memory. Now you've come back to the hospital. You'll have to stay here until you get your memory back. We couldn't possibly permit a man to go home who was unable to recognize his family or friends. It looks like you're going to be here a long time to be treated, but we have been thinking of one possibility. If, after treating you here, we still cannot bring your memory back, it may be necessary to use very drastic methods. You have heard a great deal about how people sometimes recover their memories if they are taken back to the place where they lost them. If there is no other way to get this memory back, it may be necessary for us to send you back to Germany, back to the combat zone, into battle, in order that you can get your memory back where you lost it. We hope this won't be necessary, but we have been thinking about it."

While, of course, such things are not done with neuropsychiatric patients, nevertheless, the implied threat was there. Since in the Army men become accustomed to the idea that almost anything can happen, a tremendous fear must have been unconsciously evoked in Richard—a fear which, this time, would be our ally rather than our enemy—a powerful force which would batter down his resistance to trance and his resistance toward recovering his memory. The ethical implications in this procedure are, of course, subject to controversy, but sometimes very drastic methods are necessary in order to save a man from himself.

This was one of the few cases where fear was used as a therapeutic motive. In general, fear is not a sound drive to employ in the treatment of neuroses; however, at times it may be necessary to "shock" the patient out of his infantile retreats and make him return to contact with reality. We can then hope that reality will prove to be sufficiently satisfying to him that he will wish to remain there. Insight therapy might then be employed to reinforce its attractiveness.

This is frankly a motivational and not an insightful device. However, therapists should not write off the possibilities of the motivational approach. If it were not for the satisfying drives of reality we might all be neurotic—and if it were not for the motivational demands of society and its introjected Super-Ego standards we perhaps all would prefer to live the life of the psychopath.

The practical use of motivation as a basic therapeutic weapon, although rather spurned by the more traditional followers of psychoanalysis, has been consistently practiced with good results by those who follow the psychobiological approach of Adolf Meyer (Lief, 1948).

A fourth try was now made to induce trance in our amnesic patient by the postural-swaying method, since he seemed to respond to this much more rapidly than to the eye-fixation technique. This time, induction of trance was successful. He was seated in a chair. Eye closure was tested, then the inability to free the hands when they gripped each other. Finally, a catatonic position of the right arm was suggested. As a reasonably deep degree of trance seemed to be actually present this time, the attempt to break through the amnesia was made by regressing him to an early level, as follows:

"Richard, you're forgetting all about where you are and how old you are. You're going back through the years and becoming younger and younger and younger. Now you're only eighteen years old, seventeen, sixteen, fifteen, fourteen, thirteen, twelve, eleven, ten, nine, eight, seven, six. You are six years old and you are in the first grade of school. You are sitting at your desk, the children are all around you, and the teacher is standing in front of you. The teacher is smiling."

Richard smiled.

"Do you see her?"

Richard nodded.

"What's her name?" Richard's brow wrinkled and he looked thoughtful, so the therapist said, "Now, Richard, I'm going to count up to five, and when I say the word 'five,' her name will pop right into your mind, instantly. One, two, three, four, five." At the count of "five" he still hesitated a little, but after considerable urging, he said, "Oh, yes. Her name is Miss Jones."

"That's fine, Richard. Now, who is sitting right in front of you?" Richard again wrinkled his brow and acted puzzled.

"I don't know. I can't see."

"Oh yes, you can see. Is it a girl or a boy?"

"It sort of looks like a girl. Yes, it is a girl."

"That's fine. Now, look at her, because she's turning around to smile at you. Who is she?"

"Oh, that's Mary. That's Mary Cantor."

"Splendid, Richard. Now who's sitting right behind you?"

Richard started to say, "I don't know," but the therapist interrupted and said, "Well, turn around and see."

The patient slowly turned his head and looked over his shoulder, and then smilingly replied, "Oh, that's Bill—Bill Jordan." Then he said, "I like Mary Cantor—she's pretty. Bill Jordan—he's my best friend, too. He's a little guy, and he's got blond hair."

It was obvious by now that contact had been re-established with his prebreakdown life. The motivational strategy had been effective.

After having the patient describe somewhat further the room and some of his childhood friends, he was advanced to the age of fourteen and asked, "What grade are you in?"

"I'm in the tenth grade now."

"Who's your teacher?"

"Well, I have several teachers, but I like Miss Hendrickson best. She's got brown hair. She's not exactly young, but she isn't old either."

"Richard, who's your best friend?"

"Gary's my best friend. Gary Thompson's my best friend. I like him a lot. He and I go around together."

"Is there anybody that you don't like—that makes you angry?"

"No, I guess not. I seem to like about everybody."

"Have you got a girl friend, Richard?"

Richard blushed and stammered a little bit. Finally, rather shyly, he said, "Yes."

"Well, what's her name?"

"Oh, her name's Helen—Helen McLaren. She's nice and has brown hair."

He was then asked if he went out on dates with her, and he replied, "No, I don't go on real dates. I just go with her at school."

"What else do you like to do, Richard?"

"I like to play basketball."

A few more minutes were spent exploring the activities at the age of fourteen, and then the patient was told, "Now you're growing older again, Richard. You're no longer fourteen. You're growing up; you're fifteen, sixteen, seventeen, eighteen years old. What are you doing?"

"I'm just at home. I'm helping Dad on the farm."

"Well, how do you like it?"

"Oh, I like it a lot."

"How do you get along with your Dad?"

There was a slight, almost imperceptible jerk in Richard's manner, and then he said, rather quickly, "We get along fine."

Something in his manner indicated that this lead was worth further exploration, but temporarily it was dropped, and the patient was asked, "And how about Mother?"

"Mother's very good to me. She's a good mother."

"Now Richard, tell me more about yourself and what you're doing."

He then said, "I've got a steady girl. I'm going with her. Her name is Richie—Richie Barker. She's black-haired and very pretty."

"Well, Richard, do you think you're going to marry her?"

"Of course I'm going to marry her. I've been thinking about it for six months now, and I'm going to marry her after this thing is over."

"What do you mean by 'this thing'?"

"Oh, you know, the war. I don't think one should get married and then go away to war. What do you think?"

The therapist was noncommittal. "Well, it may have its disadvantages. What other boy friends do you have, Richard?"

"There's Howard—you know, Howard Smith, and Charles—that's Charles Phillips. We bum around together."

"All right, Richard," said the therapist. "You're getting a little older now, and you're coming up to the day when you entered the Army. This is the day when you must say goodbye to your folks. You're going to the Army. Tell me all about what's happening."

"Well," the patient began, "I don't know. Father said just to be careful. I think I'm ready to go. Of course I don't want to, but everybody is going, and it's my duty, so I guess I'm ready to go. Mother seems to be cut up about it, though. She's crying."

"All right now, Richard. You are taking basic training. Where are you?"

"That's at Camp Blanding, you know."

"How do you like Camp Blanding?"

"I don't like it at all. They march you around, put you over obstacle courses. I don't know—this Army doesn't set too well with me."

"Who's your company commander, Richard?"

"It's a Lieutenant Hennigan. He seems like a good fellow. He's a little guy, but he can take it."

"And who's your first sergeant?"

"Oh, he is Sergeant Bellou, and he's all right too, but he has to be tough. I guess that's the way it has to be." And, at this particular time, tears began to flow down the patient's cheeks.

Next, he was asked about his relations with the other soldiers, and he said, "I get along with all the boys, but I go home most of the time because I live with my wife, off the post."

He was next asked what his wife's first name was and he said, "It's Richie." He was then asked if he trusted his wife completely, and he replied, "Oh, yes. She's the only woman that I ever trusted —that is, except my mother."

"Richard, what does your wife think about your going off to war?"

"She hates to see me go, but she just won't let on."

He was then asked about his friends in the company and he mentioned one name. "Babbitt. That's the man's last name. He's sort of skinny, and the other guys don't like him very much. He's a queer kind of character. I felt sorry for him; that's why I went out with him."

"What happened after you finished basic training?"

"I went home for seven days' furlough with the wife and the family. The wife told me then that she was going to have a child. I felt pretty bad about it because I knew I was heading overseas right after that. Next I'm heading overseas on a big ship—*Queen Elizabeth* or *Queen Mary* or something—and I go to Liverpool. When I got there, the city looked all shot to hell. Then we went across the Channel to France. Then, when we got into France, we went across the country in boxcars, across Germany to some little town, over by the Rhine—I don't know what the name was. I didn't know any of the names of the towns there. We got to know the other boys in the squad pretty well. For example, there's a guy named George, and he's the squad leader. I liked him a lot. Then Doc—he was the medic—and he had a couple of friends named Hank and Bill. Well, anyway, we take off like the rest of the squads, and we meet some Jerries. We kill a few of them, and there are a lot of shells coming around."

"How long have you been in combat now, Richard?" inquired the therapist.

"Oh, it's been almost a month now."

"I see. All right. Now you're going to come up to the very day when you were hospitalized, when you were knocked out. What happened then? You're right in the thick of it now. You can see it all around you. What's happening?"

The patient began to writhe and twitch. "They're shooting. They're shooting all kinds of shells. It's just hell all the way around. I'm scared to death, but I've got to go on—I've got to go on. It's better to go on than to go back. Hey, they've got our range. Look out! Boy, that one was close. And another one—that's close too. They're all too damned close! Hit the dirt—here comes one! Kill 'em! They hit on both sides of me. Huh—that's funny. I don't know much. I don't seem to know anything. Everything's black. All in a daze. Like I'm in a dream. I guess I can see myself going back to hospital—hospital—hospital. I don't seem to know just what's happening there. Then I remember they're shipping me back to the States, then finally I came down here. Now it gets more clear."

Notice that the patient has been drawn out on various details of his life from childhood up to and including the concussion which rendered him unconscious. There are no real dynamics uncovered as to why he should become completely amnesic to the past. The fact that his wife was just pregnant, the slight indication we have of hostility toward his father, might give some clues, but essentially, the therapy so far has been merely to have the patient relive as much of his life as possible and abreact the immediate stressing incident. Because of the long resistance toward entering hypnosis and the great difficulty experienced in getting him into a trance, it was felt that it would not be a good idea to bring him out without suggesting that he remember all his life in detail posthypnotically. There was a risk, of course, in removing the amnesic symptom without uncovering and resolving basic conflicts. However, there was an equally strong risk that perhaps, the next time hypnotherapy was attempted, resistances would be remobilized and it would not be possible again to hypnotize the man. Because of the lack of success with the amytal narcosis and the limited time that would be available to work with this patient, it was decided that the risk would be greater in leaving the symptom than in attempting to remove it posthypnotically. No great guilt-provoking incidents could be elicited, and it was obvious that, if there were deep underlying dynamics which would cause him to shut out his entire past life, they were so firmly embedded in the unconscious personality structure that it would require long-term analysis to unearth them.

Accordingly, the patient was told, "Now, Richard, in a minute I am going to wake you up. When I do, you will feel very fine. I shall count slowly up to ten, and as I do, you will awaken. By the time I say 'ten' you will be wide awake, but you will remember in detail everything we talked about. You will remember your entire life, and you will remember it all very clearly and feel very good. You will not be anxious or nervous, but will have a feeling of warmth and comfort all over your body, and you will remember clearly. One, two, three, four, five, six, seven, eight, nine, ten." The patient blinked his eyes and opened them. He reached up and put his hands on his head and placed his head between his knees for a little while.

Then he shook himself and said, "My, I must have been in a very deep sleep." He looked surprised and remarked, "I feel funny. I feel different all over. I feel *good* all over! What have you done to me? Say, I can remember things—I can remember. We went over my whole life, didn't we? Oh, yes, I remember now. I remember the high-school principal, and I remember my history teacher."

Step by step, all that had been recovered under regressed trance was reviewed with the patient. He went on to add a number of other details to prove that his amnesia was now gone, describing the various stores on Main Street in his home town. He said, "There's the store that belongs to me. It belonged to my father, and he gave me the money for it. He gave it to me. I'm going to operate it when I go home. Dad's got quite a lot of property around, too," and he described various houses which his father owned and rented. Then he discussed how happy he had felt when his wife first told him that she was going to have a baby. He kept shaking his head, smiling and repeating over and over how much better he felt. There seemed to be no evidence of dissociation. Previously there had been a very slight tic or twitch in his face. This, too, had apparently disappeared. He then continued to elaborate his combat experiences in detail and to describe what happened while he was in Germany.

This session occurred during the morning. That afternoon the patient kept coming around to the office and repeating that he didn't know just what to say. He felt he ought to say something. He felt so much better. He felt different, etc. He appeared to be very thankful and would continually smile, shake his head, and then smile again. However, toward the evening, he did complain of a headache.

It was planned to try deeper uncovering therapy. Accordingly, he was told he would be retained in the company for a while until some of the underlying reasons why he had lost his memory were disclosed. He appeared to be happy, and agreed to this. However, it was very obvious that there was deep resistance to having any of these reasons disclosed, because upon four subsequent sessions, hypnosis was attempted and failed each time. This was apparently the body's way of preventing the emergence of the true reasons for his condition.

Since he seemed to feel very much better, and no other neurotic symptoms appeared, he was discharged because of a personality of basically hysterical type. Prior to his discharge, he was rechecked on the abstract words in the Jung Word Association Test, and he was able to give good, clear-cut associations, showing a very distinct improvement. He was also checked each day regarding his memory for the details of his life. He retained his memory and appeared to be fully recovered from the amnesia.

In the case of Richard we have illustrated another of these short-term treatments in which the patient and his immediate family were satisfied, but not the therapist.

Chronology of the Case

The patient was hospitalized for amnesia following shell concussion during February, 1945. He was admitted to Welch Hospital on June 9. On June 12 he was transferred to a regular treatment company in which he remained until August 2 except for a month's furlough at home. During this period he had only group therapy, with the exception of the attempted narcosynthesis which failed. On August 2 he was transferred to the Special Treatment Company, and the crucial session was held August 7. One other session was held on August 14, and he was discharged to civilian life on August 23.

Follow-up Note

The misgivings voiced above were not unfounded. About thirteen months later, and long after this chapter was written, the therapist received a letter from the wife of Richard Billings. It underlines the reservation made at the end of the chapter as to the complete success of the treatment.

Dear Sir:

My husband received your letter some time ago, but refuses to answer it.[1] So I will.

You were inquiring about his condition. He is just fine, has had no trouble at all. Maybe a few headaches when he first returned but that is all. I think drinking was mostly the cause of them. You see sir my husband is mean *very* mean. Those who are good have to suffer.

---

[1] We must assume that Richard has not forgiven the therapist for "dragging" him back to reality and destroying his regressive retreat from family responsibilities.

He went to a specialist in M——— the Dr. found nothing wrong with him. His mother tells me that he is just as well as he was before he entered the service. . . .

I hope what little I have told you will help some boy to return to civilian life normal and very happy. . . .

CHAPTER 12

STUTTERING

"G-g-g-ood m-m-m-m-orning. The c-c-c-c- the c-c-c-c- the c-c-or-p-p-p-ral said y-y-y-y- said y-y-y-you w-w-w-w-anted to see m-m-m-m-me." While Jeffrey Miller was "squeezing" out this message his facial muscles were screwed up like a contortionist, and the right eyelid was quivering in a grotesque dance.

He was indeed a sick man. On first entering the Special Treatment Company at Welch Convalescent Hospital, he could hardly speak a coherent sentence. Perhaps his condition was best described in the admission note written by the examining psychiatrist. It read as follows:

This 21-year-old white Pfc with two years of service was transferred on May 14th from the Receiving Detachment to the NP Admission Company with a transfer diagnosis of Anxiety State with Hysteria. On admission he complained chiefly of pain in his feet and of stuttering.

Throughout his life this individual has been nervous. He had a speech defect in his earlier life, which he was able to conquer before he left high school. Upon going to OCS [Officer Candidate School] in the Army this recurred, and at the present time it is much worse—so much so that he is barely able to speak or make himself understood. He can hardly speak a single sentence, but he is able to bring out individual words. He states that he has been nervous through his life and has always been subject to what he calls "attacks of extreme melancholia" which are probably attacks of depression. He classifies himself as a very temperamental type of person with violent likes and dislikes. It was difficult to go into any further history with this individual because of his speech difficulty.

He is a fairly well-developed, well-nourished, white male who has a thin, sallow complexion. He showed marked compulsive twitchings of his head and his eyes. His speech defect was more in the line of a compulsion than of an hysterical stammer. He showed no tremor or sweating of the hands. He was not anxious for a furlough but was more desirous of being helped.

This individual is pretty sick at the present time and has been for a long time. One month of combat apparently aggravated his basic condition to the state where he is now no longer capable of coherent speech. He appears to be a highly immature, moderately insecure, inadequate individual who has had deep underlying basic conflicts associated with his stammer. It is felt that he is in a great need of specialized therapy, and it should be moderately successful, in view of his intelligence and his motivation. While he appears meek and mild, it is obvious that this man has very marked aggressive tendencies. However, they seemed well repressed. He is to be transferred to the Special Treatment Company in the 3rd Battalion where it is recommended that he be given hypnoanalysis or hypnotherapy or, if these have been unsuccessful, that he be given a trial of narcosynthesis. The program that is ordinarily given will be of no benefit to this individual. He needs specialized attention. He is not recommended for furlough at the present time.

It was on the 28th of May, 1945 when Jeffrey was first given suggestibility tests and found to be hypnotizable. The progress note states that "he responded slightly to postural swaying and entered a light hypnoidal trance in about five minutes by the eye-fixation method. He was not amnesic to suggestions given. The patient stated that he had this same difficulty in civilian life and that it had been 'cured' by methods using hypnosis. He readily accepted suggestions that he be given hypnotherapeutic treatment and accordingly is being transferred to Company F at this time."

On the 3rd day of May, 1945 Corporal L., the Psychiatric Social Worker in the company, interviewed the man and reported this first meeting as follows:

The patient was tense, flushed, and tremulous but cooperated in a pleasant way. He states that he feels more emotionally upset and has more difficulty with stuttering than on his admission to the hospital. He feels that he has accomplished nothing worthwhile here except in sketching and painting. He states that group psychotherapy has merely "gotten me worked up." The patient appears more tense and flushed than on admission. His speech and facial tic are also worse. He stated his resentment and frustration at still being "a damn private" in the Army. Everyone expected him to be an officer. All his friends are. He was humiliated by that. He thinks that causes his speech trouble in part. His speech difficulty makes him feel "humiliated." "It is a vicious circle." He has not yet gone home on furlough, and he does not want to. He feels he can only recover out of the Army. He would only wish to be in the Army if he were "doing important work," by which he means primarily being an officer. He seems to set a high premium on "being an officer" apart from the responsibilities, though he is sensitive and rejects that idea evasively when it is carefully suggested. He feels nothing in common with men in the barracks and is somewhat seclusive there. He says that things "run in a circle." When he says that, he moves his head and jaw in a vertical circular manner, almost convulsively, trying to speak. He says that his trouble is "driving me mad." He feels he may "shatter like glass" at any moment.

Later that same day the patient was seen by the therapist and was placed in a light trance in about ten minutes. He was interviewed under trance and stated that he was tense and depressed but had no headache. He also said that he dreams of "everything imaginable" and that he had very little appetite. While under trance he did not have a severe speech defect, and the tic in his right eye was greatly alleviated. He was given posthypnotic suggestions to the effect that he would emerge from the trance without any speech defect for a period of twenty-four hours. On first coming out he spoke quite clearly, but after a period of ten minutes reverted to his original blocking and facial tic. Trance was so light that he was not amnesic but stated he remembered everything that had been said.[1]

The patient then described an incident at the age of eleven while he was visiting his parents, who lived at an educational institution. The Physical Education Instructor gave him hypnotherapeutic treatment for his speech defect at that time. He thought that it cleared up after about three months. He remembers distinctly what was told him under trance, and apparently the treatments were only a direct suggestion against his symptoms, constantly repeated two or three times a week. He has had this speech symptom since the age of six, and his mother told him it happened when he first went to school. It returned again frequently, although there was a period of time while he was in college when he did not experience it much. This also coincided with the time he started going with girls, as he said that "he felt more easy around them at that time." He was relieved from Officer Candidate School because of his speech defect. He was most amiable and cooperative. There was little external sign of anxiety.

The following day Corporal L. again saw the patient and reported:

He came in today in usual insecure manner. He was stretched out on the bed and given instructions and practice in progressive relaxation. He was very cooperative and seemed much relaxed at the end of the period. His speech was very noticeably better. Two phrases came out without any blocking. He states that he thought of nothing during the period until he looked at a map on the wall and saw the town of St. Lô.

---

[1] This is a good example of the common mistake in hypnotherapy of assuming that a deep stage of trance has been reached, deeper than is actually the case, and making suggestions too directly and dogmatically.

He said he is fascinated and repelled whenever that comes up. (He was captured there.) Discussing his symptoms, he revealed that he sometimes has a muscular jerk of his whole body when he lies in bed. He notices that, since combat, he often loses his train of thought and sometimes has to stop speaking because of it. He says he talked with his mother about his trouble, and she remembered that his stuttering started when he entered school at the age of six or seven, and stopped when he left home and entered college.

During the following week, Corporal L. saw the patient regularly. Because of his obvious antagonism to Army officers, it was felt unwise in the beginning of the treatment for us to try too many hypnotherapy sessions. The first objective was to adjust the man to the Special Treatment Company, to socialize him among the other men, and to break down a great deal of his resistance and hostility so that he might accept hypnotherapy treatment. It was obvious that his maladjustment was deep-seated and of long standing and, although aggravated by his Army service, represented something much more fundamental to his personality structure.

During these sessions Corporal L. brought about a lowering of hostility and a lessening of tension through progressive relaxation and treatments of verbal catharsis. He also uncovered very valuable leads as will be noted from the following progress note written on June 5:

> The patient stated today that he feels slightly more relaxed than previously. Part of this may be due to his improving rapport with the personnel. The patient does not yet talk freely of his feelings. He responds to direct questioning and sometimes volunteers information. He spoke of his father always being away from home. He said that when he did come home, he always praised Jeffrey's success in school, and the patient believes that may account for his own high valuation on success. It was noted today that speech troubles began when he started to school and that his younger brother was born about that time. His brother is very active and aggressive and much better at sports than the patient. Jeffrey believes he himself is not coordinated. He notes that his whole family is "high-strung and fly off the handle easily." He states that he had a bad temper when a very small baby and used to hold his breath until he was purple. When a little older, however, his family told him that he was a model child. He would sit on the floor with a magazine and quietly look at it for hours. Tracing the history of his troubles, Jeffrey revealed that he had never completely recovered from the speech blocking. In college he stuttered under stress. Then it gradually increased before induction, during basic training, and became especially strong during OCS, and he was sure that it was only the

speech that caused his failure there. It continued to get worse. After evacuation from combat it became much worse and has continued so up to the present time. The patient says his regiment was used as "bait," and all but ten died as a result. He feels lucky to be alive. He expresses resentment at being used as "bait" and denies any kind of guilt feelings about leaving combat. Returning to his relation to his brother, he revealed that they often quarreled and fought. Work in progressive relaxation was continued. It was discovered that the patient could talk in a guttural tone without much jaw movement and have no speech blocking at all.

The therapeutic leverage in this case was greatly facilitated by the teamwork of the psychologist and social worker, who approached the patient from different viewpoints. The social worker, using a nondirective approach combined with progressive relaxation, achieved a considerable release of the patient's hostility toward Army officers —hence, father-figures. This prepared the way for the psychologist to establish a sufficiently close relationship so that hypnosis could be employed.

On June 11 the patient came in to see the therapist and was given an orientation discussion preparing him for hypnotherapy. Some of his doubts regarding hypnosis were clarified, and two points were stressed to him: first, the importance of motivation in getting well; and second, the necessity that he should have a desire for getting well stronger than a desire for getting out of the Army. He accepted this consciously, although he found it very difficult. Then it was mentioned that another important matter would be the "dynamics of the illness, which we would have to uncover together." He seemed to seize on this phrase and remember it. It became an important factor later in the therapy. He was quite cooperative and friendly but appeared somewhat depressed. His speech difficulties had shown little improvement since the first session. It was felt that he was sincerely desirous, at least on the conscious level, of receiving therapy.

That this apparent rapport with the therapist and friendly manner were mostly on the surface is obvious from a note written the following day by Corporal L.:

> The patient states that his hatred of the Army is constantly increasing. "If they would give me a Colonel's commission, I would still hate it." Then he states, "It's so darn rough." He does not think he can ever recapture his pride in the Army. "I didn't realize the draftee's part before." He thinks his father is very foolish for enlisting and going overseas. Work in progressive relaxation is going very well, and the patient is extremely cooperative.

On June 16 another note by Corporal L. stated:

> The patient came in today in a less cooperative mood. His speech
> was worse again, and he did not want to talk at all. Progressive re-
> laxation went badly. Resistance appeared which showed that he did not
> want to cooperate, though he went through the motions. After that, he
> brought up the matter of wanting to get out of the Army and confessed
> that he felt strongly that this was preventing any help from the treat-
> ments. He stated that he felt he could not be helped till he knew he
> would get out. He could not say so directly, but it was obvious that
> he was uncomfortably aware that he did not want to get well until he
> got out. He argued that he was no good to the Army because of his
> condition.

That same day the patient was seen by the therapist and given the
Jung Word Association Test. Most of the disturbances appeared to
be focused about problems of home and family. This was interesting,
since his complaints and attitudes centered largely around Army life.
He seemed very depressed. He was placed in a light trance and
stated that he dreamed he was on a battleship and was fighting air-
planes with an AA gun [2] but could not hit anything. He could not
associate to this dream. We might infer from this, however, that he
had considerable doubts concerning his masculinity if the gun is
being employed as a masculine genital symbol.

He was then regressed to the age of six, where he described an
incident in which someone had taken his lunch away from him the
first day of school and thrown it away. He said the children laughed
at that. "I tried to go into the street and get it, but the teacher would
not let me. I was very angry." This was apparently about the time
his stuttering first started.

On June 19 the patient was placed in a light trance after fifteen
minutes of metronome sedation and given posthypnotic suggestions
that he could talk clearly. On coming out of trance, however, there
was still considerable defect in his speech, although it was improved.
He appeared to have made some progress and seemed to feel better.

A conference was held between Corporal L. and the therapist to
summarize the case as it was known at that time, to determine disposition, and to plan the next step in the therapy. From various
interviews with Corporal L. it seemed obvious that underlying his
condition was an unresolved Oedipus situation, a deep-seated hostility toward his father, considerably repressed.[3] It had been noticed

---

2 Ack-ack or anti-aircraft gun.
3 The dream of the AA gun shows his frustration and his attempts at expressing aggression which don't "hit anything." The dream also indicates possible feelings of symbolic

that his stuttering symptom throughout his life had always emerged in such a way as to frustrate the wishes of his father, especially in regard to his academic success, and the stuttering had always achieved the purpose of increasing sympathy and attention from the mother. It was furthermore obvious that this hostility to the father had been transferred to all father-figures, especially Army officers, and that the authority of the Army and its disciplinary measures were associated to the deep-seated repressed hostility toward his father. Considering the severity of the symptom complex, the powerful antagonistic motivation toward getting well in the Army, and the underlying dynamics, it was obvious that therapy might or might not be successful if the man were discharged to civilian life. It was impossible if the patient considered that its success would result in his return to duty. Accordingly, it was felt he was of no further value to the Army, and it was determined that his chart would be closed with the recommendation for medical discharge. This was tantamount to discharge since the local CDD Board made a practice of accepting the recommendation of the company professional team on this matter in nearly all cases.

The following steps in therapy were now decided upon:

1. The patient was to be informed that he would be recommended for CDD (Medical Discharge) on completion of his treatment and that the success of the treatment would have no bearing on this point.
2. Attempts would be made to bring about some insight on his part into the underlying Oedipus situation and the inner meaning of his symptom.
3. Direct suggestion would be used to increase further the motivational power tending to pull down the symptom structure.

Accordingly he was informed at once concerning the decision about his final disposition. This it was felt would have the effect of reducing the underlying hostility toward all Army officers and would increase rapport and consequently the patient's hypnotizability. It had that effect.

Jeffrey was informed of his disposition on June 21, and the following day Corporal L. noted in the chart: "Patient was told yesterday that his disposition was discharge. He has appeared greatly

---

castration. Father had always succeeded where he had failed, and hence his "gun" was not as good as father's.

relieved since then, and there has been some relief from his speech blockage. He was more cooperative than before about relaxation treatment."

At about this time the group therapy session in the company had been discussing the matter of "psychodynamics." The importance of insight and how it could effect a change in the patient's body had been a matter of lively debate within the group.

This had enhanced Jeffrey's interest in his own dynamics. A model of the neurotic mechanism presented in Chapter 3 had been constructed and was used as a demonstration in the group therapy. This concept seemed to appeal greatly to Jeffrey. Since the secondary gain factor was now largely out of the way and his rapport with the therapist at a new high peak, a more reintegrative session could now be undertaken.

Accordingly on June 23 the following significant interview took place. The conversational account presented is a close approximation of the discussion although not a word-for-word transcription.

An indirect suggestive opening stressing symptoms.	W (Watkins) : You seem to be feeling somewhat better now, Jeffrey.
Obviously the patient could not have been cured if we attempted to keep him in military service.	J (Jeffrey) : I feel worlds better. You don't know what a relief it is to know that I won't have to stay much longer in the Army. My nerves just can't stand it.
Still stressing symptoms, a topic of major interest to neurotics.	W : Your speech seems somewhat improved. In what other ways do you feel that you have advanced?
	J : I've been terribly blue. You know I was even thinking of suicide at one time. I felt that was preferable to staying in the Army any longer. Even though I still stutter I feel a lot happier inside, and I don't have headaches.
Already some evidence of symptomatic relief.	W : Do you think that you are going to get well now?

First indications of *insight*. Group therapy discussions have apparently sown a fruitful seed.

J: I believe I will be a lot better, but I have been thinking about that. Didn't you say that there were "dynamics" back of our nervous sicknesses? Do you think I have special dynamics back of mine?

Nondirective agreement and return of the "lead" to the patient.

W: It seems quite possible. Why do you ask?

J: Well, I've stuttered most of my life, and maybe if I understood why I stuttered, I could get over it entirely.

W: That's possible. Tell me about when you first stuttered.

J: The first time I had trouble talking was when I entered school. I don't remember it, but my mother tells me about it.

Pushing toward significant parental relationships, Mother (less traumatic) first.

W: Were you quite closely attached to your mother before you went to school?

J: Oh yes, I was with her a great deal. I missed her terribly when I was away at school.

W: What did father think about your going to school?

School, which was highly approved by Father, began with an insecurity incident, the time when the other children took his lunch. They laughed at him, and the teacher, a person in authority, thwarted his wishes to protect himself and retaliate.

J: Father wanted me to go to school. He was very anxious to have me go and make a success.

W: Did your speech get any better after a while?

We have no information as to what was the precipitating stress at this time.

J: Yes, it improved in the later grades, but I remember it broke out severely when I was about eleven. Dad was at the ——— College, and he took me to the physical education instructor. The man would put me in a light trance, something like we've been doing, and then say

Apparently using only simple direct suggestion.

over and over again, "You are going to talk more clearly. You are going to cease stuttering."

Direct suggestion has temporary efficacy.

After about two months of that I did quit—for a while.

W: And then?

Note temporary effect of direct suggestion treatment.

J: And then it broke out again severely at the end of high school. I remember that, because it stopped me from being valedictorian of the high school class.

W: Tell me more about it.

Relation of father hostility to symptoms begins more clearly to emerge.

J: I worked hard to get good grades so that I would be valedictorian. You know, I always did that. It pleased Dad a great deal. I know he was quite anxious to have me make a success and be valedictorian. And then just before the end of school I broke out into this stuttering and someone else had to deliver the valedictory address. I was certainly disappointed. It was a big disappointment to Father, too.

The stutter succeeds in disappointing Father.

W: And when did it improve again?

The symptom improves after leaving home—and Father.

J: It got considerably better when I went away to college.

W: Did you leave home and go away to school?

J: Yes, I was by myself for the first time.

W: When did it again get worse?

J: About the time I was inducted into the Army.

W: Did you want to go into the Army?

J: Well, yes, that is, I thought it

Desires to enter the Army appear to be more Father's standards introjected than his own.

was my duty. I wanted to go in and become an officer like my father wanted and be a success. I didn't realize what being an enlisted man was like. But it improved somewhat until I got into OCS. I wanted so badly to become an officer, and Dad had his heart set on it. Then the stuttering came back again, and I was washed out.

Again the stutter thwarts Father's wishes.

W: When did your next attack of stuttering occur?

J. has actually brought out dynamics but fails as yet to grasp their implication.

J: After I had been in combat some time and was wounded, the stuttering came back so severely that I was of no further value to the Army. What do you think caused my stuttering all the time?

W. reassumes initiative in guiding J. toward understanding.

W: Do you remember in group therapy we once said that our symptoms have a purpose. They accomplish some objective or aim.

J. rejects at first. Resistance prevents "seeing."

J: That doesn't make too much sense here because all that my stuttering has done is to make me fail in everything I wanted to accomplish.

W. continues attack with leading questions.

W: Perhaps the things you wanted to accomplish, or thought you wanted to accomplish, were not really so important to you as you believed at the time. Where did you get the great desire to accomplish these things?

Insight begins to dawn.

J: Why, from Father, of course. He always—say you don't think —no, that would be foolish.

W. somewhat nondirective.

J. states basic proposition of the dynamics but rationalizes and still fails to grasp entire significance.

W. does not press issue at this time but builds up another "dynamic" toward the "insight point."

The implications of this are obvious.

Temporary distraction of "mother-dynamic" has lowered anxiety previously initiated as "father-dynamic" was being approached. W. now returns J. to "father-dynamic" which is definitely near the point of insight.

J. further externalizes hostility and ends with another rationalization.

W : What was it you were thinking?

J : I was just thinking that I failed in about everything my father wanted me to do, and that it was always my stuttering which came and made me fail in that. And yet I think a great deal of Dad. I'm sure I would want to do what he wanted me to accomplish.

W : Think back. Whom were you closer to, your father or your mother?

J : Oh, Mother, of course. She would come to my rescue in any little family argument and always sympathized with me when my stuttering and nervousness became so bad.

W : And Father?

J : Well, he was a little severe at times, and I didn't approve of his going away for long periods because that made Mother feel bad. I guess I always resented him somewhat. I wanted him to go away on the one hand, so I could be with Mother more. At the same time I felt a little angry at him for hurting Mother. But you understand, of course, that there was nothing more to it than that. I wouldn't do anything to hurt him, really.

W. aims a direct blow.

W : But you did do something to hurt him.

J.'s resistance is mobilized into a question.

J : What do you mean?

W. presses advantage and ends with a direct response-demanding question.

W : You failed in everything in which he wanted you to succeed. Doesn't it seem a bit odd that your stutter came about most conveniently to sabotage what he wished?

J.'s resistance weakly evades.

J : You don't mean that I faked the stutter?

Aiming for complete closure.

W : Of course not. But perhaps while you consciously wanted to succeed, nevertheless, because of resentment and hostility toward your father which you could express in no other way, you unconsciously wanted to fail, and by failing through your stutter you were symbolically striking back at him.

Over the hump. Resistance breaks. J. now seizes insight as eagerly as before he resisted it. Outpouring of verbalization. J. faces and extends insight.

J : Say, that's right. I never thought about it that way before. I did fail at everything he wanted me to do. Perhaps I didn't really want to achieve all those goals that he set for me. Perhaps my own ideas and ideals were different, and I had never been able to strike out on my own. I always took what he wanted me to do and tried to do it. Maybe underneath I didn't really want to, so I failed. I really didn't want to leave Mother and go to school in the first grade, and so I stuttered. I didn't want to be valedictorian of my class. At least I knew if

Father wanted me to be so very badly, that I would hurt him more if I failed than if I succeeded. I didn't want to enter the Army so I stuttered. And by failing to become an officer I hurt Dad, too. That's the reason, isn't it, why I stutter? Of course, that's the "dynamics." Isn't it?

Attention now directed to "mother-dynamic."

W: Well, at least that's part of them. Now whenever you stuttered, what did Mother do?

J: Why, she used to sympathize with me and keep me home from school.

Nondirective encouragement to continue.

W: She sympathized with you and kept you home from school.

J: [*rather cautiously*] Maybe that was a way of getting more attention and sympathy from her. Yes, I suppose it did have that effect. That would make me continue to do it, wouldn't it, Doc?

As before, mild rather than enthusiastic agreement strengthens J.'s conviction in newly realized insight.

W: Yes, it's quite probable that that could be true. Can you recall anything else about it?

A very common rationalization offered by neurotics.

J: I hadn't mentioned this before, but you know my mother stuttered when she was a child. You don't suppose that maybe there is some inheritance in this?

It is handled without direct contradiction.

W: There could be, but it isn't probable. But the fact that your mother stuttered may have some bearing on your stuttering just the same.

J : How's that?

W : Did you ever have a movie hero?

J : Of course.

W : And did you feel sometimes that you would like to be just like that person?

J : Sure, I know.

J. is a bright patient. Identification can be suggested by indirect implication.

W : In telling me that your symptoms arose to make you fail in what your father wanted you to do, you really were saying that unconsciously you didn't want to be like him.

More insight.

J : (*picking it up quickly*) But I did want to be like my mother, and so by stuttering I was sort of following her. Is that the idea?

W. agrees and restates dynamic implication.

W : Yes, that sounds like an important idea. By stuttering you could identify more with your mother.

The material evoked in the preceding discussion was now reviewed with the patient on a more directive basis with greater explanation and elaboration. (See table on page 154.)

The neurosis then, in the form it "chose," stuttering, is a solution of Jeffrey's internal conflict. It achieves his academic and military failures by an illness which "hurts" father and "woos" mother— satisfying the two neurotic needs in Factor 3. It permits him to keep repressed the mother-fixation and father-hostility, Factors 1 and 2, which he does not want to face and acknowledge as part of him. The neurosis takes a symptomatic form which identifies him with the mother—she, too, stuttered, and Jeffrey wants to be "like her." Finally, it accomplishes his release from the hated military service.

Following the integrating of this insight into the patient, he was placed in a light trance and given a posthypnotic suggestion calling for the disappearance of his symptoms. When he came out of the trance he claimed that he felt very good and that he had entered a deeper trance than ever before. It was observed that there was no speech defect nor was there any tic left in his face. This session obviously could not have been possible during the earlier stages of his therapy or treatment. By informing him of his disposition and approaching discharge from the Army, a degree of rapport had been established sufficient to permit discussion with him of the nature of his dynamics and sufficient to induce a deeper degree of hypnotic trance. Following insight, direct suggestion against the symptoms under a deep trance was much more effective than previously.

STATUS OF INSIGHT INTO DYNAMICS NOW REACHED BY PATIENT

Factor	Significance
1. Repressed father-hostility	Caused by overdominating, and mistreatment of mother
2. Fixation on mother	Caused by overindulgence by mother; further reasons not yet uncovered

3. Neurotic needs
  (a) To express hostility toward father
  (b) To secure more affection from mother
	These had not been recognized by patient; they had been repressed

The strength of the above factors explains *why neurotic symptoms must be established*. They are the predisposition. The patient's Ego has been weak and unable to face consciously these forces within him. Accordingly it must accept some kind of neurosis as a solution. The neurotic mechanism is "cocked"

4. Initiating stresses
  (a) Going to school and leaving close maternal association
  (b) Impending valedictory speech which requires facing audience
  (c) Induction into Army with its severe (father-like) discipline
  (d) Officer Candidate School
  (e) Combat
	Each of these stresses aroused the symptom complex at some time or other; each in turn served to "pull the trigger" of the neurotic mechanism, and the stutter would break out again as a result

5. Identification of patient with mother who herself had stuttered as a child	This may explain why the neurosis "chose" the form of stuttering

6. Additional factors
  (a) Hostility toward father expressed as hostility toward Army discipline and Army officers (father-figures)
  (b) Failure at OCS symbolically expresses hostility toward father by unconsciously indicating that patient "wanted" *not to be an Army Officer* (like his father)

Jeffrey left that day in a very happy frame of mind and with no noticeable symptoms. During the next week it was noted that he significantly increased the amount of time he spent in art class, time which resulted fruitfully in a number of paintings. He became much more sociable with the other men and developed into quite a missionary for the hypnotherapy treatments among some of the more hostile members of the group.

The day following the preceding session Corporal L. wrote in the progress notes,

> The patient was heard yesterday entering the barracks and joyfully telling another patient, "I know the dynamics now." In the last twenty-four hours there has been a striking improvement in his speech and a very positive attitude toward life. All the symptoms, he says, have disappeared now. The patient was shown today that he could consciously control his speech. He produced a tic of his eyes, and his scalp, initiated his speech blockage deliberately, and found that he could eliminate it that way. It was also suggested that he silently recite to himself, visualizing a free, full flow of speech.

The final progress note on June 25 states:

> The patient was placed in trance four times by *fractionation.*[4] Each time he was under trance he was given repeated suggestions tending to alleviate his symptoms of stuttering and facial tics. He entered a deeper trance progressively. At the end of the session he stated that he felt very good. There was only the slightest residual trace of his facial tic and no evidence of stuttering. He will be ready for disposition in another week. He left in a happy mood, whistling quite briskly.

"Good morning. The Corporal said you wanted to see me." There was not the slightest trace of a break in the voice of this smiling soldier.

"Yes, Jeffrey, I believe it's been two weeks since you left the Company. I heard you were still on the Post but leaving for home in a day or so."

"That's right, Doc, I'm going tomorrow." Was that a single faint twitch over the right eye? Apparently not—it wasn't repeated.

"I just wanted to see you before you left—have any more trouble with your stomach?"

"No, I feel fine—no stomach trouble, no stuttering, no headaches. I never would have believed it."

---

[4] A method of increasing trance depth by repeatedly putting the patient into and bringing him out of trance (Vogt, 1892).

"Well, best of luck.   Let us know how you are getting along."

"I will."

He did. A note to Corporal L. several weeks later reported that Jeffrey still had—no stomach trouble, no stuttering, no headaches.

When a loss of symptoms is accompanied by some insight into their meaning, we have reason to hope that something truly constructive has been done for that patient. In the case of Jeffrey Miller we utilized a certain degree of insight as well as motivation in alleviating his symptoms.

Chronology of the Case

The patient was hospitalized in the middle of November, 1944, after one month of combat. He was admitted to Welch Hospital on February 2, 1945, and retained in a general company without individual psychotherapeutic treatment until July 3, when he was transferred to the Special Treatment Company. While in Company F he was seen at six sessions by the psychologist and six by the social worker for individual therapy and was discharged about August 1. There was no evidence of symptomatic improvement until after July 3, when he started receiving individual therapy.

CHAPTER 13

SUICIDAL DEPRESSION

It was June when young Hilton was first referred to the Special Treatment Company. Staff and patients alike were feeling the warmth of the early summer and the hope that the war was at last approaching its end. Soon we would all go home. But there was at least one who was untouched by the general wave of optimism. Hilton was thinking of death.

The referring psychiatrist wrote, "We are badly worried about him. He has that deep, depressed, melancholic attitude which, although apparently not psychotic, makes us feel that he is on the point of committing suicide. Watch him closely and, if you can't help him, he will have to be shipped immediately to a general hospital."

The psychiatric note made on this patient at the time of entrance into the hospital stated:

On admission, he had no real complaints, except that he felt very tired and depressed and suffered from crying spells. This soldier has always entertained the idea that killing was wrong. Throughout his life, he has been a rather passive, dependent individual, who was inclined to turn the other cheek rather than fight back. He has always considered himself a sort of sissy and weakling. When he got into the Army, he felt that it would make a man out of him. He performed very well and experienced about sixty days of combat in France and Germany. A review of his record indicates that, under sodium amytal, he admitted to three rather dramatic incidents—the first, where he bayoneted a sleeping German; the second, in which he machine-gunned another German; and a third, involving his own buddy who was killed next to him after having been shot through the stomach. He was wounded in December and was admitted to an evacuation hospital in France. Shortly after this hospitalization, he became depressed and suffered crying spells. He complained of headaches and of difficulties with eating. He is able now to eat a little better, and his headaches bother him somewhat less, but he remains constantly depressed, easily fatigued and cries frequently. Apparently, he has a strong religious sense, and he also has a very keen sense of failure, for it was when we were discussing failure that he began to cry bitterly. It is felt that he can best gain by being placed in the Special Treatment Company in the Third Battalion. I feel that it is extremely important that we rehabilitate this individual, who appears to have a good civilian background, and who has an excellent education.

Hilton shuffled into the therapist's office, a pale, wan, thin individual, with expressionless face. He slumped forward in his chair, and said nothing. He appeared, indeed, to be a man who placed no hopes in this world. His staring eyes looked blankly out into space, and a sad expression of complete resignation and defeat covered his face.

"Hilton," began the therapist, "tell me what makes you feel bad."

After a long pause, the patient replied, "Oh, I'm all right, I guess." The tone of his voice was flat. Another thirty seconds elapsed, during which neither the therapist nor the patient spoke.

"Do you have headaches, Hilton?"

The patient slowly nodded. "Yes, my head hurts."

"Anything else?"

"There's a ringing in my ears."

"How about your eating?"

"I can't eat."

"Do you lose your meals?"

Again the patient merely nodded.

"How often?"

"Most of them, I guess."

Throughout the initial interview, the patient never took the lead. He mentioned symptoms only when pressed. He made no attempt to exaggerate. There is much more hope for a patient who can externalize his resistance, his hostility, and his anxiety—one who will talk about his symptoms, who will even consciously exaggerate them —than for one who refuses to discuss them.

It is not easy to read what is in a man's mind. Something about his entire manner, his complete lack of hostility, almost waved a red flag, warning us: "Look out for this man; there's something dangerous here. He is unable to direct his hostility outward, so it is being turned back inward against himself. Here is a man who has lost all interest in the world; lost all interest in the things about him. He is not concerned with getting well. Here is a man who could easily enter a psychotic depression, perhaps commit suicide. This is a man who says nothing about it and is likely to do it."

A few days prior to his assignment to the Special Treatment Company, Hilton had been given a Rorschach examination. The psychologist in charge summarized as follows: "This configuration is indicative of a severe, constrictive depression. The personality is overemphasizing control and exercising rigid control in an attempt to cover up the insecurity and instability. There are no evidences of suicidal tendencies at the present time. This would appear to be a reactive depression, severe. There are no evidences of psychosis at the present time."

This examination was, indeed, reassuring. However, the Rorschach, like any other clinical test, is not infallible, and, in the judgment of two psychiatrists who had been observing the case and the social worker assigned to the company, this man was a severe suicidal risk. It was obvious that therapy must be initiated at once, and that this patient must be most carefully watched. It also seemed necessary that he be brought somewhat out of his introvertive shell as soon as possible to the extent that he could form identifications and attachments with individuals and establish a certain degree of rapport with the therapist. Accordingly, two of the more likeable and well-adjusted patients were called into the office and asked to help indirectly in the therapy, somewhat as follows: "Fellows, this new boy, Hilton, who's just come in—you know, the little, short, thin fellow—is pretty upset. He feels bad, blue, discouraged, and is a lot sicker than he looks. In fact, he is so sick that we are a little afraid that he might hurt himself before we have a chance to help him. I wonder if you boys would do a great favor for me. Stick around close with him for the next few days. Don't let him wander off by himself. Try to draw him out and make a friend of him. Take him over to the post theater and show him around the camp. Get him interested in some games with you. Take him to mess with you. He needs your help, as well as mine. Do you get what I mean?"

The boys "got it" and were only too eager and glad to help by providing some support for the new patient.

The next step was to relieve, if only on a temporary and superficial basis, the headaches and the severe depression. This would help to tide the patient over until deeper dynamics could be disclosed. It would also aid in establishing a closer relationship between therapist and patient. Accordingly, the patient was given suggestibility tests, to which he responded favorably, and was then placed in a deep trance by the eye-fixation method in about five minutes. After it was determined that he had entered a sufficiently deep trance he was given suggestions of euphoria and other suggestions tending to alleviate his headache and his tinnitus. He emerged from trance stating that he felt much better, that he did not feel blue, and that he had no headache. He was completely amnesic to all suggestions made.

Notice that suggestive therapy was utilized, not to try to cure the patient, but to give him temporary support and to prevent a possible suicide until such time as the underlying maladjustment might be uncovered.

In a progress note recorded the next morning by Corporal L., the Psychiatric Social Worker of the Special Treatment Company, there was further evidence that the fears of suicide were not groundless. He reported: "Patient was extremely tense and rigid in manner. There was much blunting of emotional tone. He seemed fearful of questioning. He said that he felt confused much of the time. He admitted that he often feels suicidal and confused."

During the next day, the therapist was unable to see the patient. Corporal L. held a session with him and observed that he was more at ease, though he still held himself stiffly. The report continued,

> He says he worries much about his health. He has palpitations in bed; often feels he is going to smother. He has bizarre battle dreams and recalls one, when he was on the front lines. His mother came up in a car, and he was struggling to get her to safety. [As in most war neuroses, earlier family maladjustments are involved. Here we see conflictual material involving Mother intermingled with battle anxieties. Combat stress often provokes earlier conflicts.]
>
> In another dream, he lay in a trough, bleeding from a stab-wound, and his own blood was engulfing him when he woke up, smothering. He spoke excitedly of his combat experiences. He was wounded at night, was removed from combat, and broke down later in England. At that time, he says, "I didn't care what happened to me." Finally, in England, he had hallucinations. A beautiful young woman's face appeared constantly before him. He never told anyone, because it "scared me." He says that, often now, when he lies in bed, he hears a voice whispering his name, as though it were calling him. He says that he did well in combat and killed several Germans, but "was in a daze most of the time." He "went wild" and behaved recklessly several times. He feels that he did his part, but has guilt feelings about one incident, when he was ordered to withdraw. A man was in a hole near him and called to him. This buddy stated that he was wounded. After a short time, there were no more answers, so the patient withdrew without investigating. Later on, this other man was found dead. The patient admitted guilt feelings regarding this. When questioned about his childhood, he said he had enuresis until seven. He had or almost had St. Vitus' Dance at seven. At that time, he temporarily lost the use of his left arm. He was out of school for one year. He suddenly recovered from that and played in athletics in high school. Then, the patient

was questioned about his family. He was the youngest of six siblings. *He said his mother often quarreled with his father. At this point, the patient suddenly became very flushed and tense and moved restlessly. He ran a hand through his hair, and could scarcely speak. He seemed exhausted.* He was reassured and told that we would talk further at another time.

At this particular period, there suddenly came a very acute shortage of psychiatrists in the NP battalions. Company F, the Special Treatment Company, had not had one available now for nearly a month, and the therapist, being the only professional officer in the company, had been acting in that capacity, with the backing of the psychiatrist who was Battalion Commander. Now, still another psychiatrist was temporarily transferred out. With only three company psychiatrists on hand to take care of six NP companies, the therapist was temporarily requested to assume additional responsibility. The Special Treatment Company at this time had a rather small number of patients in it, and so the therapist was asked to act in the place of a psychiatrist for Company D also, until a replacement could be secured. These additional responsibilities meant cutting in half the amount of time available for special treatment patients. Since the psychiatric social worker had reported that Hilton was more relaxed and less tense, it was nearly a week before the therapist was again able to see this man.

At this time, the social worker came in with the report that Hilton's severe depression had returned, that it appeared to be in a most dangerous and acute stage, and that in his contacts with the other patients, Hilton had disclosed his great attachment to his mother and hinted at, but refused to admit, hostility toward his father. While claiming to be very fond of his father, he would emphasize the fact of his father's brutal mistreatment of the mother, and he would do this with a flushed, tense face, a writhing in his chair, and a clenching of his hands. This appeared every time his attention was directed to his home and family. Furthermore, at this point, the patient's actions in avoiding other soldiers in the company, his increased seclusiveness, and his entire manner warned of an immediate suicidal attack. Something drastic needed to be done, and done at once. The temporary relief of the posthypnotic suggestions had subsided. The temporary identification with new buddies in the company had been inadequate. The basic maladjustment was now emerging in an acute and dynamic stage. It was time for some decision to be made and action to be taken; yet any action involved a great risk.

Consideration of Therapeutic Strategy

Let us see what were the possibilities: The patient could be administered further reassuring suggestions and continued superficial treatment. If this failed, there would be a dead man in the company, with tremendous disruption of morale among all the other patients, not to mention a probable military investigation of the NP division and increased restrictions on all therapy.

We could "pass the buck" professionally, declare the patient too sick for treatment in a convalescent hospital and return him to locked-ward treatment in a general hospital. This would result in a freeing of our hospital from the responsibilities involved, but by breaking what little attachments and faith he still had would probably have provoked a psychotic breakdown in the patient.

Probing under hypnotic trance might uncover the basic causes. This appeared fraught with the same dangers that involved the first possibility, in that something would be partially uncovered, partially loosened, yet not adequately resolved. Then because insight would be only partial, the unstructured anxieties might manifest themselves at night or during some other unguarded moment in evoking a suicidal attempt or, perhaps, even a homicidal attack directed against another patient. Suicides during the process of psychotherapy are not unknown.

There was still a fourth possibility: that through an abreaction, the conflict might be suddenly released, the repressed anxieties and hostilities drained off, and the personality structure relieved of its stress. This, too, had its dangers. It might provoke a psychotic attack. It could initiate an amnesia, and if inadequately resolved, could also lead to suicide shortly afterwards. If this method were attempted, it meant that *the patient must not be left alone until we could be certain that the abreaction had been successful,* that real insight had been secured, and that the major maladjustment had been resolved.

There were also other obstacles. Where was this abreaction to begin? Our knowledge of the internal dynamic structure as yet was extremely spotty—only a few hints as to where the true heart of the conflict lay. We were in much the same position as a surgeon who is brought an acute case where an operation is necessary but, there being no X-ray reports available, the exact location of the pathology is not known and can only be inferred. Yet the severity of the symptoms demands that we operate at once. After considerable discussion with the social worker, who had been closest to the patient, it was decided to try the fourth method.

From what was known of the dynamics so far, it seemed probable that there was an unresolved Oedipus situation, a strong fixation upon his mother, and great internalized hatred and hostility of his father for the father's mistreatment of his mother. Since the individual was a passive type who was afraid to kill and an individual who had always been taught to repress his hostility, it was probable there was a great desire to kill his father. This desire could not be faced, so the aggression was then directed inward against himself. By eliminating himself, he would not perform the crime of patricide, actually; yet, because there was probably also an identification of himself with his father, in killing himself he could *symbolically kill* his father. This meant that, in the act of suicide, he was psychologically eating his cake and having it at the same time. K. A. Menninger, in Chapter 2 of his book entitled *Man Against Himself* (1938), describes more in detail how this mechanism can operate.

We did not know with certainty that this was the true situation; yet, all evidence received so far fell in line with this hypothesis. It was further possible that the patient might have identified one or more of the enemy he had killed in combat with his father and thereby further increased his guilt feelings, which were now being manifested in the severe depression. At any rate, here we were faced with a situation which must be dealt with immediately.

Hilton was called into the therapist's office and, without further preliminaries, the psychological scalpel was deeply inserted:

"Hilton, why do you want to kill your father?"

Hilton exploded. With an hysterical burst of crying and weeping, he started pounding his hands together. Tears flowed copiously. His whole body was one mass of tremors as he writhed in his chair. The drive that his entire being had striven to conceal from himself, that had been repressed, and that he was even willing to take his own life to escape facing, had now been instantly and brutally forced upon his attention. Except for his hysterical sobbing, Hilton was speechless. It was some fifteen or twenty minutes later before the convulsive weeping attack began to subside, perhaps from sheer exhaustion, and then the therapist began to talk to the patient, using the most quiet and reassuring manner possible.

"Did you think you were the only man in the world who ever felt like killing his father? Lots of boys have felt that way, but it isn't really wrong or bad. After all, you didn't commit a crime; you only felt like doing it, and refused to admit it to yourself. You've probably always hated your father a great deal, and at this late stage in your development, you probably never will be able to get along with him; yet it's a lot better if you will face your hostility; admit it honestly to yourself; talk about it, realize that it's there; accept the fact and don't try to push it down inside you.

"And now, let's go a little further, Hilton. Because you couldn't even recognize you wanted to kill your father, you couldn't get rid of all those feelings, so you directed them against yourself. I'll bet you were even planning to kill yourself. Is that right?"

The patient looked up and nodded.

"Were you planning to kill yourself in the very near future?"

Again, the patient nodded. The deep sobbing had quit, and there was now only a soft, quiet flow of tears.

The therapist continued, "I imagine you've felt very insecure and inadequate all your life. Being thwarted at home, unable to resist your father and protect your mother as you thought you should, you have probably felt that you were not a real man. By going into the Army you could prove to yourself that you were a man. As you were killing enemy soldiers, perhaps you were even killing your father symbolically. Maybe you saw in the enemy soldier an image of your father, and at that time took considerable satisfaction in killing. Then, after you went away to the hospital, down deep inside, you began to feel guilty about the killing, because you felt as if you had been a father-murderer. Is that right?"

The patient nodded and then said, "Yes, that is right. That's what I've been doing, all the time," and for the first time a slight smile, almost a smile of understanding, came over his face, and he took out a handkerchief and wiped away the tears.

At this particular moment, the company returned from one of its afternoon activities and began to stomp into the barracks, so the therapist suggested: "Let's go for a little walk. What do you say? We'll walk around the post and talk."

Hilton eagerly agreed to this, and so for another hour the patient and therapist strolled up one street and down the next while Hilton began, at first gradually, hesitatingly, later almost with an outburst of enthusiasm, to verbalize his childhood experiences of mistreatment at the hands of his father, the outbursts of indignation at the brutality meted out to his mother, his helplessness and feelings of inability to fight back against his father and to protect his mother. He further voiced great, intensive hostility to the Army and Army officers, whom he identified with his father.

As the story of his inadequacies, insecurities, and repressed hostility emerged, the tenseness and the depression gradually left him. Toward the end of the session, he began to laugh and smile, even to relate humorous anecdotes of his past life. He began to talk about his interest in sports and athletics, his desire to be a teacher, to be a teacher of vocational agriculture, and he began to ask about various schools and what the possibilities were in this field.

At this point, he was told about a decision which had already been made concerning him in the light of his condition and of his basic personality structure. This was to the effect that his chart would be closed for discharge and he would not be returned to military service. He appeared to be greatly relieved at this. However, since this point had not been previously mentioned, it had had no effect upon the abreactive relief and subsequent gain of insight. It was felt that this was now the time to further capitalize upon his reawakened interest in life in general.

Accordingly, he was asked, "How would you like to find out something about various colleges and universities, and which ones have good courses in vocational agriculture?"

Hilton's face lighted up. "Do you mean that on this Post I could find out something about that?"

"Why, certainly. We have a vocational guidance department, with skilled counselors to help you, men who are university-trained. They also have a fine library here, with catalogues from all the various universities. You can find out which departments are strong. Then you can write, get their catalogues, and find out how much it will cost you. Assuming there is no red tape and unnecessary delay, it is quite probable that you could enter the fall session. You don't want to go home, do you?"

Immediately the patient replied. "I'm not going home. I see now I can't get along at home. While I don't think I'll ever get to the point where I would want to kill my father, I know now I can never get along with him and that I'd better go away. Don't you think it would be a good idea for me to go clear away—not even go back to my home state, or to the South—but out to some other part of the country and start all over again?"

"That sounds like an excellent idea," the therapist agreed.

Here is evidence of a really positive insight on the patient's part. What was needed now was a beginning on an entirely new basis and in a new environment. Seldom did one find a patient who showed so much insight into the environmental factor which produced his maladjustment. Prior to the understanding and insight received, moving away from home would have been a sheer escape reaction. Now, correlated as it was with the understanding of the motivation behind it, it became instead an intelligent move. If you catch malaria in a swamp-infested region, move somewhere else. If your tuberculosis is such that you cannot live along the Northeastern coast, move to a dry Western climate. And if you feel frustrated, insecure, thwarted, and hostile in the home environment, build yourself a new home somewhere else.

So, at the therapist's recommendation, Hilton wrote several Midwestern universities which were known to have strong departments in vocational agriculture. During the next few days the social worker and patients in the company reported him to be an utterly changed boy. He took an active part in group therapy sessions. He began to be interested in other patients' problems about him, and he confided to the social worker, "You know, if I'm a teacher, I can be helping other people that need it—like I once did." He took an active interest in the education classes. He began to make various articles in arts and crafts, which he would bring back proudly to demonstrate in the company.

Four weeks after entering Company F, the patient was released and sent for discharge from the service. He still had occasional headaches and was bothered somewhat by battle dreams, but most of his anxiety and tenseness was gone. There was no more severe depression. He began to gain weight and did not lose his meals. By his manner, his actions, and what he said, there no longer appeared to be any suicidal risk. The psychological operation, drastic as it was, seemed to have been successful.

Review of the Case

In a later consideration of this case and its therapeutic strategy, a number of factors come to mind. The hazard of precipitating a psychosis or suicidal reaction was real. The general Ego strength as shown by the ability to overcontrol on the Rorschach is an indicator that the patient can withstand considerable anxiety. This is a reassuring finding. However, the use of such direct precipitation of a conflict is certainly questionable if the therapist is treating out of a hospital setting or under conditions where immediate control or restriction is not possible. Many techniques used under the press of war conditions would probably be deferred in favor of less active tactics if one had more time and less load of patients to treat. The case, however, was considered to be one of those more successfully treated by brief active therapy. Hypnosis here was used only as a palliative measure and for interviewing when the therapist did not wish to precipitate too much stress until more of the personality structure was understood.

During any therapy the clinician can minimize the chance of failure, but always he is forced to take a certain margin of calculated risk. That's why psychotherapy is sometimes a hazardous game—a gamble with life and death.

Chronology of the Case

The patient was wounded on December 4, 1944 and developed his depression afterwards while hospitalized. He was admitted to Welch Hospital on May 5, 1945, and transferred to the Special Treatment Company on June 26. He was seen by the therapist for a total of five sessions and was discharged from the Hospital about the end of July. The crucial session was held July 6.

CHAPTER 14

PHOBIA

In the doorway of the brightly lighted main barracks of Company F leaned a solitary figure—apparently all the other patients had gone out for the evening. The therapist had stopped by his office for a moment and was about to go out the back door when the lone figure turned around.

There was something in the staring eyes of this boy which caused him to stop. "I don't think I've seen your face before. You're new in the Company, aren't you?"

In a timid voice the thin, sallow patient replied, "Yes, sir, I just came in yesterday."

"It looks like the rest of the boys are out. You staying in tonight?"

The soldier wrinkled his brow. "Well, you see, sir, I don't know any of the fellows here yet, and"—there was a slow, hesitating pause—"and I don't like to go out by myself."

"You'll get used to that. I think you will probably like most of the fellows in this company. Why don't you go down to the Service Club? It won't take you long to get acquainted."

There were slight tremors in the boy's hand, and he bit his lip. "It isn't that, sir—it's just that I can't go out alone in the dark."

"You can't go out alone in the dark?"

"Well, I can if I force myself, but I'm afraid to."

The therapist sat down on a cot. "You're afraid to? Tell me more about it."

"Yes, whenever I'm out alone in the dark I have the feeling that people are slipping up on me—somebody—I don't know who it is, but I get clammy all over. I get so damn scared, I start running. I'd rather just not go out at all in the dark."

"Does it bother you when other people are with you?"

"No, it's just when I'm alone."

"What's your name?"

"Paul Jordan. I was in Company E. They sent me over here and said maybe you could help me."

"Is there anything else besides your fear of the dark which troubles you?"

"Yes, sir, I have headaches, a great deal—right here." The patient put his hand up to the frontal region of his head.

The therapist then recalled that he had agreed to accept a patient from Company E who was reported as having a phobia of the dark and who had been found to be hypnotizable. There was no time, however, for therapy this evening.

"Jordan, if you would like to go to the Service Club I'm headed that way. Would you care to walk with me?"

"Yes, I would like to, sir." Jordan and the therapist strolled toward the Service Club.

The next day was the 6th of August. A meeting was scheduled with Jordan for the afternoon. At that time the patient claimed he had always been afraid of the dark. He could not remember back to a time prior to the existence of this fear. However, he believed that it had become much worse during his combat experience. He described his fear as so intense that he couldn't possibly sleep in a room by himself.

Jordan was placed in a light trance by the eye-fixation method. However, he was rather slow to respond, and it took some twenty minutes of suggestion to secure even partial hand levitation. On emerging from trance, he said that he could hear some buzzing, and he exhibited partial amnesia for what had occurred in trance. He did not recall the motion of his arm, nor could he remember questions asked him, but he did feel that he had heard talking in the distance, and he complained of pain in the head. He was placed back in a moderate trance in three minutes by the postural-swaying method and given a posthypnotic suggestion to alleviate his headache.

On emerging from this he was amnesic to the entire period. Here was a good example of a case that responded much better to postural swaying than to the eye-fixation technique. Since the purpose of this first hour was only to determine the degree of hypnotizability, no attempt was made to explore further.

Before we discuss the next three significant sessions, the reader may be interested to know why this particular case was chosen for one of the chapters. It was an interesting one because, first, the major symptoms had existed for years; and second, symptomatic relief, apparently through insight, came with surprising rapidity.

On August 10 the patient was placed in a light trance after ten minutes of suggestion. The waking method was used. After he had exhibited the phenomena of arm anesthesia, catalepsy, and hand levitation, attempts were made to interview him under trance. Immediately, strong resistance occurred, and he refused to talk. It was apparent that, although hypnotizable, he was afraid to talk under trance. Accordingly, he was awakened, and the session was conducted in the conscious state.

"What do you remember, Paul, about your early childhood?"

"I remember something that my father did to me when I was very young."

"Your father?"

"My stepfather."

"Do you want to tell me about it?"

"I remember when I was a little boy about five years old. I was playing with my sister. We were—well, we were doing things that we weren't supposed to be doing—you know what I mean." Paul looked at the therapist through the corner of his eye to see whether he was being shocked.

Apparently reassured on this, he continued, "He caught both of us together, and he punished us."

"How did he punish you?"

"He put us in a closet and shut the door. It used to scare us."

"Was the closet dark?"

"Yes, it was terribly dark, and my little sister—she used to cry until he would let us out."

"Do you think maybe it's your father that you are afraid of in the dark?"

"I don't know. I think that sometimes, but I don't see the connection."

"Is there anything else you were afraid of?"

"Well, I had many bad dreams. There was one in which there was something like a dragon. I also remember I used to work in a picture show, and I would see a great many murder pictures. Then I would be afraid to go home afterwards."

"Do you remember any particular one?"

"No, I don't recall any particular one now."

"Can you tell me more about your father and mother?"

"They never did get along. They were always fighting and arguing. I think Father would get drunk at times. I was always very fond of Mother, and I felt that Father might try to kill her."

"Did their relationship get better or worse?"

"Well, it got worse for quite a while, but there was a recent reconciliation. They get along much better now."

"What else do you remember?"

"I remember that we lived in an apartment house. Upstairs there was another couple who did a great deal of arguing. They would fight—just like my folks—and one day the lady tried to kill herself—poured Lysol all over her. I watched the medical men carry her limp body out. I guess I was about nine years old at the time."

"Why did you say they argued 'just like' your folks?"

"I don't know. For some reason, thinking about my folks reminded me of the people upstairs."

"Did you ever think that something might happen to your mother—something like what happened to the lady upstairs?"

"I never thought of it that way before. Maybe I was afraid that my mother might do something like that—or my father would do something like that to her."

The rest of the hour was devoted to routine discussion, which uncovered no other promising lead. At the end of the session it was suggested to the patient that he do some thinking along the line that he might be afraid of his father in the dark—that his fear was associated with his having been locked in the closet with his sister and his belief that something might happen to his mother. It was obvious that a strong Oedipus conflict was involved in this man's neurosis. There was the punishing father—the father who might hurt his mother, the father who punished sex play with his sister, locking them both in a dark closet where they were frightened. In one conscious interview a promising element was emerging.

Since it was time for the end of the hour, the patient was given some reassurance as follows: "Jordan, regarding your fear that your father might hurt your mother, didn't you tell me that they had become reconciled now?"

Jordan replied, "Yes, they get along fine now."

"So you don't have to be afraid that your mother is going to be hurt any more. You might, however, do some thinking along the line that your stepfather is involved in your fear of the dark—that fundamentally the person you fear creeping up on you in the dark is really your father—your father who might punish you for sexual activities. We won't attempt to go any further at this time, but think about it. The next meeting we will explore the matter in more detail."

The next session was held on August 20. He had been thinking about the possibility that he was afraid of his father in the dark and reported that his thoughts on this seemed to relieve the fear.

"Would you like to tell me about your first experiences with sex?"

"I remember when I was around twelve or thirteen years old. I was working in the theater, and I saw a woman undress in a backstage room. For some reason it made me very scared."

"Yes?"

"Then, when I was eighteen years old I had an affair—I was afraid of VD afterwards, because I didn't use a rubber. I don't remember anything else important about it now. —Oh, yes, I do remember that I was afraid to sleep in our house after the woman upstairs had committed suicide."

"The woman committed suicide?"

"Yes, didn't I tell you when she poured Lysol all over herself? It killed her. I remember hearing her scream. And I was afraid to leave my mother alone at night after that. I was afraid that my father might hurt her. Still I didn't think that he had enough courage to do it.

"That makes me think of something else which just happened recently. I was up in Jacksonville the other day, walking down the street. As I passed a bar a soldier came out with a bottle of liquor in his hand. This happened about a week ago. It was fairly late at night. And this guy pulled out a knife and made a pass at me. Even though there were a lot of people around, it brought out all my old fears again. I got clammy all over."

"Does this experience, which happened to you a week ago, make you think of anything that occurred in your childhood?"

"Yes, I remember when I was twelve years old. There were some Syrian boys that lived on the street. One of them was calling me names. I hit him on the elbow with a stone. I remember his old lady came out, and shouted, 'I'll have my older boys kill you.' She came down and raised hell to Ma. Then I remember Mother talked to her and sent her home. But I was scared for the next few days. I was scared that maybe the big boys would hurt me. Nothing came of it though. This was about the same time that I was afraid my father might kill my mother.

"And now I think of something else that happened then. I saw a man all cut up in front of a bar. Somebody had slashed him. That's almost like what might have happened to me if this soldier had cut me. Now why do you suppose I thought of the incident with the Syrian boys and the man who was cut up when you asked me to associate to what happened in Jacksonville?"

"Maybe all of these things were linked together. They may all have something to do with your fear of the dark."

"I don't believe I have thought of the fight with the Syrian boys for years."

On the following day another session was held. Jordan claimed that he felt a great deal better. He had not noticed his fear of the dark much since the first meeting. He also said that since the discussion yesterday he had been able to recall clearly the incident in Jacksonville involving the threatening soldier without becoming fearful of this memory.

He was placed in a light hypnotic trance, which he entered with some resistance. It was suggested to him that he could remember many things of which he had not previously spoken—matters relating to Father and Home. He spoke with considerable resistance and blocking.

"I can remember my stepfather coming home drunk as he could be. He would yell at us—beat us hard. I remember once he beat me because I didn't clean the yard. Then I went into the park, and I was afraid he was going to chase me through the park."

"Did your father know you went to the park?"

"I don't know. I don't think so. Whenever he would come home in the evening drunk, he would beat us. I would run out and hide in the park."

"Was that after nightfall, when it was dark?"

"Yes, it was dark. He used to beat us—only Mother would get mad and make him quit. I think he beat me more than anyone else in the family. He beat my sister too."

"Why do you think he beat you and your sister more?"

"I guess it was because we weren't his children—the other members of the family were. My real Dad died, you see."

"Was there anything about your stepfather which you admired?"

"I didn't like anything about him. I was always afraid of him. He never did want me. I thought I would leave when I got bigger, but I was afraid to leave him with Mother. She would take my part, and that would start a quarrel, and then he would get mad. I was afraid he would hurt her."

"Did you ever feel responsible for their quarrels?"

"Yes, I did. Sometimes I was afraid that maybe he would hurt her because of me. He made me feel—sort of guilty-like, especially when I would run away into the park and hide."

"How old were you when this happened?"

"I was in the fifth grade of school."

"Did you think your father might chase you and catch you in the park?"

"No, I don't believe I thought of it, but. . . ."

"But what?"

"But, you know, I believe it was about then that I first began to be afraid in the dark. Father would tell me I could not go through the park, but I would go anyway. He never did follow me—but then, he might have." Jordan sat quietly for a while engrossed in thought.

"What would happen if he caught you doing something he had forbidden you to do?"

"He would put me behind the door, or in the closet—the dark closet."

"I believe you told me you used to dream about being chased by a dragon. Can you tell more about it?"

"Yes, I remember that I would go in one direction, and I would meet the dragon. I'd turn around and then go in the other direction—I would also meet the dragon. It was always when it was dark. I would wake up in a cold sweat—just like I feel when I go out at night."

"What do dragons make you think of?"

"Something bad."

"And what does something bad make you think of?"

"My old man—he's bad. What good does it do to think of one thing after another?"

"You know, Jordan, dreams are really stories told in symbols. Things that are in dreams, objects and images, stand for something else. Now you mentioned about being afraid of the dragon. And when I asked you to think of what a dragon meant you first told me it was something bad. Then you said that something bad made you think of your father. Who do you suppose the dragon in that dream is?"

"I suppose it is Dad. It's my stepfather."

"And what would the dream be saying then?"

"I suppose it means that I'm afraid of my father in the dark. That's it, isn't it, Doc? I've been afraid of my father in the dark all the time."

The emotional eagerness with which Jordan seized this new insight indicated that a significant inner change was occurring in him. As the matter was discussed further, there prevailed an affective excitement throughout the patient which was in great contrast to his previous apathetic manner.

He was now told that he would wake up from trance and remember distinctly everything that had been discussed while he was asleep. He opened his eyes, and his face began beaming. He eagerly described more incidents involving the punishing father. Gone was the hesitant, resistant manner which had marked his first responses to questioning under trance.

There now occurred a heated discussion in which all the following points were accented:

1. His inability to go out alone and attend the dance—Father would disapprove of any sexual relations which might develop and would punish him
2. His escape from parental wrath by running away—in the dark at night—into the park, with the obvious unconscious fear that Father would follow and catch him there
3. His father's punishment of his disobedience by putting him in a dark closet
4. His fear that the father might hurt his mother. This point was emphasized by his identification of his parents with "the couple upstairs," the lady who had so many bitter arguments with her husband "like Mother and Dad," and who committed suicide in a gruesome fashion through the use of Lysol

It was eight o'clock the next morning. The therapist had just started planning the day's sessions when the door burst open, and Paul came rushing in.

"Hey Doc, it's gone."

"It's gone. What do you mean?"

"My fear of the dark—I'm not afraid any more. I went out last night, and for the first time in years I didn't seem to be afraid at all. I remember once when I thought I was going to get uneasy, I said to myself, 'It's just Dad that I'm afraid of—and I'm not afraid of him any more. He can't hurt me now.' And then the fear disappeared—I didn't have it. I was out quite late, and I didn't have the slightest sign of it. You know, that's the first time in years that I wasn't scared in the dark."

Two days later, August 23, Jordan was called in for another check. Again he reported the same thing. He had been out late each night, "testing myself," as he described it. He had gone walking alone—there was no trace of fear. The phobia had simply vanished.

During the next week the patient stopped in almost every day to inform the therapist again, "It's gone—I'm not afraid any more." He seemed almost unable to comprehend the change, and he kept constantly "testing" himself.

Undoubtedly there were many deeper factors which it would be desirable to resolve. Yet it is significant that for the first time in this patient's illness his very severe phobia, which had lasted at least eight years, had disappeared. Paul Jordan could walk alone at night. No longer did the unconscious fantasy of a punishing father threaten him in the dark.

On August 30, 1945, his chart was closed, and two weeks later he was discharged to civilian life. Not once during this three-week period was there any tendency for the fear to return.

Review of the Case

The case of Paul Jordan illustrates the fact that at least some neuroses may have a comparatively superficial dynamic structure. Paul had suffered long and severely from his phobia, yet it was relieved by brief treatment and a few simple insights achieved with the aid of hypnosis. Apparently he feared the dark as a direct displacement of his fear of the father, a fear which could not be manifested because of the hostility and consequent guilt which was aroused. His understanding of this displacement as revealed by the dream of the dragon was seemingly enough to relieve the symptom. There may be many of such simple neuroses where a short-term active psychotherapy which concentrates on the enucleation of one or two conflicts may bring adequate relief without the long and protracted "working-through" of deeper material by the analysis of transference reactions and other analytic procedures. It is in this area where hypnotherapy promises to make its greatest contribution.

Chronology of the Case

The patient was hospitalized in December, 1944, for psychoneurosis, anxiety state, after twenty-six months of service including ninety days of combat. He was admitted to Welch Hospital on April 23, 1945, and transferred to the Special Treatment Company on August 5. At that time he did not show any severe battle anxieties; his phobia of the dark was the only pronounced symptom. He was seen by the therapist for a total of five sessions. He was discharged from the hospital about the middle of September, 1945.

CHAPTER 15

PSYCHOGENIC SKELETO-MUSCULAR REACTION

"An eye for an eye, and a tooth for a tooth." Nowhere is this applied with greater vengeance than when a man's own Super-Ego becomes his judge, jury, and executioner.

Harry Weber sat writhing in the chair, pain engraved on his entire face. His dark eyes stared mutely at the therapist as if pleading for a relief which he could not find from his suffering.

"Doc, it's no use. This has been going on for months. I can't stand it any more." He reached around and rubbed the lower region of his back. "Can't you do something about it? Can't you take the pain away? How about these hypnotism treatments? Some of the boys say they stop headaches. Can you take my pains away?"

The therapist cautiously refrained from making any promises. "I don't know, Weber. We can try. Sometimes the treatment helps —sometimes not. We can never be sure in any one case. Would you like to see if you can enter an hypnotic sleep?"

Harry's face brightened. "I'll try anything—absolutely anything. I can't sleep. I can't sit down. I can't lie down. I can't walk. Nothing but these sharp pains all the time. I'm going to go crazy if they don't stop."

The patient entered a trance rather easily, reaching about twenty on the Davis and Husband Hypnotic Susceptibility Scale (page 70). He was given direct suggestions under trance to the effect that he would have a general euphoric feeling and that the pains in his back region would become much less. This was accompanied by massage of the afflicted area. He emerged from trance stating that he felt better than he had for a long time—that there seemed to be practically no pain in his back. His attitude was quite positive toward being helped. Rather optimistically the progress note on this patient dated 3 April 1945 states, "Prognosis on this case is good."

But Harry's troubles were much deeper, and the direct suggestion treatment for his back pain had but a temporary effect. On April 12 he came in complaining of a return of severe pains in his back. He wanted another hypnotherapy treatment. Again direct suggestion was used. After fifteen minutes of suggestion he came out of trance to report that his back felt much better, and that nearly all the pain was gone. He was requested to return the next day, as it was felt that he should be interviewed under trance in an attempt to uncover some of the dynamics while his pains were temporarily less intense.

Session of April 13, 1945

Harry was interviewed today under hypnotic trance, and the following interesting material emerged.

"Tell me about your mother?"

"Mother was very beautiful. I don't remember much about her. She left my Dad when I was only three years old."

"How did you feel about it?"

"I think she should have stayed with him. It was her place to adjust."

"What happened to her?"

"Oh, she married a number of other times. She didn't seem to care much about me. She left me."

"How did this make you feel?"

"I always felt deserted. I always wanted a mother. I never had one."

"And how about your father?"

"I got along well with Dad. We were very close together. He raised me."

"How did you feel about not having a mother in the family?"

"I always felt rather inferior. I always felt insecure. The other boys had mothers, but I didn't. My mother had gone off and left my father. I guess she just didn't want me. Maybe I wasn't good enough for her."

The therapist made no attempt to reassure the patient at this point but permitted the fullest clarification of his feelings toward his mother.

"How did you get along in school?"

"I didn't do very well."

"How do you mean, you 'didn't do very well'?"

"I got kicked out of school."

"Why did that happen?"

"Another boy and I got into a quarrel, and the teacher said it was my fault. They threw me out, but they didn't expel the other boy."

"Do you think they should have expelled both of you?"

"Well, he started it. It wasn't my fault."

The therapist made no effort to check the validity of this story or to question him further regarding responsibility. The important point is that the patient felt he had been discriminated against.

"And then what happened in school?"

"I didn't go back to that school. I went to another one."

"Why did you go to another one?"

"Because I was afraid that after I had been expelled—even though they would let me come back—the teachers wouldn't be good to me. The other boys would poke fun at me. I felt inferior. I felt like I wanted to crawl away and hide by myself; so I didn't go back to the same school."

"And then what happened?"

"Well," there was a pause, "they sent me to the reform school." This last was blurted out as if it were a very painful admission.

"Do you want to tell me why they sent you to the reform school?"

"I stole some candy. I was with another boy. He got me to do it. We stole the candy all right, but we got caught. They sent me to the reform school."

"How did you feel about going to reform school?"

"It was really good for me. I learned a lot about getting along with other people, but it still made me feel bad. It made me feel inferior."

"How was that?"

"Because then, I always knew that I was a reform school guy. That made me different from other people. It made me not as good as other people."

Further exploration along this line did not uncover anything else that was significant. The pattern of insecurity and inferiority, however, had already been well established.

Harry was next questioned about his relations with his wife. He said that they had not been as good as he would want them, chiefly because, "she has always had her way, and I always give her her way." At this point there seemed to be a strong resistance toward talking further. Accordingly, he was given direct suggestions to ease the pain in his back. On awakening he claimed that his back felt much better.

The session was finished, but Harry kept sitting in his chair—he obviously didn't want to leave. He had something he wanted to reveal. That which could not be forced out under trance was now eager to emerge spontaneously in the conscious state. This is an interesting phenomenon for hypnotherapists to observe. Something is "kicked loose" under trance and dislodged from its structuration but does not actually emerge under trance conditions. The patient, having entered trance with resistance and suspicion, has discovered that the therapist is not trying to pry too far. Therefore, there is a new manifestation of positive attitude. Rapport increases. When this happens the wise therapist will not conclude the session. While the patient is in this state he should be encouraged in a nondirective manner. There were a number of cases in which the most significant material was disclosed, not during trance, but immediately after the patient had awakened.

Harry Weber sat fidgeting. There was a great deal of tension. The therapist directed some harmless questions to see whether this might start the stream flowing. It did.

"Harry, what kind of a person have you always wanted to be?"

Harry broke down at once into the deepest sobbing. Tears flowed like rivers.

"I want to be like my buddy. I always wanted to be like him. He's the real kind of guy. Why did it have to happen to him—why couldn't it have happened to me?"

"What happened to him?"

"He got killed, and it should have been stopped—somebody should have stopped it. Why did a good guy like that have to die when a heel like me has to live?"

"Would you like to tell me about it, Harry?"

"We were at the front. I was a paratrooper. It was a little after D-Day. We had jumped and landed. We just had consolidated our position, and the Captain told us to advance. There was a machine gun nest up ahead. The whole squad was pinned down. The Captain told my buddy and me to go up, sneak around the side, and heave in a hand grenade. We got up real close to their position." (All this description was accompanied by violent twisting in the chair, crying, writhing, "washing" of the hands, and tremendous anxiety.)

"We were getting right close—there was a little rise between the machine gun and our position so they couldn't hit us. We had cover, but I guess they must have spotted us. Anyway, they threw a grenade—one of those fire grenades. My buddy was about six feet from me. The explosion blew me back on the ground. It threw me down on my back, and I couldn't get up—I couldn't move. It set fire to my buddy. He was only six feet away. I should have got up, gone over, and put the fire out—but I didn't—I couldn't. I just lay there on my back—and he burned up. God, I heard him screaming."

Harry stared up, his eyes pleading for understanding, sympathy, and reassurance. One could see written all over him, "Tell me, Doc, that I wasn't responsible—that I wasn't a coward—that I wasn't guilty. Tell me that my back was really hurt—that it was impossible for me to get up and help him."

Then he continued, "He burned up—don't you see—he burned up, and he was the grandest fellow in the world. He's the kind of guy that I always wanted to be like. He was a real he-man. He wasn't afraid of anything. Why did it have to be him instead of me? I guess I wasn't much good as a man. I wasn't a very good soldier, but he was a good soldier—a real soldier."

Harry was given reassurance. The deeper significance of this incident was missed at this time by both the therapist and the patient. Here the solution of the case was actually within our grasp. The rationalization offered him at this time, however, was only supportive in nature and a golden opportunity was wasted. It is at a time like this where the passive, nondirective approach fails to capitalize the therapeutic potentialities.

The discussion was next directed back to events which preceded this traumatic incident.

"Tell me, Harry, how long had you been with your buddy?"

"We'd been together ever since we left Fort Benning. We'd always been in the same outfit, but you know my back was always weak—even before the explosion of the grenade."

"Tell me about it."

"When I was in Benning I jumped, and I wrenched my back. I twisted and sprained it, but I didn't go on sick call. I just gritted my teeth—didn't say anything to anyone about it."

"Why didn't you?"

"Because if I had they would have washed me out of the paratroopers, and I just *had* to be a paratrooper."

"How did you get to be one?"

"I volunteered. I'm not too big, so they barely let me in."

"And why did you want to be a paratrooper?"

Harry misunderstood the question. "Oh, when I enlisted in the Army."

"You enlisted, did you?"

"Yes, I enlisted, and I asked to be sent to the paratroopers. It seemed like that was a real he-man job, and I didn't want to get kicked out. I couldn't go back and face people if I had been thrown out of the paratroops; so that's why I just taped up my back and didn't say anything. It hurt some all the time, even when I was in combat, but it didn't hurt really bad. It didn't hurt bad until after I was blown over on the ground, and my buddy got killed. Ever since then it has just been torturing me all the time." Harry began to cry again, and writhe about uncomfortably in his chair. As he appeared exhausted, he was given reassurance, and the session was concluded.

The next day, May 14, Harry was sent to the Infirmary and an X ray was taken to locate a shell fragment that still remained in his hand. He returned very bitter at his medical treatment—claiming that he had been pushed around. Then he burst into tears. He intimated that he may have "blown his top" and said a number of things he shouldn't have. Accordingly, the therapist scheduled another session immediately. At this time the patient disclosed a recent incident which had brought about considerable stress and caused an increase in his back pains.

His small son had undergone an operation in a hospital, and Harry had recently been given a furlough to go home. For twelve days and nights this patient had sat by the bedside with his son. He seemed utterly exhausted, physically and mentally. There was deep depression and anxiety over his face. He complained of very severe suffering in the back region. He was placed in a trance and given suggestions to ease the back pains. This time when he awakened— even though he was amnesic for the suggestions given and though they had been repeated under trance for some ten minutes—he reported that his back was just as sore as before. It was apparent that the symptoms were not going to respond much longer to direct suggestion alone.

Harry Weber's home was about a day's journey from the hospital. On May 17 the company commander reported him AWOL. He returned the next day and came into the therapist's office. He was a worn, haggard, tired man. Where before he looked sick, now he looked almost like a skeleton. The deepest depression had enveloped him. He had gone home one evening expecting to return before morning and found conditions at home very bad. After a misunderstanding with his wife he stayed AWOL the next day and instituted divorce action. His back pains were worse than ever, and he was in such a state of anxiety and depression that he was confined immediately to quarters for the remainder of the day. Plans were made for intensive therapy.

The case was discussed with Captain R., battalion psychiatrist, concerning the advisability of "adjusting" the memory of the traumatic situation. It was planned to place the patient back in hypnotic

trance and have him abreact again the incident in which his buddy
was killed. The therapist would then take the role of his commanding officer, the captain who had ordered him to take the machine gun
nest, and arrive on the scene just after the fire grenade had exploded.
Then while the patient was lying on the ground and wanting to help
his buddy put the fire out, the "captain" would order him to stay
down under cover. This "adjustment" might relieve his severe guilt,
remove his feelings of cowardice, and transfer responsibility for his
buddy's death to the "captain." Perhaps this would ease his punishing back pains.

Session of May 21, 1945

When Harry reported today he had severely increased back pains.
He was very depressed and discouraged. It was planned to have him
abreact the traumatic incident and "adjust" his memory of the situation as planned.

An attempt was now made to induce trance. Ten minutes of sleep
suggestions were given—another ten minutes—another ten minutes.
Thirty minutes had elapsed.

"Doc, I'm not the least bit sleepy. My back hurts—I can't go to
sleep."

Another attempt was made. This time he entered a very light
hypnoidal state. As soon as the therapist directed a question to him,
he immediately opened his eyes and was wide awake. Obviously a
period of negative transference had set it. Here was a patient, previously hypnotizable, who now, on the eve of the planned "psychological operation," suddenly became inaccessible. He left the session
without any alleviation of his back pains—and greatly discouraged.
Equally so was the therapist.

Session of May 25, 1945

Harry reported today, feeling somewhat better in spirits. He had
reached an understanding with his wife, but he still suffered from
the severe pains in his back. Again repeated attempts to induce
hypnotic trance were unsuccessful. There was much evidence of
negativism—he simply could not be hypnotized. What a thwarting
situation! Enough of the dynamics were now known to do something constructive. An "adjusted memory" under one more abreactive trance might turn the trick. Now, just when the crucial part of
the therapy was to be applied, he could no longer be hypnotized.

Another discussion on the case was held with Captain R. The only thing left to do was to review the dynamics as they appeared at the present time with the patient in the conscious state. It was also decided to initiate his discharge from the Army. He was a man much too sick to be retained in the service. The tenuous nature of his marital relationship was such that if it were not mended by his return home the entire neurosis, even if relieved by insight, would be re-invoked. It was also felt that if he could be told that he would be discharged from the Army, there might be a return of the positive transference so badly needed. Therefore, he was informed that he would be discharged from the Army shortly, and another session was scheduled.

Session of May 29, 1945

Harry's depression had subsided because he knew that he would be released from the Army. Also, a recent understanding with his wife had reduced the stress. However, he still suffered from the pains in his back. These had not retreated in the least.

Harry reclined on the cot in a despondent manner. He had given up the fight. The therapist sensed this was the last chance—this was *it*.

"I want to talk to you today, Harry, about a young man that I know. This is a young fellow who has always been fighting himself. Lately he's also been punishing himself." Harry lay quietly—there was no response on his haggard face. The therapist spun the following story—dramatizing it at times.

"This young man had always been afraid of the world and afraid of people. He has always felt very insecure and inferior—inferior to the next guy. And why did he feel inferior? Well, for a lot of reasons. When he was a young boy about three years old his mother left him and his father. Of course, it wasn't his fault that his mother left. It was the parent's fault. Nevertheless, he felt rejected, and he believed that his mother didn't want him. He felt that he was not as good as other people. So he first started feeling inferior way back there when he was three years old.

"Then when he was older, he got into trouble in school. It wasn't his fault, but he got expelled from school. That also made him feel inferior—made him feel even more inferior than he did before." Harry began to listen intently.

"And this boy became afraid of other boys in school. He was afraid that they would poke fun at him because he had been expelled from school. That made him feel still more inferior—so much so that he went to another school instead of returning to the first one.

"Then he got into still more trouble. Because of an attempt at stealing he was sent to the reform school. That made him believe he was a marked man—he was a criminal—he was really inferior— he wasn't as good as the next person. And it made him feel so bad, so afraid of life and other people, that, as he grew older, he had to do something to prove he was a man. He was afraid that other people wouldn't accept him as a man or recognize him as being as good as anybody else.

"Because he had to prove to himself that he was as good as the next person, he tried to do more than his strength would allow. He tried to do something over and above what he should have."

Harry broke in. "What was that—what did I do?"

"Well, for one thing, he had to enlist in the Army. He couldn't wait until he was inducted like the rest of the men. He had to enlist ahead of his time. Not that there is anything wrong with enlisting, but you see this boy had to prove his manhood so much that he en- listed, not just in the Army, but in the paratroopers. He had to be a big shot. He had to be a paratrooper, even though he wasn't quite strong enough to go into the paratroops. He had to prove to himself that he was a better man than the next guy because inside he felt so inferior. And then when he was at camp, and he was called upon to perform feats of physical strength that were beyond his endurance, he drove himself until he injured his back. It wasn't a severe injury. Nothing was broken—only a little sprain, but it started things off. He was afraid that he would be washed out of the paratroops—some- thing that he couldn't stand—something that would make him feel terribly inferior; so he just taped up his back. He didn't go and have the doctors take care of it like he should have.

"About that time, he found a buddy. He met the kind of a guy he would like to have been. He found a fellow who didn't have any fears like himself. So he identified with this buddy. He became very closely attached to this fellow. He hero-worshiped him. Isn't that right?"

Harry didn't say anything—he only nodded. The tears were streaming down from his eyes.

"And so when he went over to France, he had a buddy who repre- sented the kind of fellow he always wanted to be. Then when he got into combat he and his buddy were ordered to go up and clear out a machine gun nest. The breaks were against them. There was an explosion, and he was blown over on his back. His buddy was set on fire. And when he was blown over on his back, he suddenly felt weak. He didn't feel strong enough either physically or psychologically to get up, go over, and put out the fire on his buddy—he couldn't make enough exertion or effort to do so. Maybe he was even a little afraid to get up because he didn't feel strong enough to go through the storm of bullets which the Jerries would fire. Anyway the important thing is, that in his own eyes, he felt that he hadn't done his best. He felt that he was a coward, and he blamed himself for his buddy's death. And down inside him that part of him that's unconscious, kept saying over and over again, 'You're guilty. You murdered your buddy. You're guilty of the death of your buddy.' But it was his unconscious, down inside of him, that said those things, not he, himself—nor anybody else. He couldn't recognize that. He wouldn't want to recognize it. It would cause him too much anxiety. So he pushed it down and kept it down where it was unconscious. He didn't recognize that he felt he had been cowardly and was responsible for his buddy's death. He couldn't face that fact out in the open—in his conscious mind.

"But when a man thinks he is guilty, sometimes his body punishes him. Another part of him recognizes that he feels guilty; and so he is his own judge—and his own executioner. That other part, his conscience, punishes him. It makes him suffer, and it is going to make him suffer right where he is weakest. Where was this boy weakest?"

Harry mumbled, "In his back—that's where I was weakest. That's what I had strained."

The therapist agreed. "That's right. It was the back that was the weakest part of you. That was the part which you had strained. That was the part of your body you had been blown over on. That was the part which you felt had let you down at the crucial time— had kept you from helping your buddy when he needed it. So that was the part which had to be punished. It was the back that was wrong. It was the back that was guilty. Because if the back had been stronger, it would have got up, carried you over near your buddy, and helped save his life. So it was the back that must be punished. The back must be punished for the guilt feeling you had. And so, having driven yourself as a child in order to overcome these feelings of inferiority, the only way they could be satisfied now was by a severe punishment of the back. The back must hurt. Therefore, the pains came into the back."

For an hour and a half this type of "insight feeding" continued. It was insight, not pulled out on a nondirective basis—it was insight crammed in by a completely directive manner—relying for its power only on the persuasive ability of the therapist, and the strength of the transference relationship.

Harry listened and did not talk much. At times he would shed a few tears. But he listened intently—and he understood. At the end of the session he looked up at the therapist with a smile on his face and said very simply, "You're the first man that has ever understood me—everything that you said is true. That is just what happened to me." Then he got up rather quietly and walked out of the office.

The next day was May 30. There was a light knocking at the door. When the therapist opened it, Harry Weber's face was seen wreathed in smiles.

"Doc, I feel grand. The pains are all gone—I haven't got any back pains."

The therapist was bowled over. He had felt that there had been some true insight at the end of the previous hour, but that the symptoms would dramatically disappear within twenty-four hours did not seem possible. Yet, on discussing it further with the patient, it was quite apparent that the depression and the punishing back pains had gone. Harry reported that the back still felt slightly stiff and sore. But the sharp pains which had been there up until the 29th of May, and with which he had suffered for a period of months, were gone.

Harry Weber remained in the company about a week and a half and spent another week in the discharge company before finally leaving the Army. During these two and a half weeks he was seen on various occasions by the therapist. Each time he smiled and was most profuse in his thanks. He affirmed at all times that there had been no return of his back pains.

Yes, when a corrective emotional experience has been achieved through insight, the symptom structure can collapse. But this insight must be real. It must be an emotional insight. It must involve a re-integration of the inner energy structure of the human organism. Something of this nature must have happened in the nervous system of Harry Weber.

Chronology of the Case

The exact dates of this patient's breakdown, hospitalization, and previous service are not available, but he was seen by the therapist first on April 3, 1945. Ten therapeutic sessions were held between that date and May 30, 1945. The crucial session was held May 29.

CHAPTER 16

TREMOR

In the treatment of neurotic disorders it is the unexpected which often happens. May 23, 1946 was just such a day. The therapist and an officer patient were engaged in a crucial session. The patient was a physician, a battalion surgeon, who insisted that his hysterical tremor was a Parkinson and was submitting to psychotherapy very reluctantly. This man, harboring a great reservoir of inhibited hate toward a former superior officer, was throwing himself into an emotional abreaction under deep hypnotic trance.[1]

A light tap was heard at the door. Underneath it appeared a small note. "Miss K——— would like you to call her on the phone as soon as possible." Miss K——— was one of the Red Cross workers who counseled separatees before they left the Hospital.

Since the case load for that day was both quantitatively and qualitatively heavy the therapist had intended to answer this call at the end of the afternoon, but at three o'clock another knock sounded on the office door.

This time it was a long, tall, lanky soldier who stood there, nervously fingering his cap and shuffling about.

---

[1] For professional and ethical reasons this case, one of the most interesting, cannot be completely presented here, but a few points are of especial interest to professional readers. The patient was so hypnotizable that at each session he entered a deep trance in less than three seconds by the eye-fixation method. During this hour he was encouraged to "murder symbolically" his enemy. He had previously stated his conscious wish that he could "have the man on my operating table." Accordingly, under a deep trance he was now being given this opportunity. He was given a pillow and informed that this was the officer he hated. He was then given an imaginary scalpel and told that he was completely free to do as he wished. For fifteen minutes this patient, a powerful man, tore at the pillow, stabbing it repeatedly, and with the utmost satisfaction on his face shouted a stream of epithets while he secured his "revenge."

The therapist kept prodding for the fullest participation, physiologically and psychologically, until, with beads of sweat pouring down his face, his shirt wringing wet, the man nearly collapsed from sheer exhaustion. After giving him a few minutes' rest, still under trance, the therapist tried to make him again enact the murder scene. He replied, "I don't feel like it any more. The hate is all gone."

He was then told that he had symbolically killed his enemy and now could release his hate. The relation of the repressed hate to his symptom was pointed out. Finally, memory for the entire abreaction and the interpretations were stuck posthypnotically, and the matter again integrated on the conscious level. Following this session there was a great improvement in his major symptoms.

This case illustrates the previously-mentioned contention—that abreactions are successful when exploited by the fullest physical and psychological participation while under trance, followed by insight and reintegration at both the trance and the conscious levels.

"Miss K——— said for me to come and see you."

Already in the office another crucial case, an obsessive-compulsive patient bordering on schizophrenia, was waiting, so the therapist, perhaps with some impatience, replied, "If you'll wait I'll see you later in the afternoon."

It was four o'clock, just time enough to transcribe the notes of the day's sessions before retreat, when the obsessive-compulsive left and the therapist again recalled the tall soldier who was patiently waiting outside.

"Come in. What would you like to see me about?"

The soldier exhibited extreme bashfulness and timidity as he slumped back into the chair.

"Well, it's about this." He held out a pair of hands which trembled in a slight but distinctly noticeable manner.

"I'm getting out of the Army, and I was talking with Miss K——— today about veterans' benefits when she noticed the shaking in my hands. I've had it about two years, but I never told the doctors."

"You say you're getting out of the Army?"

"Yes—that is—I'm already out. I'm scheduled to leave tomorrow and go home."

"You're leaving tomorrow? Didn't you ever call your doctor's attention to your hands before this?"

"No, I was an orthopedic patient, wounded in the leg, and I've had the trembling ever since that time with the BAR." [2]

"What about the BAR?"

"Miss K——— asked me that too after she noticed my hands trembling. I told her the incident. Then she said I should come up and see you before I left the Hospital."

"Suppose you start from the beginning and tell me about it."

"I was one of the oldest men in the outfit. We had a lot of casualties and they kept sending us replacements. One time we didn't have any BAR man and the lieutenant—he was new—insisted I take the BAR. I didn't want to. I didn't know anything about the gun, but he ordered me to take it and while I was trying to see how it worked the damn thing went off and mowed my buddy down. They took him away to the hospital. It was shortly after that when I first noticed the trembling in my hands."

"Why didn't you call your doctor's attention to this symptom? Wasn't it important to you to get some treatment for it?"

---

[2] Browning automatic rifle.

"Oh, yes. I realize now how important it is. You see in civilian life I'm a professional athlete—play basketball and football—and I'm sure now the trembling may keep me from earning a living that way again. But it seemed foolish at first to worry about it. I thought it was just the jitters—that it would go away by itself. Then of course when I was wounded, getting my leg fixed was more important. I've been wanting to go home and I thought that if I brought up the trembling it might keep me here longer. Miss K———, though, thought I shouldn't leave the Hospital without having you look at it."

What a problem to be thrown into the lap of any therapist! Four-fifteen in the afternoon. In less than twenty-four hours this patient would be on his way home. His medical charts were now closed and unavailable; no psychiatric social history; no psychological tests; no initial psychiatric examination; no authorization for treatment—no nothing! Just a tall, gawky, bashful lad asking that the impossible be done at once.

The patient—let us call him George Winkelman—looked down at the therapist with a questioning expression. "Can you find out what's wrong?"

The therapist made no reply. He just sat quietly for about a minute. Snatches of many different ideas were running through his mind: No neurologicals—maybe the condition is organic. No Rorschach—wonder if he's got an hysterical-type personality? Parkinson?—could be. What's his family background—stable or unstable? Wonder if he's hypnotizable—might help the condition with some direct suggestion. But he's had it for two years; sounds pretty chronic. I can't do anything! Well, maybe it *is* hysteria! What are the dynamics?—Maybe guilt over shooting his buddy with the BAR? Why the hands?—One holds a BAR in the hands. Would have to punish the hands—punishment would interfere with earning a living —playing basketball—couldn't make shots—important to him. Ought to make a try. Insight would have to come rapidly even if this theory is right—got to do it in one session. Maybe an abreaction? No time for careful, slow exploring. Must induce narcosis. Amytal or pentothal?—D. (the psychiatrist) has already gone home. Got to be hypnosis—is he hypnotizable?—can't spend several sessions finding out—even one hour. He's got to be highly hypnotizable— must go under at once—must be able to abreact—the dynamics inferred must be the right ones—the participation must be thorough— must get over the insight—must, must, must! Too many "ifs"—it can't be done.

"Winkelman, did you go to college?"

"Yes, I did, sir."

"Ever take any courses in psychology?"

"I took one in general psych."

"Did you ever see a demonstration of hypnosis?"

"Yes, the professor put a boy under for us."

"What did you think about it?"

"I was greatly impressed."

"Have you ever been hypnotized?"

"No."

"Do you have any fears or misgivings about hypnosis?"

"No."

For five minutes the therapist sketched over hypnosis, neurosis, hysteria, the usual reassurance and orientation, which ordinarily took an hour or so. The patient listened and seemed most co-operative.

"How about it, Winkelman? There's just an outside chance—if we only had a few weeks to work with you, even several hours. I can't promise a thing—there just isn't enough time—but if you're willing I'll be glad to try."

"I'm willing to try anything if it might help."

The patient was given the arm-drop suggestibility test—he responded positively.

The eye-fixation method of trance induction was started. In five minutes the eyes closed. In another minute or two anesthesia could be induced in his arm. No time for preliminary exploring, testing limits, testing trance depth, mapping sensitive areas, etc.

"Winkelman, you're back in France. The new lieutenant is handing you a BAR. Your buddy is beside you. The lieutenant wants you to be the BAR man for the platoon. Your buddy stands here." (The patient was placed in the middle of the room and touched on the right side to indicate the position of his buddy.) "Now Winkelman, the lieutenant is starting to talk to you. 'Winkelman, you're the oldest man in the company. You've got to take the BAR; can't trust one of these green replacements. Here!'" (The therapist thrust an imaginary BAR into the patient's hands.)

Winkelman scowled and began to protest. "Hell, I don't know anything about a BAR. Never handled one before. Why have I got to take it? I'll bet some of the new guys have had BAR training."

"'Winkelman, I said you're to be the BAR man. Now you shut up and take it or I'll court-martial you. That's an order!'"

The patient "took" the "BAR," began to fuss with it, and mumbled oaths against the "lieutenant" under his breath.

"I've never handled one before. How does the bolt work? What's this thing for?"

" 'Go ahead and work the bolt. You're going to handle it, you might as well learn how to use the piece.' "

The patient took hold of "the bolt" and rammed it home. Instantly he jumped back, grabbed his own leg, threw the "BAR" down, and held his arms out toward the right side.

"Artie, Artie, what have I done to you! I didn't mean to do it! Are you hurt? Speak to me, Artie! Please speak, Artie! I didn't know it was loaded. Oh God, what have I done!" A flood of tears poured down his face.

The therapist eased the patient back into a chair and began reassuring, explaining dynamics and relieving guilt. The manner was the same as that used in treating Harry Weber (Chapter 15), but less time was used. Unlike the case of Weber, the reassurance and insight were being delivered with the patient under deep trance. This continued for five more minutes. A smile of understanding came over the patient's face as the therapist concluded, "And now since you realize that for two years you have been condemning yourself with feelings of guilt for shooting your buddy, you will be able to lose those guilty feelings. You won't have to punish your hands any more. You will wake up like a new man, understanding what caused your hands to tremble. That is why they will be steady and without tremors. I shall count to five and you will wake up. 1-2-3-4—5."

Winkelman opened his eyes. "Look, Doc, my hands are steady." He held them out. Not a trace of tremor disturbed their control. "That's wonderful. How did you do it? Oh yes, I remember now. I've been punishing myself for having shot my buddy, haven't I? That's what made my hands tremble. But now I don't feel guilty any more. I understand. It was just an accident." For the next few minutes the patient continued with profuse thanks, but his expressions of gratitude could not possibly have increased the satisfaction of the therapist. Perhaps the "remission" was temporary, mere suggestion. Perhaps, but it had all the earmarks of a cure through insight—an emotionally corrective experience. Time alone could tell.

"Don't you think it would be a good idea to go back and talk to Miss K———— before you leave the Hospital? Let her see your hands as they are now. I'm sure it will please her." (Miss K———— reported that the next day he was symptom-free, happy, and exhibiting good insight into the causes of his disability.)

It was 4:45 P.M. (1645 as the Army would put it)—just forty-five minutes since Winkelman had first walked into the office.

Chronology of the Case

Nothing is available on the patient other than that reported here. His chart had been closed, and his records were no longer in his company. The next day he returned to civilian life.

CHAPTER 17

CONVERSION HYSTERIA

Arthur Jones was discussing his symptoms. "Yes, Doc, I do have headaches. They come over my right eye. I used to have fainting and dizzy spells, and when I was wounded I got numb pains all through my shoulders and arm. Then the hand lost all its feeling. See, I can't straighten my finger out." Arthur extended his left hand with the third finger sticking out at right angles from the rest of them. No amount of force could bend it back in line. Art smiled as he looked at the warped hand—no sadness—no sign of worry—no irritability—no bitter denunciation—just a smile. He then mentioned the ringing in his right ear, the profuse sweating in his hands, the prickly feelings throughout his arm, and the occasional battle dreams.

Art was an hysteric. But all of his anxiety had not been converted into a single disability. There was still some of it floating freely— not structured into a symptom. That is why, in addition to an hysterical paralysis, he also had the headaches, the stomach trouble, and battle dreams.

It was the middle of July when Arthur arrived at Welch Hospital. The examining psychiatrist on admission noticed, "He is a rather thin, undernourished, asthenic-looking individual above average in intelligence—answers questions readily and coherently. Gives the impression of being sincere and truthful—well oriented in all spheres —judgment and insight unimpaired. Memory both recent and past is good. No malignant psychiatric trends. Denies delusions or hallucinations. Appears to be rather suggestible." This was true. When he arrived in Company F, he was found to be quite easily hypnotizable during an initial study.

Further evidence that he was not a pure hysterical case but that there were unstructured anxiety components in his personality was made more evident by the company social worker, who on first interviewing him July 31 wrote the following note: "The patient appeared on an interview today to be phlegmatic, preoccupied, moderately depressed. He was pleasant and cooperative. He did not elaborate his complaints. Symptoms that he noted were partial paralysis and anesthesia of the left arm, headaches, right frontal, back pains when he uses the left arm, loss of weight, enuresis, and battle dreams. He cannot concentrate and complains of poor memory. He expresses desire to get out of the Army and is disgusted with military things."

Session of August 2, 1945

On the 2nd of August the following interview under trance was held. Only forty seconds were required to place him in a moderate trance by the eye-fixation method.

"How have you been feeling lately, Art?"

"I seem to be sorta tense—my head bothers a good deal."

"I want you to forget all about where you are and go back, back, back, in your memories until you are only seven years old."

Art "went back" to the age of seven. He named his teacher and all the children sitting in his row in school. Then the interview was continued.

"Do you fear anybody?"

"I'm afraid of people."

"Why?"

"I don't know. I'm just afraid of them. I'm afraid to talk to them."

"Are you afraid of any particular people?"

"I'm afraid of Dad."

"Why?"

"He's always getting after me. I don't know why. I want to stay at home, and he wants me to go out and play all the time."

"You want to stay at home—how do you mean?"

"I don't like to go out and play with the other children. I want to go in the house and play by myself."

"Why don't you like to go out and play with the other children?"

"I'm afraid the other boys will hurt me."

"Do you ever play with them?"

"Yes, but they are all bigger than I am, and they run over me."

"What does Daddy say about it?"

"He tries to tell me I'm a sissy." Art sobbed lightly. "I don't want to see him, or nobody—I just want to be alone."

"What does Mother say?"

"She helps—no, she's on Dad's side. She says for me to go out and be like the others."

The patient was then regressed back to the age of five. At this point he developed a twisting of the head and a jerking and quivering of the whole body. There was very heavy breathing. He would

hardly talk at all. Since no material could be elicited at this age he
was regressed still further back to the age of four. At this level he
gave his nickname. Then he stated once more that he feared his
Dad, but he didn't know why. He kept shaking his head and twisting
about.

"Would you like to tell me how you feel, Art?"

Art shook his head and remained silent.

"Have you seen something real bad—something that you are
afraid to talk about?"

The patient turned away. "Yes."

"I won't tell anybody about it, Art. Wouldn't you like to trust
me with it?"

"No, it's very bad." (No amount of persuasion could get him to
talk about it.)

He now mentioned his fear of people because "they hurt you" and
then refused to discuss the matter further.

Art was given suggestions to alleviate some of his symptoms. He
emerged from trance amnesic to all that had occurred. He claimed
that he felt better. He had no headaches, although he was a bit dizzy.

On August 8 the social worker reported that Art was "transfer-
ring and identifying with the therapist but was very slow to identify
with the group." Art described to Corporal L. his preoccupation
with battle, chiefly a very traumatic situation in which he was
wounded and removed from combat.

His platoon had been holding a position on a hill for about thirty-
six hours. The Jerries came over in waves. He killed many of them
with his machine gun. Then his buddy was killed, and he was the
last survivor of his platoon. He remembered killing a certain
German soldier. The helmet fell off, and he saw long black hair.
He felt sure that it was a woman. This made him extremely upset.
Shortly afterward he ran out of ammunition. The next thing he
knew he was looking into the barrel of a "burp gun." He was shot
in the shoulder. He lay on the ground for about three minutes filled
with overwhelming fear. Suddenly a mortar shell landed near by
and struck a tree which fell over on top of him. That was the last
he remembered until he "came to" in the aid station. Corporal L.
made the following significant notation at the end of this session:

"The patient sweated heavily as he talked but displayed no other
anxiety. His emotional tone improved, and he became very friendly,
showed insight and did not resist interpretive comments, but applied
them as best he could. It was felt that the man has remarkable ego
strength in view of very predisposing family factors."

Corporal L. followed the last significant session with another the next day. It was apparent that Arthur had received some relief from the cathartic description of his battlefield experience. He felt much better and had lost his headache. He had abreacted this same incident once before under sodium pentothal a month or so after removal from combat. The notes on this showed that he was still conscious after having been struck by the tree. He could see his buddies being bayoneted while he was lying there. Apparently the trauma of the event had rendered him amnesic rather than unconscious to what transpired. Art recalled on questioning that he had often dreamt of sleeping men being bayoneted. Corporal L. noted that the patient might have guilt feelings because he was "not sure that his buddy was dead, and he did not rise to protect him." Art did have a .45 caliber pistol on his right hip which he did not use.

During this same session Art recalled that once before he had fainted in combat—they had to take him back to the first aid station. He was gone from his outfit over night. But he returned the next day and found that the Germans had counterattacked and killed several of the men. They might not have been killed, he indicated, except that the machine gun which he left had jammed and could not be used to protect them. He felt that he was guilty—if he had been there he could have repaired the gun at once. This feeling of guilt drove him to volunteer for at least two dangerous missions "to make up for it." He was always fearful that he would faint at a crucial moment and that this would cost the life of someone. One time he fainted while out in the cold, guarding a dugout, but he recovered before anyone knew of it. He said that he had always been "ashamed" of fainting. Corporal L. concluded the session by giving the patient further reassurance.

Sessions of August 10 and August 17, 1945. Regression

On August 10 the therapist again saw Private Jones. He appeared to be in much better spirits. The airing of his guilt feelings, the cathartic release of his battle experiences, and the reassurance had had a very beneficial effect. This was increased at the meeting by telling him he would be recommended for discharge from the service as soon as he was well enough, and "the faster you get well, the sooner you will be able to go home."

The patient was hypnotized twice, and both times he was given suggestions to straighten out his third finger. The finger could be straightened under trance with considerable difficulty, but would not remain so posthypnotically. However, it was much more manipulable than previously, and the spastic resistance was considerably less when he emerged from trance the second time. He said that his hand had a prickling sensation in it. He was able to move the fingers almost normally.

Evidence was being unearthed to the effect that Arthur's problems were much more deep-seated than was at first apparent. Behind his traumatic battle experience revolved a whole system of childhood phobias, insecurities, sex maladjustments, and family difficulties. On August 17 deeper therapy was initiated. It was noticed at this time that his hand was straight, there being only a slight bending of the third finger. There was no sign of vomiting or stomach difficulties, but he still experienced headaches. He suffered one dizzy spell on August 15.

Arthur was placed in trance and regressed to the first grade, naming the teacher and a large number of the children in the room as a check on regression.

"Tell me more about your fears."

"People."

"What about people?"

"They hurt me—everyone hurts me."

"How will they hurt you?"

"They will hurt me."

"Are you afraid of your father?"

"He talks, and he gets after me."

"Why?"

"I don't know why—he just talks."

"How long have you been afraid of Dad?"

"A long time."

"What about Mother?"

"She gets after me, too. I'm afraid of her some."

"Why?"

"She will get after me, too."

"What will Dad say?"

"He will tell me to get out."

"What do you mean, 'out'?"

"I mean out of the house."

"Don't you like to play?"

"I like to play, but I don't like to be told—Mother and Father would talk real low together, and they would talk about us."

"Did you ever see anybody do anything really bad?"

He tightened his lips and spoke with difficulty, "No."

"Who do you like best in your family?"

"I like Joan. She's my sister. She's all right."

"Is Joan pretty?"

"Yes, she is very pretty."

"You are going to go back and become younger, younger. You will now be only four years old. You are a little boy four years old playing in the yard."

Arthur pursed his lips. He wouldn't speak but gritted his teeth.

"What's the matter? Are you afraid to talk, Arthur?"

"Yes, I don't want to talk."

"What are you afraid of?"

"Dad."

"What about Dad?"

"Daddy talks bad to me. He said that I was a sissy."

"Do you want to tell me more about it?"

"Joan and I were playing in the house—we were playing dresses. We were putting on our clothes and taking off our clothes too, and Daddy got very angry and said that it wasn't nice."

"Is Joan any different from you?"

"Yes."

"How?"

"She is littler."

"Does she have the same parts on her body?"

"No."

"In what way is she different?"

"She is different." (Arthur did not want to discuss the matter further.)

"Did you touch her?"

"No, I just looked."

"How old is Joan?"

"Three."

"Did Daddy slap her or punish her?"

"Yes, Daddy did."

"Why?"

"For messing up her clothes—and she messed up Mommy's clothes too."

"Do you mean that she wet her clothes?"

"No, she tore a hole in them."

"Did you ever play again with her when she didn't have her clothes on?"

"No."

When Arthur was next regressed to the age of three his lips became very tight. He denied that he had any fear, but he would not respond much to questioning. He said, "I like Mommy, and I like Daddy, and I play with Joan." He was then advanced to the age of five. At this regressed age he still would not talk. Accordingly, he was awakened, being given suggestions to alleviate his headaches just before he emerged from trance. He woke up and said that his head felt much better. He was quite amnesic to all the material discussed.

From what has been disclosed so far, we would infer that the patient has been rejected by both his father and his mother, and that his libidinal impulses have been turned toward his sister. There may have been incestual desires toward her, but these have been well repressed because of the father's punishment of the children when they were playing without clothes. This has undoubtedly affected his later attitude toward sex and love.

Alpert, Carbone, and Brooks (1946) have shown the value of repeated abreactions in releasing repressed anxiety. In his discussions Arthur had secured considerable cathartic relief from guilt feelings and anxiety associated with the traumatic incidents of battle. However, it was felt that these would be more adequately and completely resolved if experienced under hypnotic trance.

Session of August 20, 1945. Abreaction

The following session took place on August 20. Arthur was placed in a deep trance merely by being told that he would be sound asleep by the time the therapist had counted up to twenty.

"You're back in battle now, Arthur. The shells are all around. You're right in the thick of it. What's happening?"

"I'm in a church. The eighty-eights [1] are firing. They're hitting everywhere. I'm down in the cellar, and a shell hits upstairs. Somebody is hurt. I can hear 'em holler. I wonder if it is one of the boys I know?"

"Now, what do you do?"

"I don't go up. I'm afraid to go up. I'm afraid if I go up that another shell will come along and knock me out too. God, I wish they'd quit hollering. I should go up now—I'm supposed to go up and help, but I'm afraid to, and it's dark—those eighty-eights are hitting. I don't want to go up. Here comes another." The patient ducked.

---

[1] 88-millimeter cannon.

Then he suddenly relaxed and continued, "That was another shell. It made a direct hit—wiped out everybody upstairs. They're all dead."

"Were there many buddies of yours among them?"

"They were all my buddies."

"Do you think that you could have saved them?"

"I don't know—I might have. I should have tried. I shouldn't have stayed down here."

"Did you finally go upstairs?"

"Yes, everyone was dead. It was all quiet. I wanted to get away. So I went down into the town and moved through the houses along with another buddy of mine. There was a Jerry in one house, and I threw a grenade at him. Then I rushed in. When I got in there I couldn't find the Jerry anywhere. He had been wounded, but he sneaked out the back—and then . . ." Arthur's eyes began to cloud up with tears.

"And then, what?"

"And then my buddy, Bill, came in, and the Jerry shot him. Why didn't I get the damn Jerry in the first place. I should've known that I hadn't really killed him. He was still sneaking around. If I'd have been more careful, Bill would be alive today. Bill, he shouldn't have got it. The Jerry should have been dead."

"How does it make you feel?"

"It makes me feel bad—very bad." Arthur began to cry. The therapist made no effort to inhibit the release of anxiety but instead encouraged the patient to relive the incident to the fullest. He was then given reassurance and rationalizations to the effect that it was merely the breaks of war which caused his buddy's death—not his own lack of responsibility. Arthur was encouraged then to continue his story.

"Then we went on and took some more towns."

"Let's go to the place where you were just before you were wounded."

"There are shells all around. I'm scared to death. The Jerries are coming. There is a great deal of hollering and screaming. They are getting closer, and I can see a Jerry looking straight at me." At this point the patient became so paralyzed that he couldn't move. "I can't grab my rifle quick enough. The Jerry shoots me right here— right here in the shoulder." Arthur stroked the left shoulder with his right hand.

"And then I lay still. Just as quiet as I can. I know that this is going to be my last moment. I know that the Jerry is going to stick me with a bayonet. Just then a mortar shell comes. I guess it knocked the Jerry out. It blows up a tree. The tree falls over and hits me on top of the head and on the back. Then I don't remember anything. I don't remember anything until I'm back in battalion aid station."

At this point the patient was brought out of the trance, and all the material uncovered was discussed with him in the conscious state. At first he did not remember it, but after it was suggested to him complete details returned. The incident involving the people upstairs in the church and the death of his buddy were rationalized to him. This eased his guilt feelings. He was told that he could not have prevented it; therefore, he should not feel guilty.

He was once more placed back in deep trance, and the following suggestions were given to him. "When you wake up, Arthur, you will feel a lot better. You will not have any headaches. You will feel calm and relaxed because you have been able to get off your chest something that has been bothering you for a long time. You will understand that it wasn't your fault that the other people and your buddy were killed. You couldn't have stopped it—that was just the breaks of war. You will understand this and accept this insight, and you are going to remember everything you discussed while you were asleep. You will not forget it because you won't have to hide it from yourself any more. You can remember it, and then just let it go. You won't worry about it any longer."

When he came out of trance he said that he felt much better. Once more the material disclosed was reviewed, and this time it seemed to have considerably fewer anxiety-provoking features.

Session of August 24, 1945. Projective Techniques Under Regressed Trance

On the 24th of August Arthur came in stating that his head had felt a lot better and that he had suffered no nausea attacks lately. There was still some pain in the left shoulder when he exercised. This was his only remaining symptom.

So far, all the therapy had been along superficial lines of reassurance, direct suggestion, catharsis, and abreaction. Very little had been done to explore further the obvious predispositions in his personality structure. Now "depth techniques" were employed for the first time. This particular session illustrates the opportunities for uncovering psychodynamics through the use of such projective methods as the Thematic Apperception Test.

The patient was shown several pictures from the TAT under the following conditions: first, when normal and not in a trance; second, when he was under deep trance and regressed to the age of 13 (in the seventh grade of school); and finally, when he was regressed to the age of six (in the first grade of school). The difference in his responses to these pictures at the different age levels proved to be most interesting.

The test was not given entirely in the standardized manner. It was found necessary to probe the patient in order to encourage him to construct a short story about each picture.

RESPONSES TO THE MURRAY THEMATIC APPERCEPTION TEST PICTURES

PICTURE 1

(SMALL BOY SEATED AT TABLE LOOKING AT VIOLIN IN FRONT OF HIM)

Normal, Not Under Trance.—

A (Arthur) : This kid wanted to play the violin. His father got it for him. He is looking at it, and he is starting to learn. He learns to play it and becomes a master at the violin.

Under Trance Regressed to Age Thirteen.

A : A boy playing a violin. He is finished and puts it down.

W (Watkins) : What happens to the boy when he is finished?

A : He goes on inside and plays.

W : What does he play?

A : Baseball.

W : Whose violin is it?

A : His.

W : Does he like to play it?

A : No.

W : What did he get the violin for?

A : They gave it to him.

W : Who?

A : His folks.

Under Trance Regressed to Age Six.—(The following statements were elicited only after continuous questioning and prodding.)

A : Boy going to play. He is a good boy. He don't do anything bad. He does not like people. They are bad. They all the time get after him. He plays that thing. It makes noise.

W : How does he play it?

A : He rubs.

W : Does he like it?
A : Yes.
W : Why?
A : People don't like him.

PICTURE 3BM

(FIGURE OF INDEFINITE SEX SEATED ON FLOOR WITH FACE BURIED IN COT;
REVOLVER-LIKE OBJECT ON FLOOR NEARBY)

Normal, Not Under Trance.—

A : Is this a boy or girl?—This girl [patient identifies with femi-nine figure] has been mistreated by someone and has gone over to this sofa and is crying. She wanted to go out, and her folks would not let her, and she is crying now. So they finally let her go out, and she has a good time. Then she comes back.

Under Trance Regressed to Age Thirteen.—

A : Boy.
W : What is the boy doing?
A : Sleeping—tired.
W : Why?
A : Studying.
W : What?
A : History.
W : Does he like history?
A : No.
W : Does he like anything?
A : Yes.
W : What?
A : Arithmetic.
W : Does history studying always make him go to sleep?
A : No.

The patient refused to give more responses to this picture at this time.

Under Trance Regressed to Age Six.—

A : Boy. They don't love him.
W : Why not?
A : They did whip him.
W : Why?
A : 'Cause.
W : Why?
A : He won't go out.

W : Why?

A : 'Cause.

W : Why?

A : 'Cause he don't want to. He's afraid. People will get him and hurt him.

PICTURE 8BM

(RECLINING FIGURE BEING OPERATED UPON; GUN ALONG ONE SIDE OF PICTURE; YOUNG BOY, APPARENTLY DREAMING, IN LOWER PART OF PICTURE)

Normal, Not Under Trance.—

A : This kid has been dreaming about becoming a doctor. This shows his dream. This man has been shot, and they are removing the bullet. They are not using any anesthetic. This kid here dreams about relieving pain; so he invents ether and becomes a great man.

Under Trance Regressed to Age Thirteen.—The patient completely rejects the picture.

Under Trance Regressed to Age Six.—The patient again completely rejects the picture.

PICTURE 13MF

(WOMAN COVERED WITH BLANKET, BUT WITH BREASTS BARE, LYING IN BED; MAN STANDING IN FRONT OF BED, FACING AWAY, WITH ARM OVER FACE)

Normal, Not Under Trance.—

A : This couple were married a good while and lived pretty happy. One night they got into an argument; so he killed her. Now he realizes what he has done, but he does not know what to do.

W : What was the argument about?

A : Well, he is dressed, and she is not—maybe he came in drunk, and she got after him for being in trouble.

W : How does it end?

A : He commits suicide.

Under Trance Regressed to Age Thirteen.—

A : Woman in bed. She is in bed. He is going to bed.

W : To do what?

A : To sleep.

Under Trance Regressed to Age Six.—

A : No! No! Bad! Woman!—Seeing bad things.

W : Why?
A : Don't know.
W : Because she is not dressed?
A : Yes.

PICTURE 15
(WEIRD-LOOKING OLD MAN STANDING IN GRAVEYARD)

Normal, Not Under Trance.—

A : This old man is standing on the grave of his wife. He was married, and they were very happy and devoted to each other; so he comes to visit her grave. Pretty soon he kicks the bucket too, and he joins her.

Under Trance Regressed to Age Six.—

A : No! Graveyard! No—no—no! Scared—back! [The patient pushed the picture away from him, rejecting it.]

PICTURE 18GF
(ORDINARILY USED IN TESTING GIRLS AND WOMEN; TWO FIGURES OF INDEFINITE SEX, EMBRACING OR FIGHTING ON STAIRWAY)

Under Trance Regressed to Age Six.—
A : Bad! Hurting—no—no! Daddy hurts Mommy.
W : Why?
A : No!
W : Where did Daddy hurt Mommy?
A : In bed at night.
W : What does he do to her?
A : He beats her up.
W : How do you know?
A : I saw them.
W : How does he beat her up?
A : He on top—she hollers.[2]
W : What did he do to her?
A : I don't know—dunno—dunno.
W : Did they see you?
A : No, I ran out.

---

2 Children who witness parental sexual intercourse often interpret it as an act of aggression by father against mother.

W : How old were you?

A : Five years old.

W : Where were they?

A : Under the covers.

W : Why did Mommy holler?

A : I don't know—the bed squeaks. I felt bad.

W : Would they be angry with you if they knew you saw them?

A : Yes.

W : Would you be punished?

A : Yes.

W : Did they know that you saw them?

A : No.

W : How did it make you feel?

A : Bad. I don't want to get married.

W : Why not?

A : I don't want to beat nobody.

Before he awakened from trance, suggestions were given to ease the pain in his shoulder and arm. He woke up claiming that he felt good.

Session of August 30, 1945

Six days later on the 30th of August the final treatment session was held. He had been feeling a great deal better, with only one headache about three days previously. He had been eating well— there was no sign of nausea, and he had been sleeping easily. The feeling and movement had been completely restored to his arm and hand. The third finger was straight and had the same movement and flexibility as the others. The hour was spent in a conscious integrating interview.

He was shown that one of the reasons he feared people was because of the parental punishment inflicted upon him as a child when he preferred staying in the house to playing outside with the children. The guilt of observing parental sexual intercourse as disclosed in the Thematic Apperception Test was also discussed. In the conscious state he did not clearly remember that particular incident, but he recalled the ultramoralistic viewpoint held by his parents toward sex, and he discussed at great length how this had prevented him from seeking the affection of girls and had caused him to avoid marriage. He was given reassurance about his feelings of inferiority. It was pointed out to him how others in his group had the same feelings. He seized upon this idea—he had always believed that he alone felt inferior.

Before the session was completed he was placed back again in deep trance. All the material previously uncovered was again discussed—including some interpretations of its significance. He was then given suggestions to the effect that he would feel greatly relieved—that he would not experience his fears in the future, that he would accept the insight, would understand it, and would always remember the incidents which had been uncovered.

On awakening from trance he seemed to accept all the interpretations offered. He remembered clearly the incident involving the sex relations of his parents. He claimed that he was feeling very fine. He was unable to mention any particular symptom that disturbed him at all.

During the next few days he showed no return of anxiety, nausea, headaches, or pains in the shoulder or arms. He had gained complete flexion and contraction in the previously warped left hand. There was no trace left of the paralysis. At this time all psychoneurotic patients were being discharged from the service. Accordingly, Arthur went home and did not return to duty.

Summary of Psychodynamics

Feelings of inferiority, inadequacy, and frustration had been developed in a young boy through overstrict parental handling. Because of punishment of sex play with his sister and fear at observing parental sexual intercourse, he developed an attitude which made it impossible for him to adjust to members of the other sex and seek normal sexual outlets in marriage. In battle there were very traumatic incidents which showed clearly the overly strong Super-Ego structure and the tremendous feelings of guilt engendered because of the death of certain buddies for whom he felt responsible. Here was the *predisposition,* and here was the initiating *stress.*

Now why did it take the form of an arm paralysis? We do not know of any specific psychological dynamics which would convert the anxiety into a paralysis of the left arm and spastic condition of the third finger. The patient was actually wounded in the arm and struck on the shoulder by a falling tree during the most traumatic incident of his battle career. This may have caused sufficient organic pathology to start the symptom. We know that hysterical symptoms commonly "take over" pre-existing or minor organic pathologies and become fixated on them (White, 1948).

In the treatment of this case we find many therapeutic elements cooperating: progressive relaxation, catharsis, abreaction, recovery of amnesic material under trance, recovery of early childhood traumata through hypnoanalytic and projective techniques, reintegration, reassurance, and direct suggestion.

When Arthur Jones first entered Company F on the last day of July he was one of the sickest men in a group already consisting of the severest psychoneurotics in the hospital. He was discharged less than two months later, symptom-free as nearly as could be observed. During this period he was seen by the psychologist for a total of six therapeutic sessions and for approximately an equal number by the social worker.

CHAPTER 18

CAMPTOCORMIA

Sometimes a psychotherapist, in adjusting damaged personality structure, must operate within narrow limits. On one side he is confronted with overpowering Id drives, while on the other, pressures from a highly developed Super-Ego greatly restrict his area of operation. The case of Edward Farley was an outstanding example of the limitation such restrictions place on therapy.

Edward's body was bent almost double. He walked about with his chest nearly parallel to the ground and was able to look ahead only by bending back his neck at a most uncomfortable angle. The examining psychiatrist noted, "He has had two attacks similar to this in civilian life, and he feels this is the worst." The psychiatric history also contained the notation that "in civilian life he could get relief only by going to a chiropractor. His condition, he states, was aggravated because the orthopedic men who treated him tried to straighten his back while he was in an upright position. He believes that the only way to work on his back is to have him lying flat on a hard surface." Orthopedic clearance had already been secured, and the hysterical nature of these symptoms was summarized in the psychiatric reports with a recommendation that "this patient be transferred to Co. F of the 3rd Bn. without further workup."

It was September 23, approximately three months after the condition had first started, when the therapist met Corporal Edward Farley. Edward was cooperative and friendly. He responded positively to all suggestibility tests. A light hypnoidal trance was induced as a check, and he was accepted for treatment in Company F.

The next day, before the transfer of the patient could be secured, the therapist was called by one of the post chaplains.

"Lieutenant Watkins? This is Chaplain W."

"Yes, sir, can I help you?"

"I believe you're going to have a patient, Edward Farley, who has a severely twisted back. He's one of the boys in my religious group, and I've been talking to him lately."

"That's right, Chaplain, he is being transferred to our company."

"Well, Farley's getting very discouraged. He's been here some time and also in other Army hospitals. He doesn't think they're going to help him any. He claims that he was once cured of this same difficulty by a chiropractor and asked permission to go off the post and secure chiropractic treatment. Do you think he should?"

"Chaplain, Farley has a severe conversion hysteria. Yes, I believe the chiropractic treatment might straighten out his back, but it would be only a symptomatic cure. We're going to make a study of his case and try to get to the root of the difficulty so as to prevent its return. It would be much better if he could have some confidence and wait until after we have a chance to do our best. Can you encourage him to be more patient?"

The Chaplain replied, "Oh, if you're going to do some individual therapy with him, I agree that it is best for him not to complicate matters by going off the post. I'll advise him not to do anything for the time being."

"Thanks, Chaplain, and I'm glad you called."

On September 27 Edward, having been transferred to Company F, was called in for his first treatment. He was placed in trance by eye fixation and then he was given an additional ten minutes of sedation under the metronome. While under this trance his back was massaged. He was told that it would slowly straighten. Eventually it relaxed until he was able to lie on his stomach full length with the back completely straight. Next, while still under trance, he was asked to stand up. When standing, his back could not be straightened but remained in the severely warped position. On emerging from trance he was amnesic to all suggestions given and was quite friendly. The progress note for that day ends with a significant remark, *"He seems overly eager to talk about his family and children."*

The next day, September 28, Edward was placed in a deep trance, and under trance his back was straightened while he was standing. What a temptation to any therapist! How easy it would have been to say, "And now, Farley, I am going to wake you. When you wake up your back will be straight and strong like it is now, and you will feel very good." Farley would have awakened a straight man— no longer a twisted hunchback. He would have been delighted and happy—"cured" in these two treatments. Yes, indeed, what a temptation!

But we did not know what was behind his twisted condition. Had this temptation been followed, there would have been a temporary remission of his symptom, but it would have recurred at some future stress. This warped back was solving some extremely deep-seated problem. The loss of it might evoke a panic state. There was only one thing to do.

"In a minute I shall wake you up, Farley. When I do, you will not remember anything about your back being straightened. It will be bent over and twisted just as it was before you went to sleep."

Farley was seated and awakened, completely amnesic to all that had transpired. It was reassuring to know that the symptom could be manipulated under hypnotic trance, and it was comforting to the therapist to feel that at any session he could "cure" the patient. But this was the third attack of camptocormia, and there was meaning behind this illness, a meaning which required resolution. A series of uncovering sessions would be required.

Session of October 1, 1945

The following interview was conducted with the patient in the conscious state.

"Farley, tell me a little about your family."

"Mother died a number of years ago. They drained two or three quarts of water out of her, and the doctor said that if she had been all right, she might have been paralyzed for the rest of her life."

"Were you quite close to your mother?"

"Oh, yes, I was very fond of her. It was a terrible blow to all of us when she died."

"How did you get along in school?"

"I didn't do too well. It seemed rather tough. I would rather have been home with my mother."

"I believe that you had other brothers and sisters too. Whom were you most attached to?"

"There was an older sister. She always took care of me."

"And Father?"

"My father is a very, very intelligent man. He was the boss. All he had to do was say it, and we did it."

"Did he ever punish you?"

"I don't remember, although he did slap some of my brothers at times. He talked to me, and I would do it, but he wasn't ever mean. I wasn't ever afraid of him. He had a business of his own, and he would come home every night."

"Would you like to tell me more about your mother?"

"Mother was easy-going and fun. She was kind to all of us. I remember that she had scarlet fever once—once when she was pregnant. Of course they told me about that. I was the youngest."

"Did it bother you a lot when your mother died?"

"Yes, somewhat, but I think even more of her since."

"How did you like school?"

"I went to a parochial school. I liked spelling most of all. I liked religious instruction too."

"You are married now, aren't you, Farley?"

"Yes, about two and a half years. My wife is a wonderful woman. She came from a good family. As Dad always preached to do, 'pick a wife like your mother.' She doesn't cheat on me, and I don't on her. I'm proud to say so."

"Would you like to tell me about the time when your back was twisted before?"

"The first time, I fell down and strained my back rather suddenly. It was in August. I went eight weeks to a chiropractor. It didn't seem to get any better, and then all of a sudden it straightened out during one particular treatment."

"Was anything unusual happening in your family at this time?"

"No, nothing particular."

"Did your wife take care of you?"

"Yes, she did—that is she was pregnant at the time."

"How far along in the pregnancy was she?"

"Oh, our child was born in the following November."

"I see—and when did you have the second attack?"

"The next time it happened in February. I slipped on a grease rack."

"How long did your twisted back last this time?"

"It was crooked for three weeks, and I took chiropractic treatment all the time. It got straightened out just three days before I was told to report to the Army for a medical examination. The doctor at the induction center said that they would X ray it later. It was not considered to disqualify me for service."

"And now what happened, Farley—this last time?"

"I was doing KP duty—carrying a heavy bucket of water. Anyway, I fell—couldn't get up. When I got to the hospital my back was twisted—like it is now."

"What about your outfit? What happened to them?"

"We were on the alert many times. It was about the fourth or fifth time, I guess—when I was hospitalized. I couldn't go with the bunch. They went overseas. I guess it was four or five weeks after I entered the hospital."

"Farley, I would like to talk to you about some personal matters. It isn't because I'm trying to pry, but only because if you want me to help you I have to examine everything in your life which might have some bearing on this problem."

"I understand, sir, and I don't mind talking about anything."

"All right, how do you get along with your wife—I mean sexually?"

"We get along OK."

"What do you mean 'OK'? How often do you have relations?"

"When we were first married it was every night for a few weeks; then it settled down to two to three times a week."

"Did you ever worry about having children? Were you or your wife ever fearful of a pregnancy?"

"No, my father always said, 'Let them come. God will take care of them.'"

"Did you ever feel like you would like to use some device or method to prevent your wife from conceiving?"

"Oh no, that wouldn't be right. My religion teaches that one should never use anything unnatural. I'm a good Christian, and we don't do that."

"I see. Now Farley, do both you and your wife enjoy these relations?"

"Yes, we enjoy them—that is—I—think she does."

"Did anything ever happen of a sexual nature which brought you unhappiness?"

Farley paused a moment and then remarked, "Our second child—he came at the end of seven months."

"How did that happen?"

"My wife strained herself lifting something, and the baby was born two weeks later."

"Did that ever discourage you from having more children?"

"Oh, no, I would like to have six or eight children—that is, if my wife can stand it."

"Don't you worry about your ability to support a large family?"

"No, I never worried about that. God will take care of them."

Deep trance was induced by the eye-fixation method in about thirty seconds, and the patient was given suggestions posthypnotically tending to relieve the pains in his back. The back was once more straightened under trance but returned again to the twisted stage before he was awakened, and he was given suggestions that he would be amnesic to all this—but that he would feel encouraged about the treatment.

When Edward came out of the trance, he said that he felt much better—that there were no pains in his back. He was most jovial and friendly. It was apparent that a high degree of rapport was established.

The next step was to try interviewing the patient under trance to see if more pertinent and significant material could be uncovered. The following session disclosed more clearly some of the dynamics behind the back condition.

Session of October 3, 1945. Horizontal and Vertical Exploration Under Regressed Trance

The patient was regressed under trance to the age of seven, where he identified his teacher and named a large number of children in the room.

"Edward, how do you like your teacher?"

"Oh, I like her all right."

"What is your best subject in school?"

"Spelling."

"Are you afraid of anyone?"

"No, I'm not afraid of anybody. I like my buddies real well."

"Do you like Mother or Dad best?"

There was a cautious pause. "Mother, I guess."

"Why?"

"Because I'm closer to her."

"Have you ever been scared or frightened?"

"No."

"How do Mother and Daddy get along?"

"They get along well."

"Have you ever seen them fight?"

"No."

"Now, Edward, you are going to forget about being seven. You're becoming younger, and younger, and younger. You're six, five, four, four. You are now four years old." (Tests were given to check adequacy of regression.)

"Does your father ever punish you for anything?"

"He just scolds me if I am a bad boy."

"How do you mean—a bad boy?"

"I wouldn't go to the store—my mother told me to."

"Did your father spank you for that?"

"No, he just scolded me."

"Are you ever afraid of anything?"

"Sometimes I'm scared of the dark. I don't like to be by myself."

"Why not?"

"I remember when I was put alone in a room to sleep. I thought I heard some one upstairs trying to get me—it might be a robber." [1]

"Do you sleep in your own room?"

"No, I sleep in Mother and Dad's room."

"Have you ever been awakened and heard them arguing or talking—or doing something?"

"No, I go to sleep and sleep all night."

"Edward, you're going to be able to remember what happened to you at any age. Tell me, how long did you sleep in your parents' room?"

" 'Till I was about eight or nine years old."

"What made you stop?"

"There was a baby sister coming, and they moved me into the room upstairs."

"I thought you were the youngest?"

"I am now. My baby sister died when she was a few years old."

"How did you feel about moving out of your parents' room?"

"I didn't like it. I felt better, though, when I got upstairs with my sisters and brothers."

"Did you ever feel funny about sleeping with your sisters—'cause they were girls?"

"No, I always knew they were my sisters, and I never thought about such things."

"How long did you sleep in your sisters' room?"

"Until I was twelve years old."

"And then?"

"And then they moved me into a room with some of the other boys."

"Edward, you are going to become younger and younger. You're going back now to the time when you were three years old. You're going to remember distinctly everything that happened then. What do you like to do?"

"I like to play with toys. I want to ride a bicycle."

"Do you ever do anything that Mother doesn't like?"

"No, I always listen to Dad and Mother."

"Do you worry about Mother?"

"Yes, I worry a lot about Mother."

"Why?"

" 'Cause she might get sick—she might get old and die."

---

[1] It was common for the patient under regressed trance to shift back and forth often between the present and past tenses.

No other significant material could be found at the age of three; so the patient was encouraged to tell more of his family life in general.

"Edward, did you ever worry about your mother having so many babies?"

"No, she had twelve, and I always figured that she would pull through."

Edward shifted his position in his chair and squirmed rather uncomfortably.

"How many do you think you want to have in your family?"

"Six or eight, maybe more—if my wife can stand it."

"Edward, we are going to the time when you were sixteen years old. Would you like to tell me about what happened then?"

"I remember I went with a girl. She was a very good girl and came from a very good family. I wanted to marry her one time. I always figured that I could get her."

"What do you mean 'get her?'"

"Oh, I mean I could take her to the movies whenever I wanted to."

"How late would you stay out?"

"Till ten or eleven at night."

"Did anything important ever happen between you?"

"Oh no, she moved away, and I quit going with her."

"What else happened about girls?"

"The next girl I had was my wife—that is the one who is my wife. I went with her two—no, I guess three—years before we were married. She came from a very good family. She was an orphan, and she went to work with some very good people when I met her."

"What do you mean, Edward, by 'very good' people?"

"Well, good people are people who come from good families. They keep up on their religion—they live like people should. They live like my Mother and Dad did—and like I live with my wife. They treat their kids nice. They don't ever scold them. We never scold our children. We iron out our things behind the kids' back. They love each other very much, like Mother and Dad did."

"Who takes care of your children most of the time?"

"I take care of them at night, and she does during the day. I want my children to grow up to be very good."

"Whom do you want them to be like, Edward?"

"I want them to be like my wife. She is a very sweet woman. She's suffered an awful lot. She's had to put up with all of us. She has never been too well—was sick quite a good deal."

"Do you think, Edward, that maybe with her being sick it wasn't good for her to have so many children?"

"No, they were God's blessing, and like father said, she is blessed by the Lord in taking care of the children. We have a great faith. I pray a lot. I am a good Christian—both my wife and I are."

"Now, Edward, in a minute I am going to wake you up. When I do you will not remember anything we talked about, but your back is going to be straightened sometime next week. I will let you know later the day it will happen." When Edward emerged from trance he was amnesic to all the material disclosed.

Let us take a moment to summarize the dynamic implications that have emerged thus far. From his overeagerness to praise his father it is probable that there is some deeply repressed hostility. There is obviously considerable identification of his wife with his mother. There is also, apparently, a deeply repressed unconscious dread of large numbers of children and pregnancies. Because of his religious indoctrination he will not face this fear—even in the trance state. His religious structure is so strong that not only would he never consider practicing methods of birth limitation, but he would not even recognize in himself the fear of repeated pregnancies. How all this is connected with his twisted back we do not yet know. But it is obvious that behind this lovely façade of happy home, wonderful wife, "good" parents, and devout religion all is not well.

As mentioned before, the hypnoanalytic procedure had been from simple, superficial uncovering techniques to deeper methods. The first session was held in the conscious state. The second was an interview under trance. The third involved a continuation of the inquiry, this time with more complex uncovering methods.

Session of October 4, 1945; Dissociated Handwriting Under Trance

Edward was placed in a deep trance. After adequate checks of depth he was seated at a table and his right hand was dissociated from his body through inducing paralysis and the hallucination that it was no longer connected to him. He was then questioned, and the hand wrote the answers.

W: What do you worry most about, Farley?

The Hand: WORRIED ABOUT MY WIFE.

W: Why?

The Hand: SHE WAS OPERATED ON GOITER AND BOTHERS ME FOR SHE IS STILL LITTLE NERVOUS.

W: Tell me more about it.

The Hand: SON WAS JUST 4½ POUNDS WHEN HE WAS BORN AND ONLY 7 MONTHS OLD.

W: Do you feel at all guilty? Do you feel as if you were responsible?

The Hand: YES I AND MY WIFE ARE RESPONSIBLE FOR OUR CHILDREN AND WE WANT TO GIVE THEM THE BEST CARE THAT A FATHER AND MOTHER SHOULD GIVE THEIR CHILDREN.

W: Do you think that you have ever sinned in any way?

The Hand: NO I AND MY WIFE ALWAYS LIVED UP TO OUR FAITH.

W: What thoughts do you have that might be pushed down inside you—thoughts that only the hand can write about?

The Hand: WORRY ABOUT MARY. FOR I AM TOO FAR AWAY TO HELP HER OUT WHEN HER AND THE CHILDREN DO GET SICK OR VERY BAD COLDS.

W: Is there something down deep in Farley which he does not know—something in him which he thinks might be bad? What is it?

The Hand: I WORRY AN AWFUL LOT ABOUT MY BACK FOR I AM WORRIED IT WON'T GET BETTER. THIS IS THE THIRD TIME AND I'M WORRIED ABOUT WHAT MIGHT HAPPEN TO IT LATER.

W: What is the real reason that the back is twisted?

The Hand: THE BACK IS BAD BECAUSE I LIFTED TOO HEAVY AND WORKED THE REST OF THE DAY OUT. IT SEEMS LIKE A BONE WENT OUT OF PLACE OR THAT THE MUSCLES WERE SO TIGHT THAT I JUST WASN'T ABLE TO GET UP AND THE MORE I WORKED ON IT THE WORSE IT PULLED ME OVER.

W: Farley is a good man; but perhaps sometimes he thinks of things that his father would not approve. What are some of these deeper thoughts?

The Hand: WELL, DAD ALWAYS WANTED US TO MARRY A GOOD CHRISTIAN GIRL AND HAVE A WIFE JUST LIKE MOTHER WAS AND ALSO TO NOT BUM WITH A BUNCH OF FELLOWS THAT WOULD DO WRONG.

W: Did you ever have any wishes not to marry the way your father wanted?

The Hand: NO I ALWAYS THOUGHT I WOULD BE LIKE DAD AND TRY TO MARRY A GOOD GIRL AND RAISE A GOOD SIZE FAMILY.

W: Is there any possible reason why you do not want a large family or are afraid of a large family?

The Hand: WELL, MY LOVING WIFE HAD A VERY SEVERE OPERATION AND WORRIED THAT TOO MANY CHILDREN MAY CAUSE HER TO GET MORE NERVOUS AND SURE DON'T WANT NOTHING TO HAPPEN TO MY LOVING WIFE.

W: What might it do to her if she does get nervous?

The Hand: SHE MAY BECOME ILL AND DIE TO BE A VERY YOUNG WOMAN LIKE HER MOTHER PASSED AWAY WHEN SHE WAS QUITE A YOUNG GIRL.

W: Why did her mother die?

The Hand: I DON'T KNOW. HER MOTHER DIED AFTER SHE HAD THE LAST BOY WHO DIED WHEN HE WAS ABOUT 4 YEARS OLD.

W: Are you afraid that your wife might get sick and die if she has more children?

The Hand: NO, I WOULD NOT SAY THAT BUT WITH THAT GOITER OPERATION BECOMING MOTHER TOO OFTEN MAY BOTHER HER.

W: What does Farley fear may have caused his mother to die?

The Hand: MOTHER WE ALL THOUGHT DIED BECAUSE THEY TAPPED HER IN THE STOMACH AND GOT TWO QTS OF WATER FROM HER AND THE DOCTOR SAID IF HE OPERATED ON HER IT MAY CAUSE HER TO BE PARALYZED.

W: Did Farley think it might have something to do with having so many children?

The Hand: NO, I ALWAYS THOUGHT AFTER MY SISTER WAS BORN MOTHER WAS VERY HAPPY AND LOOKED A LOT BETTER THAN EVER HAD. I DON'T THINK IT WAS CAUSED BY HAVING 12 OF US.

W: What kind of operation was it?

The Hand: SHE WAS OPERATED ON AN INWARD GOITER [now referring to his wife] AND HAD SEVEN TUBES TAKEN OUT OF HER NECK AND IT WAS A VERY DANGEROUS OPERATION AND SHE WAS VERY NERVOUS AND SHE WAS CAUGHT IN TIME FOR IT WAS GETTING WHERE IT WAS BOTHERING HER HEART AND EYES WERE POPPING OUT AND IT WORRIED ME FOR SOME TIME.

W: Did it make it worse because your wife was pregnant?

The Hand: AFTER HAVING THE FIRST BOY WHO WAS 6 MONTHS OLD IT BROUGHT OUT THE GOITER BUT SHE WAS FEELING OKAY AND WHEN THE DAUGHTER WAS BORN SEEM TO MAKE HER FEEL A LITTLE BETTER.

W: Were you afraid that her nervousness might affect her mind?

The Hand: NO I WAS NOT TO TO SURE WHAT IT MIGHT CAUSE FOR THE WAY THE DOCTOR SAID THAT IF SHE WOULDN'T HAVE TAKEN CARE OF IT WHEN SHE DID SHE WOULD HAVE HAD A WEAK HEART AND WOULD HAVE DIED A LOT EARLIER MAYBE WITHIN TWO MONTHS.

W: Did the doctor ever advise you against having more children?

The Hand: DOCTOR SAID AFTER DAUGHTER WAS BORN IT WAS OKAY TO HAVE MORE CHILDREN FOR IT WOULD HELP HER NERVOUS SYSTEM OUT AND THAT IS WHY WE THOUGHT IT WOULD BE SAFE TO KEEP UP WITH OUR FAMILY.

W: Has Farley ever been afraid of having intercourse?

The Hand: WELL, FARLEY IS A VERY GOOD CHRISTIAN AND SO IS HIS WIFE AND THEY NEVER USE ANYTHING TO GO AGAINST THE CHURCH BUT THEY DO IT FAIRLY REGULAR ABOUT AS OFTEN AS A REGULAR MARRIED COUPLE WOULD DO.

W: Have you ever wanted to do something you shouldn't do? Or have you ever been afraid that you would? Let's put it this way, has Farley ever wanted to do something that he shouldn't do?

The Hand: HE THINKS THAT HIS WIFE CAN STAND IT BETTER SINCE SHE HAD THE GOITER TAKEN OUT. WELL I BELIEVE HE THINKS IT WOULD BE BETTER NOT TO DO IT TOO OFTEN.

W: Why does he think that he should not do it too often?

The Hand: HE DON'T WANT TO HURT HER IN ANYWAY OR CAUSE MORE TROUBLE WITH THE OLD OPERATION.

At this point the session was finished, and the hand was reassociated to the personality. With great prodding the admission had been secured that Farley did have fears connected with sexual intercourse and having large numbers of children.

Next, the patient's back was straightened under trance. He stood perfectly straight and took a few steps. Then the back was returned again to the twisted position. He was given suggestions of euphoria and told that next week "we will straighten out the back." He was also given suggestions to make him amnesic to the entire interview. He emerged from the trance in a happy mood and remarked about his back still being bent but did not complain of any pain. He was given further reassurance about going home "as soon as the back has been cured." Motivational pressures were being built up for the eventual loss of the symptom.

The next day another delving session was held using still more intricate methods. It was obvious that Farley's true feelings were very deeply repressed. The dissociated hand gave only the slightest hint toward admitting there were misgivings about having a large family.

Session of October 5, 1945; Projective Technique Under Trance —Identification with Heroes

Farley was placed in a deep trance and then told the following:

"Today we are going to make up stories. You are a great writer. There is an imaginary man by the name of *Fordham*. I want you to make up the best story you can about him and his life. This is all just imaginary."

Edward commenced talking. "This man, Fordham, is a baseball player. He manages the game and pitches for them. He is a very good manager, but he has trouble because he can't win no pennant. He can't imagine why he doesn't have a good baseball club, but he just felt that he should win the pennant. It makes trouble at home with his wife and kids because he gets very crabby with them. He likes his children and his wife very much, but with his mind on the ball game it makes him nervous, and he worries and gets cranky at home. He may fly off the handle once in awhile, and his wife tries to keep him in good spirits. She talks to him and asks him why he can't be more lenient with the kids."

The therapist broke in with, "How does this affect the personal relationship between the couple?"

Edward replied, "He may be a man that likes it a lot. She may be a cold, frigid woman. She's not tickled about it. She wouldn't say 'no' because she loves him so very much. He suspects though that she doesn't really enjoy it. She may not get warmed up as he does about it. He may *go* way before she's really hot, then she might get warm that way, and by that time he is all through, and she is disappointed."

The therapist asked, "Do you think this man, Fordham, knows or recognizes this conflict down inside of him?"

There was a slight pause. Edward wrinkled his brow, and then emerged with, "It's very possible that he doesn't know what is going on inside him. He gets more sure because she can't get hot at the same time. If she had told him this before they got married it would have changed their life. He would still love her, though."

"Do you think that this man might have had sex relations with his wife before he married her?"

"He was very fortunate the first time to get her out at the same time. He wanted it a great deal, and she didn't want to give it to him; so he worked her up until she was ready and gave him what he wanted."

"Did they use any contraceptives or protection at that time?"

"Yes, he probably used a rubber. Most fellows—a lot of them use a diaphragm or the rhythm system. Myself, I wouldn't use either of them. We take our chances, and if the Lord blesses us with a child we are glad to have it."

The patient continued for some time on the viewpoint toward birth control held by his religious group. He then was returned to the story of Fordham.

"Do you think that they had relations many times?"

"They were probably good people, and they probably didn't have relations more than five times, and if they did they probably used a rubber because they didn't want no scandal in the family. You know how people talk."

"Do you think that this Fordham man might have felt guilty?"

"Well, it may have hurt him because he may have seen blood, and because he had been taught—he knew that he had broken it because of the blood, and it kinda bothered him, and it worried him that they might have a baby in spite of the rubber, and people would talk about it."

"What do you think Fordham and this girl probably did?"

"They may have talked it out, and maybe they loved each other a great deal anyway, and so they figured that they would get married sooner or later, and maybe they ought to get married right now, because if the baby was born in eight months or so nobody would talk, but it would be very bad if it came very soon after they were married."

"Do you think that Fordham might have married this woman without being quite sure that he was in love with her?"

"Well, it would have been in advance a little bit, but if the woman liked him well it would be all right."

He then rambled at length about how loose some people were in their sex relations and about how bad it was. He was asked if "this man, Fordham," thought his wife might have had relations with some one else before he married her.

He was very hesitant on the point. "Well, if they were any kind of man or woman they would have ironed that out before they were married." At this point there was considerable evidence of deep anxiety and heavy breathing.

"Do you think Fordham ever cheated on his wife?"

"Well, he might have cheated on her, because he was a big baseball man, and he traveled around a good deal, and there were many temptations in this occupation."

With some hesitancy Edward continued, "He may have found a girl who was very fast and had what his wife used to have, and if he were fast he would have a hard time staying away from it." (It was mentioned earlier that wishes rather than *true, objective reality* often emerge during projective dream fantasies under trance. Here is a good example. We might assume that through this projective method Farley is admitting to extramarital affairs. Yet, in a later and deeper session we find that these were only wishes to have these affairs. Actually these were controlled. To the therapist, however, either reality or wish can be a source of guilt feelings—and hence neurotic repression.)

"Now let's take Fordham after he has been married a few years and has several children. How do you think he is getting along with his wife now?"

"He should be getting deeper with her all the time—as long as she can give it to him." There was a pause. "Half the time he may not have been satisfied and thinks his wife is not all she should be. He may say she isn't up to what she used to be. It's all over—her passion. She is getting quite old. This young girl has what his wife used to have. He goes to see her and is very much tempted, but he doesn't really do anything with her."

"Supposing Fordham had broken his leg and was crippled. Do you think that might send the young girl away and relieve Fordham from his temptation?"

"She wouldn't want a man who was crippled unless he was very, very rich. Then she would want him for his money. But if he were just an ordinary guy she would leave him if he were crippled."

"If Fordham had been crippled, do you think that would prevent him from having too many sex relations with his wife and stop another source of difficulty?"

"Yes, there wouldn't be so much temptation, and he would probably stay home and be good to his wife. He should behave himself and be thankful for what he's got. If he chases after the young girl and divorces his wife, then later on the girl would turn against him because she would want a younger man, too."

The patient was then given suggestions of amnesia for all material discussed. Once more his back was completely straightened, and he was taken for a short walk around the office; then the back was twisted back through suggestion into its usual warped condition. He was given a posthypnotic suggestion to the effect that "by next Thursday your back will be straightened out normally. From that time on you will always be able to walk straight."

When he emerged from trance he could remember none of the matters discussed. He felt quite good. There were no pains left in his back. He was given the following preparation for the final straightening.

"Farley, soon we will be ready to straighten your back. I won't tell you now when it is going to be, but it will be before long. You can write your wife and tell her that you will be coming home shortly and that your back will be straight. You remember how twice before your back became warped; so we must not let you go home this time until after we have found out the real cause. We must clear the roots out permanently, so that your bent back will not return again."

"That's right, Doc. Let's find out the root, so it won't come back again."

The next session was held four days later. At that time the patient said he felt much better. The pain in his back was entirely gone, and he was much stronger. He had been able to take several long walks without difficulty.

Session of October 9, 1945; Projective Techniques under Regressed Trance

Farley was placed in deep trance, and the following material emerged.

"Do you remember the last time—we were talking about a man named Fordham? You told me a very good story about this man. Now, let's go back and make up the story about what happened to him when he was small. Tell about Fordham when he was three years old."

"Fordham, he came from a very good family. His daddy played baseball, and he wanted to be very much like his daddy. His daddy would get angry and come home and raise heck for something that didn't work out on the baseball field."

"What would he do to Fordham if Fordham was a naughty boy?"

"He would probably bawl him out the first time but whip him later."

"Do you think that Fordham might have had some antagonism and felt hostile toward his father?"

"He might not have liked him, but he respected him."

"Do you think that Fordham might have been angry at his daddy down inside—but he wouldn't let it come out?"

"Maybe so, but he liked his daddy too, and he didn't want to cause any difficulty in the family."

"Do you feel that he had some real thoughts of anger against his father?"

"Fordham may have felt some bad thoughts. Maybe he thought that his daddy might have done wrong—but his daddy was right."

"Do you think that his daddy might not have been right at this time?"

"I wouldn't say that; because the daddy is older and knows what is good for children."

Note that it has taken projective techniques under regressed trance to bring out any evidences of father hostility—hostility so repressed it could not be elicited in either the conscious state or by simple interviewing under trance. Even the dissociated hand method, previously used, did not bring it out so clearly. However, the patient immediately returns to the indoctrination of home and church—"Father is always right."

"How do you think Fordham felt about his mother?"

"He thought very much of his mother. She seemed to be like other mothers—very nice." At this time Edward became very restless and yawned a great deal.

"Do you think that Fordham, when he was a little boy three years old, was afraid of anything?"

"No, I wouldn't say that."

"Do you think that he had any unconscious fears—some that he didn't know of?"

"No, I don't think so." There was more yawning.

"Let's suppose now that Fordham is five years old. Let's tell a story about him when he was five."

"Fordham had in his mind that he wanted to be a baseball player, and his daddy also wanted him to be a baseball player. He thought that baseball was the right thing."

"Do you think that maybe back in his mind he had other ideas— you know, ones with which his father didn't agree?"

"No, Dad thought that the baseball career was very good."

"How about Fordham's relations with other children?"

"Oh, they were OK."

"Which of his brothers and sisters do you think he liked best?"

"He liked his sister best because she was always at home with him."

"Do you think that there are any other matters—like sex—that may have bothered Fordham when he was a boy?"

At this point the patient became very restless. He continued yawning but denied that Fordham had any knowledge of sex. On being questioned further whether Fordham had ever seen or heard anything pertaining to sex, or had seen or heard his parents having any sex relations, the patient merely replied, "No."

"Just imagine that Fordham is fifteen or sixteen years old. How do you think he got along with girls?"

"He probably got a girl and tried her out. He was a regular fellow, and she was a very good girl, and the girl probably refused him at first, and it may have got him very mad, but he remembered what Mother and Father had said, and then he tried again, and if the girl was not so decent, she gave in to him, and it may have made him very happy."

"Do you think that it also made Fordham feel rather guilty?"

"Yes, it may have made him guilty in some respects, but she was a decent girl, and she got the idea that her decency was removed, and he may have felt bad that he got it from this girl."

"How old do you think Fordham was when this happened?"

"I would say about seventeen or eighteen."

The patient was then advanced to the present day and asked, "What day is it now?"

He responded with, "Tuesday."

"And what is going to happen Thursday?"

"I hope to be well and straight again." There was heavy breathing.

"Do you want to tell me more about it?"

"That's the day Lieutenant W. is going to straighten my back. I hope he can make me well, and after that he is going to keep me several days to get down to the root of it. I pray every day that my back will be straight."

"That's fine, Farley. Your back will be straight on Thursday. Thursday is the day—Thursday. And now I'm going to wake you up. You will not remember what we discussed, but you will feel fine." Edward came out of trance smiling, completely amnesic to all that he had discussed.

"By the way, Farley," casually remarked the therapist, "what do you think of the World Series?" This started the patient on a discussion of baseball.

He said, "I used to play a little baseball myself. Father took me to games. I loved it a great deal."

"Did you ever want to be a baseball player, or did your father play baseball?"

"No, he never played, but I merely played it as a hobby. Father hoped that I would go into religious work, but he didn't force it on any of us. I decided against it."

"Did you play any other sports?"

"Oh, I used to bowl a lot—had a 175 average. I sure can't do it any more though. I had to quit when my back was injured."

The session was terminated. Everything that had been divulged so far indicated even deeper-lying material.

Session of October 10, 1945; Psychodramatic Projective Technique Under Trance with Multiple Characters

The patient was placed in deep trance in a matter of five minutes through use of eye-fixation and the metronome.

"Listen carefully. Can you hear me, Farley?"

"Yes."

"Are you relaxing?"

"Yes."

"At this time you are going to do something very different. You're going to come out of your body. Your spirit is soaring through the air. There are people down below. You can see them, and you know what they think. You're going to a great city. You see a young man by the name of *Findley*. He is in a great struggle between his Christian training and his baser motives. The Devil and an Angel are trying to win his soul. The Angel sees the good. The Devil sees the bad. You can see it all. You are going to act out the parts of all three—Findley, the Angel, and the Devil. This is a play. You are writing the play. You can take the part of any of the three. You can describe how each feels and what is happening. Do it to the best of your imagination."

"Findley, he is trying to live up to his folks' way of living. He is trying to keep up with his mother's and dad's way of life. He becomes a very good boy and doesn't want to do anything to hurt their feelings. He goes to church often and is very religious. The Devil is pulling against him; so it makes it a harder job for him to do what he should."

"What does the Devil want?"

"The Devil plans to do things that are bad—that he shouldn't do."

"What does the Devil want him to do?"

"He wants him to do evil."

"What kind of evil?"

"He probably wants him to go against his will and do things like taking out another woman and have intercourse with her. The Devil tried hard to get him to do it. The Devil tried hard to have him take out another woman and have intercourse with her."

"Did he do it?"

"I don't know, but he was awful close."

"What else does the Devil want?"

"He tried to get him and his wife separated."

"What ideas did the Devil try to get him to take?"

"He wanted him to do something against his wife. She would find out."

"Would she leave him?"

"She might give him another chance. He would probably have done those things against his will. He would be against his wife, and she would hate him."

"What things?"

"Going out with other women."

"Did the Devil have anything to do with his sex relations with his wife?"

"No, it was very good."

"Did the Devil make him do anything else?"

"No, Findley wanted to stay home with his wife."

"How did it make him feel inside when the Devil persuaded him this way?"

"When he learned about it, Findley tried to do better, and the Devil gave up, and he felt much better, but he was ashamed of it. He was sure that she would never find out, and he would never want her to find out how he had felt."

"Did the Devil succeed in some way?"

"No, because he was very good after that. He liked another woman very well, but his wife would find out. He was very tempted, but didn't do it."

"Did Findley break off with the other woman?"

"It was hard, but he broke off. He thought of what would happen if he didn't break off."

"What kind of man did this woman want?"

"One with money—to have a good time."

"Would this woman have liked Findley if he got sick?"

"She may not have. He was friendly to her, but he didn't have any relations with her. He may even have got to have loved her, but he had a good wife."

"Did he get to love this woman?" There was a pause.

"He was in love with her all the time."

"Did he keep this love after he returned to his wife?"

"Yes—to a certain extent."

"Did Findley love this woman more than he did his wife?"

"No, he had a different feeling about her. He loved his wife."

"What did the Devil tell Findley about it?"

"The Devil would say 'you want that other woman. She has got more. She is built better.' Findley would answer, 'Yes, but my wife has got that family touch. She is like her mother—a good woman. The other women go around with other men.' "

"And what would the Devil say to that?"

" 'Come on. Keep going. Maybe you will get what you want.' And Findley would say, 'No, I won't do it.' And Findley would go to this woman at certain times."

"How often?"

"Once or twice a week and spend a half hour or hour with her. They were very good friends before he was married."

"Did the Devil ever try to make Findley sick?"

"No, because the Angel and the voice of the Lord had the Devil overpowered."

"Was Findley ever sick?"

"No, never sick—never hurt himself, but he was always between these two women."

"How do you mean that?"

"He never said a word against his wife."

"Did he ever kiss the woman?"

"Yes, but he didn't go any farther."

"Did Findley try to solve this by staying home with his wife?"

"Yes, he stayed home more and more with his family as he should have done in the first place."

"Did the Devil do anything else?"

"No, the Devil gave up. The dear Lord gave Findley the power never to look at another woman after that."

"Now, Farley, you are going back into a deep sleep—a very deep sleep. You are floating back into yourself. You are forgetting all about Findley. You are feeling fine. What day is today?"

"Wednesday, and tomorrow is Thursday."

"What will happen tomorrow?"

"Lieutenant W. says that I will be cured tomorrow."

"Do you believe that?"

"Yes, I do—I don't think he would lie. I believe that I will be a straight man again at this time tomorrow."

"You can now go into a very, very deep sleep. You will not remember anything which we talked about, but you will feel very fine."

The patient woke up in a very cheerful frame of mind. He was amnesic to all that had been discussed. After this session the psychodynamics in the case as understood by the therapist to date were summarized and a specific therapeutic program was decided upon.

Summary of Psychodynamics

At the present time this patient's camptocormia probably represents the resolution of a conflict between his Christian training and love of his wife on the one hand and strong desires for adultery on the other. The back symptom has appeared three times—twice during the middle of his wife's pregnancy. At these times he would not be having sex relations with her, and therefore, would be more tempted. When his back is deformed, he must stay home and cannot go out. The deformity thus serves as a punishment for having had these desires, and it is a method of preventing him from getting into trouble. The minor sprain incurred during his first fall was the precipitating stress and served to turn the conversion in the direction of a back disability which would satisfy the neurotic needs. In spite of his strong religious training, there are certain unconscious resistances to having more children; so the back symptom also becomes a method of limiting pregnancy in the family because it interferes with normal sexual intercourse. There are some indications that his mother may have died because of her repeated pregnancies. His inner suspicion of this, plus his wife's poor health, are further reasons for the development of fears toward more pregnancies in the family. However, his strong religious beliefs will not permit him to recognize these fears overtly. They must be, and are, repressed. There are indications that his wife's ill health may be partly a functional adjustment toward unsatisfying sex relations and her own repressed fears of pregnancy. The warped back may also serve as a method of expressing hostility toward his father who believes in large families and who is "such a good man" that the patient could never vent hostility in any way or even recognize its existence. He thus attacks the dominating father's wishes in the only way possible—*limiting his family by an hysterical method of birth control—the camptocormia.*

THERAPEUTIC PROGRAM

1. Back to be straightened by direct posthypnotic suggestion tomorrow
2. Educational program as to the nature of an hysterical neurosis
3. Insight to be developed into the psychodynamics behind his disability
    (a) This to be done without disturbing his religious beliefs
4. Patient to be sent to the chaplain of his faith to receive reassurance that "rhythm" methods of birth control are not against the teachings of his church

5. Patient to be sent to a medical officer of his faith for instructions on acceptable rhythm methods of birth limitation

6. Patient to be given instruction on the physiology and psychology of sex and sexual relations

(a) This would be designed to improve his sex techniques and thus make the satisfaction of his own high sexual needs more acceptable to his wife

Session of Thursday, October 11, 1945

The patient was placed in deep trance by eye fixation and metronome methods in about fifteen minutes.

"Are you in the deepest sleep you have ever been in?"

"Uh-huh."

"What day is today?"

"Thursday."

"What will happen today?"

"My back will be straightened out so I can walk."

"Sit up. I will put pressure on the small of your back and then count to ten. You will slowly stand up straight while I am doing this. One, two, three, . . . ten."

Next he was told, "I'm going to count up to ten again, continually exerting pressure on the back. This will mean that you will never bend over again—never will be twisted and deformed the way you were. This will make it last permanently. One, two, three, . . . ten."

Edward was led over to the wall. "Place your shoulders against the wall. Stand up straight at attention like a soldier. That's fine. When I awaken you, you will not remember what I have said. Listen very, very carefully. I'm going to count to ten once more. This will put a great deal of strength into your muscles and make them quite strong. One, two, three, . . . ten. Now they are strong, aren't they?"

"Yes."

"I will count up to twenty-five and you will gradually wake up. You will realize that you are straight, awake, and well again. By the time I get to twenty-five you will be completely awake. One, two, three, . . . twenty-three, twenty-four, twenty-five."

Edward smiled. "I'm as tall as you are." Standing at attention, with his shoulders against the wall, he did not move for a minute. Then he shook hands with the therapist. There was a profusion of thanks.

"Why don't you walk around the barracks? Show some of the other boys how straight you are."

Edward eagerly bounced down the steps, and to the amazed eyes of the other patients shouted, "How do I look?"

Throughout the rest of the day he walked quite straight although there was some tendency toward a humping of the shoulders at times. He was always able to straighten these whenever reminded of it.

That same day Chaplain W. was contacted. The essential nature of an hysterical symptom and some of Farley's dynamics were discussed with him. He was greatly interested and agreed to give the patient suitable support during the coming week when Edward would be brought to face some rather unpleasant insight. The chaplain seemed to be especially relieved that *the treatment was being accomplished without tampering with Edward's religious beliefs.*

The chaplain agreed to the following suggestions:

1. To let the patient bring up all new points
2. To reassure him that the "rhythm" method of birth control was not against his religion
3. To give him strength and support to face the insight which would be forthcoming

Developing Insight

The next day, October 12, 1945, Edward was placed in a deep trance and given additional suggestions tending to strengthen the back muscles. He was then prepared for the achieving of insight.

"What is the next phase in your treatment, Farley?"

"To uncover the root."

"What do you mean by that?"

"There are some things which I will be surprised to find out."

"Are you prepared to face these dynamics?" (This term had been used in group therapy.) "Are you brave? Can you stand the unpleasantness?"

"Yes, I'm ready to face anything if it will keep my back straight like it is now. I can take anything you will tell me."

Farley was brought out of trance and was given some manuscript materials prepared by the author of this book to explain the principles of psychotherapy to patients. He was asked to study the matter carefully. He had already been subjected to a great deal of this material through his attendance at group therapy sessions in the Company.

Farley was no genius, but he was also no mental defective. The Wechsler-Bellevue Test reported his IQ within normal range and near to the average. He seemed quite eager to know why his back disability had developed as it did and what would keep it from recurring.

On October 14 a session was held in which the manuscript materials were discussed. The points stressed were that a symptom has meaning and significance, that it solves an unconscious problem for the patient, that it can be cured by insight (removing the dynamics spring), and that insight involves understanding and acceptance—both intellectual and emotional. Farley left the session eager-eyed. He said he could hardly wait until the next day when his own individual dynamics would be explained. This method of first developing understanding of what a conversion hysteria represented and then motivating and stimulating an interest in solving the personal dynamics was used successfully in treating several of the hysterical cases.

On October 15 all the material uncovered under trance was revealed to Farley. The progress notes were discussed, word for word, with the patient, just as they have been reported here—his obvious repressed hostility toward his father; the need for frankly recognizing this hostility; the fact that his marital relations were unsatisfactory to himself and his wife; the need for his own education in more effectual sex techniques; the possible reasons for his wife's ill health, such as her use of a functional illness as a protection against sexual intercourse and pregnancy; the meaning of his back symptom as expressed by a limitation of his sexual intercourse with his wife, thus achieving a form of birth control; the need for a frank recognition of his moral conflicts concerning his desires toward other women rather than a repression of these wishes; and his control of his desires by the development of a disabling symptom, a symptom which would make him unacceptable to the other woman and hence unable to have intercourse with her. The patient and the therapist went over and over the progress notes.

At the end of the afternoon there was a great relief of tension. Edward appeared to understand and accept his dynamics. He was able to explain back to the therapist not only the "why's" of a conversion hysteria, but also the specific "why" underlying his own symptom. When checked under deep trance he showed a surprising amount of insight into his condition. At that time he stated under trance that he did not believe he would ever have the difficulty again —because *he felt that he understood, and knew that understanding would prevent a return of the back disability.* The intellectual aspects of insight can be tested, just as in school, by requiring the patient to explain back to the therapist a conversion hysteria and his own dynamics. This test should be made both under trance and in the conscious state. Emotional reintegration can only be inferred by the sincerity with which the patient makes his explanations, the signs of loss of tension—and the final proof, permanent loss of the symptom.

On October 19 another session was spent discussing sex techniques. At the conclusion of this he was given certain literature to read with the hope of improving his own ability to control his emotions and more fully satisfy his wife during marital relations. He seemed grateful for this instruction.

The next day Farley contacted his chaplain and was reassured that the rhythm method of birth control was not against his religion. He said afterwards that this cleared up the last doubt which he had on the matter. Arrangements were made for him to go to a physician of his faith and get specific instructions in this method.

On October 22 the patient was seen by Captain S. and was given specific instruction in rhythm methods of birth control. He reported later that the doctor made many valuable suggestions and told him much that he thought would be helpful when he returned home. He was very enthusiastic and showed no trace of anxiety. There was no sign of the return of his symptom. He continued to show the same insight into the nature of a conversion hysteria and the dynamics of his own case.

And so Edward Farley walked once more as a straight man. Yet twice before he had been warped and twisted. He was straightened then by direct suggestive treatment. What assurance had we that this illness would not recur? Well, first, Edward knew what a conversion hysteria was and how it could occur. Second, he accepted himself as having that diagnosis. Third, he understood his own predisposition for such an illness, the strict demands of his highly structured Super-Ego and the powerful Id drives manifested in sexual desire. Fourth, he had been given a method of birth limitation which was acceptable to his religious faith and which, though not 100 per cent effective, would at least serve to diminish his and his wife's fears of pregnancy. Finally, he received some instructions in better techniques of sexual adjustment—methods which should result in a material improvement in his marital relations and increase the happiness of himself and his wife.

The reports of the uncovering sessions have been so long that word-for-word descriptions cannot be given of the long discussions through which this insight was achieved. Methods similar to those described in earlier chapters were employed. Suffice it to say that several long meetings were required to bring all that had been uncovered to Edward's understanding.

Just before he left the hospital Edward's case was presented at a clinical conference. The change in his condition and the status of his insight may be best described by reporting this particular meeting. Present was a group of some thirty psychiatrists, psychologists, and psychiatric social workers in the NP Division of the Hospital. In front of this group the following demonstration occurred.

W : Edward will you tell these people here what type of condition you have had?

E : I've had a conversion hysteria.

W : What do you mean by a conversion hysteria?

E : It is an illness that is psychologically caused—caused by conflicts inside.

W : Do you know what your conflicts were?

E : Yes, I do.

W : How long was your back twisted?

E : This last time I was bent over for about four months. This was the third time.

W : And what happened the first two times?

E : I had chiropractic treatment.

W : And your back did straighten with that treatment?

E : Yes.

W : Do you know why it did not continue to stay straight with chiropractic treatment?

E : Yes, I know now. I had to know the "roots" of the trouble.

W : Do you think you're going to have more trouble with your back?

E : I don't think so now—I understand why it happened.

The patient was then placed in a deep trance before the group.

W : Now, Edward, you are forgetting about where you are. You are going back, one, two, three months. It is three months ago. It is back in late July. It is now the month of late July.

With no other word Edward, who was standing on his feet, slowly began to bend until he reached the early position where his chest was nearly parallel to the floor. Notice that the back symptom was returned not by direct suggestion but by the use of regression. There are many interesting possibilities in attempting to remove symptoms without the use of direct suggestion through regressing the patient to an earlier age, one prior to the onset of the symptoms.

Nobody has yet reported trying to eliminate them through a regression—stuck posthypnotically.

Farley was questioned in deep trance.

W: Now, I want to talk over with you why it was that your back got twisted. Can you tell me why in your own words?

E: My back was twisted because I had conflicts that I couldn't solve.

W: What kind of conflicts?

E: Well, I was afraid to have more relations with my wife because she was sick, and she might become pregnant, and it was wrong to use any artificial methods to stop it. The Church says that it is wrong.

W: Go on.

E: And also, while I was at home crippled I didn't go out and get into any temptations—like chasing after any other women.

W: And what did your back have to do with it?

E: As long as I was crippled, I wouldn't always be wanting sex relations with my wife, and I wouldn't be going out and getting into trouble.

W: Do you think that you will be crippled again?

E: No, I know now why my back was bent. I will be a good husband and a good father, and I have learned how to get along better with my wife without breaking God's will. I will not be crippled again.

These words were spoken by the patient before the psychiatric conference while he was under trance. It was obvious that his insight had reached a level deeper than the conscious surface.

Another therapist, Sandler (1945), made a study of nineteen camptocormia patients in the Army. His general conclusions coincided amazingly with the factors in Edward's condition. Sandler found that there was a strong overidentification with the father; that in addition to an admiration of the father, there was a suppressed hostility against him. He also noted that most of the patients had difficulty in their domestic and sexual situations. There were sexual maladjustments and impotence. In each of these cases the sexual disturbances were either preceded or accompanied by the trouble with the back—the camptocormia was the prevailing excuse for their sexual impotence.

Edward was discharged shortly afterward to civilian life. No one could guarantee the depth of his insight, nor how long it would be retained. Undoubtedly there were many even deeper problems which were not resolved. At least this soldier had been able to achieve some insight into the nature of his illness. He had lost his symptom and had been fortified against its return.

Five months later the therapist received a card from Edward. He was still well—and happy.

Chronology of the Case

The patient was hospitalized on July 3, 1945, and transferred to Welch Hospital on September 4. He was moved to the Special Treatment Company September 23. He was seen for a total of fifteen sessions (some of them two hours in length). His symptom was removed October 10, at the ninth session. He was discharged to civilian life shortly after October 22, 1945.

CHAPTER 19

HYSTERICAL PARALYSIS

Sometimes a mild neurotic symptom will stubbornly defy years of analysis. On the other hand a severe hysterical disability may become resolved unexpectedly in a short time. There was certainly nothing mild about Barkley Masterson's trouble. For thirteen months this twenty-three-year-old soldier had been shunted from one Army hospital to another—that hand, that right hand, had three fingers clenched. Only the thumb and the index finger were free. The hand, twisted with pain, the muscles now atrophying from disuse, simply wouldn't respond to treatment. Massage, electrical stimulation, physiotherapy, heat, baths, exercise—all had been tried, over and over again. Still Barkley couldn't open his hand.

Thirteen months in the hospital does not improve the disposition of any man. Barkley was bitter, hostile, discouraged, antagonistic, and depressed.

"To hell with the Army. To hell with the doctors. To hell with all of them. Why don't they cut off my fingers and let it go at that? They've tried everything. I'll never get well—I'll never use my hand again." This was the Barkley who arrived at Welch Hospital late in September, 1945, for definitive treatment because of "partial paralysis of right ulnar nerve."

But when he reached the Hospital he did not go to the Neuropsychiatric Service. He was assigned to an orthopedic company. Why? In the middle of Barkley's forearm was a small scar—all that was left to show where a piece of shell had penetrated. Barkley thought—the nurses thought—the doctors thought—this shell fragment must have severed one of the nerves. That must be why he couldn't open the hand. That would explain why for thirteen long months this hand had been clenched—and that was why Barkley went to the Orthopedic Division.

But Barkley's physician there began to suspect that this was not an organic disability. Perhaps it was functional—an hysterical conversion. He called on the director of the NP service for a psychiatric consultation. Several psychiatrists saw Barkley, and they, too, felt that this might represent an hysterical difficulty.

239

Accordingly, he was transferred to the Infirmary and given a narcosynthetic treatment with sodium pentothal.

Nothing came of it except—but let's have Barkley tell it in his own words. Five days later at the request of the Director of the Neuropsychiatric Division, Barkley was transferred to Company F.

Sullenly he strode across the room and sat down in the chair. "To hell with it all, Doc. See that hand. I've had it thirteen months. I've been in every hospital in the Army. They've done everything they could, and it won't open. It just won't open. It's never going to open. I want to get out of the Army so I can have my fingers cut off. Let's stop all this damn foolishness. I want to go home. And then up in the Infirmary, you know what they did up there. They stuck a needle in my arm. I don't know what you got over here, but I'm not going to have any more needles. My whole left arm has a numb feeling, and it hurts like the devil. See?" Barkley held up his left arm, which appeared to be perfectly normal. "That's what caused all those pains—the needle. You're not going to stick me with any more needles up here."

"No, Barkley," replied the therapist, "we're not going to stick you with any more needles. We may not be able to cure your hand here, but you won't be stuck with needles."

"And another thing," inquired Barkley belligerently, "this is a psycho company, isn't it? What am I doing here? I'm not nuts. First, they can't cure my hand, and now they throw me into a damn psycho ward. Why can't I go home?"

"You are going home, Barkley. You're going home just as soon as possible. Nobody here thinks you're 'nuts.' You were sent here because we have had some success in treating cases like yours. In fact there are several boys in the company right now who have a similar type of paralysis. Have you had a chance to meet any of them?"

"No, who do you mean?"

"Well, now take Farley—he's the fellow who is all bent over double. His back is paralyzed so badly that he can hardly walk upstairs. He's been feeling a lot better since he came here—and you know, I think we are going to be able to cure him."

Barkley looked up and blinked. "You mean that he's got his whole back paralyzed like my hand?"

"That's right. He's even worse off than you are. He can't walk up straight—looks like a hunchback."

Barkley continued, "And you think you're going to straighten him out?"

The reader will note that, in the case of Farley (Chapter 18), at this time (October 8), we were approaching the final stages of the treatment. Any indentification that Barkley could make with Edward Farley before Farley's symptom was removed should prove to be of tremendous help.

"I suppose, like a lot of the fellows, Barkley, you feel pretty discouraged—sore—and thinking that you're just going to get the runaround. I would like to have you meet Farley and talk to him. He can tell you that you're going to get some treatment." Barkley only grunted.

After further orientation designed to establish rapport, the patient was given suggestibility tests. The progress note for that session summarized with: "He was not found to be highly suggestible and did not respond to the postural-swaying test. [This is a reassuring point worth remembering when one is frustrated in the early stages of treating an apparently unresponsive subject, since he became quite hypnotizable later.] The patient reported hyperesthesia and anesthesia in the left arm 'caused by the needle.' He was given narcosynthesis five days ago. He seemed to be quite hostile and belligerent and said that he would 'rather accept a court martial than the needle again.' He has no insight at all into his condition and resents the term 'psycho.' It was felt that there was good conscious rapport established with the patient before the end of the hour, but unconscious resistance is quite strong."

Immediately after Barkley Masterson had left the office the therapist called in Edward Farley with the hysterically twisted back.

"Edward, we've got another fellow who has just come into the company. His condition is a lot like yours—only it's his hand instead of his back that's twisted. I think that maybe you can help him."

"How's that, sir?" asked Farley.

"He is mighty discouraged, bitter, upset, and has been in the hospital a long time. He doesn't think that anybody is going to be able to help him. I know that you have been improving some from your treatment. Even though your back isn't straightened yet, it doesn't hurt like it did, and I think you know that we are going to be able to straighten it soon. I believe it would be a good Christian thing for you to do if you could go to him. Give him some reassurance. Pep him up. Make him feel that he is going to be helped."

"Yes, I'll be glad to do that, sir. I'll go see him right away. Where is his bunk?" And Farley shuffled out of the office eager to help another who had a condition similar to his.

Farley and Masterson met—Farley and Masterson talked. The results were very gratifying. The next day, October 9, Masterson came in for another treatment.

Sessions of October 9-10, 1945; Direct Suggestion to Relieve Minor Symptom

"Good morning, Barkley. How are you feeling today?"

"I'm feeling a lot better. I guess I felt too bad and sorta blew my top yesterday."

"Oh, that's all right. What made you feel better?"

"Well, yesterday afternoon I had a talk with that guy, Farley—you know the one you told me about. And I said to myself, 'Boy, if that guy can be cheerful, what the hell am I bitching about?' He told me that the treatments here were helping him a lot, and he felt a great deal better. He said, 'They'll fix you up—they'll straighten out that hand.' I don't know—it's been a long time. Maybe he's right. Anyway I feel a lot better than I did yesterday—I've been thinking, Doc. I'd even have the nerve to take the needle treatment again if it were necessary, but it sure does hurt this arm," and he twisted the left arm about.

"That won't be necessary. I told you we weren't going to use any needles on you. You can count on that. We may put you to sleep as part of the treatment, but it will be a *natural sleep*. We won't stick any drugs into you." (The word "natural" was usually reassuring.)

Trance was induced by the eye-fixation method. Eye closure and catalepsy occurred in about ten minutes. Following this he was given ten minutes further sedation by the metronome. He entered a medium trance. Note the importance of rapport and attitude in influencing hypnotizability.

He was next given direct suggestions of relaxation, euphoria, freedom from tension, ability to sleep at night, and loss of pain in the left arm only. No attempt was made to touch the spastic condition in the right hand. It is sounder strategy (*during the beginning stages of treatment*) to alleviate minor symptoms and build up rapport rather than attempt frontal assaults against the major symptom.

He emerged from trance amnesic to all suggestions and immediately became much preoccupied with his left arm. "It doesn't hurt at all." He appeared to be greatly surprised and exercised the arm for some time, observing it most intently.

Barkley was called in again October 10. He was quite jovial at this time and claimed that his left arm felt much better following the previous day's treatment. He was again placed in a medium trance. This time, however, there was every evidence of strong resistance. It required twenty minutes to induce the trance. Suggestions of hand levitation, used as a test of trance depth, failed at first, but succeeded later. Next arm catalepsy and anesthesia were suggested. Following this a direct suggestion attack under trance was made against the spastic hand. With considerable difficulty the fingers were straightened. However, he could not hold them straight without some pressure from the therapist. He was able to put them against the flat of a book and keep them straightened fairly well, but there was a great deal of tension, tremors, and a constant tendency to close them. He was then given posthypnotic suggestions tending further to remove the pains in the left arm. The anesthesia, about which he complained in this arm, was not touched. No attempt was made to suggest that the right hand would remain open posthypnotically. On awakening he did not remember any of the suggestions. He reported that there was no pain in the left arm. The session ended on a high note of pleasantry.

On Thursday, October 11, 1945, Edward Farley's back was straightened. This became a moment of rejoicing, not only to Farley, but also to many of the other patients. The severity of his back symptom had been so noticeable that small bets had even been made as to whether the treatment would or would not be successful. When it was, and Farley was able to walk among his buddies perfectly straight, there was a remarkable attitudinal change among all the patients in the company. Obvious was the effect upon Barkley Masterson, who had so recently arrived in Company F discouraged with the feeling that no possibility existed for the successful treatment of his spastic hand. Finding, as he did, a man with whom he had already identified now apparently cured brought about a tremendous change of attitude and new hope.

Session of October 12, 1945; Abreaction

It was with almost an eager sense of anticipation that on October 12, the day after Farley's "cure," Barkley came to the office for treatment. Both he and the therapist sensed that this session would be most significant. Bitterness and discouragement had turned to new hope and cheerfulness. Somebody like himself had just been "cured."

At the beginning of the hour, time was devoted to a discussion of Farley's recovery. Barkley was almost as pleased about it as if it had been himself.

He was placed in a deep trance in twenty minutes. The depth finally became adequate, but he did enter rather slowly. The therapist had previously determined to try an abreactive session; so the discussion was opened as follows:

"You may think of things which worry you. There are matters down deep inside of you which are greatly disturbing. They are now going to come out, and you can talk about them."

Barkley began to breathe rapidly. Tremors swept over his body. He squirmed and twisted about. Occasionally tears would come into his eyes, and he would grind his teeth. He lay on the bed a quivering mass of silent agitation, biting his lips to keep from speaking.

"These matters are going to rise within you. They are coming up higher now—on your tongue. Now they are on the tip of your tongue. Now your lips are opening. You are going to be able to talk."

Barkley's lips parted, and he began to murmur, "My buddy—my buddy—they killed him." This was followed by more thrashing about on the cot. Tears began to flow copiously. Continually the therapist reassured and prodded. Higher and higher mounted the anxiety.

Finally in gasping breaths, snatches of almost incoherent speech began to emerge. "I was in front of him—I couldn't help him. The sons of bitches killed him. I couldn't help him. They would have killed me. Keep going—keep going—keep going."

"That's right, Barkley, keep going."

"Where am I? What's happening? The damn Jerries, the damn Jerries are coming. The patrol—I'm point man. I'm supposed to spot 'em. I don't see nothing. Where are the Jerries? There aren't any Jerries."

"Who is behind you, Barkley?"

"My buddy—the best soldier in the Army. My buddy, he is right behind me—about twenty feet. A lot of Jerries here. Oh, damn," and in a tidal wave of agony, Barkley began to paw his face.

"Kill the sons of bitches. Too late—too late." Rivers of tears now streamed down his cheeks.

"What's too late?"

"Too late—my buddy is dead. They killed him—they got behind me. I didn't see them. I didn't see—I want him to come back. I want him to come back so very bad. Why didn't I see them first?

Why didn't I knock them out? I could have. Why didn't I—Why didn't I throw it?"

"Throw what?"

"The grenade—the grenade I had in my hand. Why didn't I throw it?"

"Did you have a grenade in your right hand at the moment your buddy was killed?"

"Yes, I was holding a grenade. I saw the Jerries pass. I could have knocked them out." (In holding a grenade the hand assumes the same position in which Barkley's hand had become paralyzed—three fingers around the grenade with the index finger holding the release.)

"Do you feel as if you were responsible for your buddy's death?"

Barkley began to kick his feet about. He turned over and pounded with his fists on the wall—weeping, wailing, crying, bawling, shouting, "I didn't see them. I didn't see them. I couldn't help it. It wasn't my fault. If I could have saved him—I wanted to save him so much."

"Did you think that if you threw the grenade you would have given away your position to the Germans? Were you afraid to throw the grenade?"

"Oh no—they knew our position. I just didn't see 'em is all. I should've seen 'em." Then he began shouting in a loud voice, "I didn't kill. I didn't kill." This could have meant either that he wasn't responsible for the death of his buddy or that he was castigating himself for not killing the Germans.

This scene continued for another fifteen to twenty minutes. The sweating, writhing, crying man on the cot poured out every last ounce of energy—screaming with his whole body that he was not guilty for the death of his buddy. Like a warehouse full of fireworks, he was exploding. The abreaction would have to continue until Barkley was exhausted—until this vast reservoir of pent-up emotion had been released. All this time he was in deep hypnotic trance.

Gradually the heaving tide of anxiety began to subside. Minutes passed, and from pure exhaustion alone the legs and arms ceased their thrashing. The blanket was so wet that it seemed impossible his eyes could have manufactured another single tear.

Once again the therapist began talking, this time in a soft, low, reassuring voice. "Barkley, I want you to listen. I want you to listen very carefully now. For thirteen months you have been condemning yourself, condemning yourself for the death of your buddy. When a man feels guilty he pushes the guilt down inside of himself.

It's like steam in a boiler. And the pressure can cause the boiler to leak at the seams. You've been under tremendous pressure. Down deep inside, you felt guilty. You felt responsible. Over and over your inside mind has said to itself, 'Barkley Masterson, you're guilty. Barkley Masterson, you have killed your buddy. Barkley Masterson, if you had only thrown the grenade your buddy would be alive today'; and so having condemned yourself you have gone on also to punish yourself. What was it that was responsible for your buddy's death? Your unconscious mind answered back, 'my right hand.' So the right hand must be punished. It must be punished by being paralyzed, because only in this way would you feel that you had atoned for your buddy's death. Only in this way could you look the world in the face.

"All the deep anxiety, all the deep fear, all the deep guilt has been *tied up in three fingers*. As long as those three fingers were paralyzed, as long as the three fingers clasped each other tightly, as long as you had a maimed hand, just that long were you able to keep the feelings of guilt down in the unconscious where you would not have to look at them—where you would not have to face them.

"You don't have to push them down there, because you were not responsible for the death of your buddy. It wasn't your fault. It's just the breaks of battle. Maybe you didn't see the Germans. One can't see everything. Neither you, nor I, nor anybody else has perfect attention and perfect eyesight. No, it wasn't Barkley Masterson who caused his buddy's death. But it has been Barkley Masterson who has punished himself for thirteen months—punished himself for a crime which he did not commit. You must remember that. You must know that—know that deeply through you. Can't you see that it really wasn't your fault?" Barkley, tongue-tied and incoherent, feebly nodded.

"And now because you are not guilty, you can open your hand. It was just the luck of battle that caused the death of your buddy. You've got to open your hand now, because your buddy would want you to do that. Open it and carry on as a good, strong soldier—like he would have wanted you to do. See, there is nothing to hold it shut any more. The fingers can come open."

At that Barkley began to open his hand. Slowly and with effort the fingers came out—straighter—straighter—straighter—straighter. The two smallest fingers, weak from the atrophy of long months of disuse, prevented the hand from being completely straight. There was still a slight bend. But once more he had a man's hand, not a warped, twisted mass of flesh—a hand that could move—a hand that could grasp—a hand with five full fingers in it.

"And now, Barkley, in a minute I am going to waken you. When I do, you will feel good all over. Your hand will be open just like it is now, and you will remember in detail everything we discussed. You will not forget it when you wake up. You will never forget. You will realize that it was not your fault—that you could not have helped it because your buddy was killed. You will never again punish yourself for something for which you were not to blame. I shall count up to ten. You will wake up with your hand wide open and remembering all. 1, 2, 3, . . . 10."

Barkley slowly opened his eyes and looked at his hand. Then he burst again into tears and buried his head in his hands. But these were not tears of anxiety, nor sorrow, nor bitterness. Barkley was crying with the relief of sheer happiness.

Finally he regained his composure and brushed away his tears with a dirty handkerchief. Smiling, he sat on the edge of the cot while he and the therapist went over and over every detail of what had happened—happened over in France—the meaning of it all— why his hand had become paralyzed—why he could not open it for thirteen months.

"Gosh, I feel wonderful, Doc. Gee, I feel as if there is a great weight off me." Barkley paused. An idea crept over his face. He rushed toward the door. "I'm going to see Farley—show him my hand is as good as his back." There was a clatter of steps down the staircase.

In this abreaction or reliving of the original traumatic episode the corrective emotional experience is administered which enables the patient to close off or complete the incomplete Gestalt of the neurosis. By a return to the emotion of the moment, followed by a more beneficial interpretation, the guilt can be released, and what has been referred to by Kubie (1943) as the "repetitive core" need no longer compulsively plague the patient in a never-ending search for fulfilment which never comes. In the traditional psychoanalytic treatment of the chronic, deep-seated, civilian neurosis this corrective experience is accomplished within the transference relationship. In the military neurosis, which is more often the product of specific and recent traumatic experiences, our insight can be achieved without such extended working through. We can "relive" in a projected fantasy because the faulty learning was acquired in a recent and traumatic experience. Where the neurotic "faulty learning" comes from early childhood fixations or regressions, it may be necessary to wait until the patient can project onto the therapist (transference) his immature, emotional feelings before he can "relive" and correct.

Conclusion of the Case

On October 18, 1945, the therapist and the patient again went over the dynamics in review, with further discussion as to the nature of a conversion hysteria.

After his hand was opened, Masterson was assigned to both physiotherapy and occupational therapy. But it was different now than it had been during the past thirteen months. Now he accepted treatment eagerly. With each passing day strength came back into the fingers.

Two weeks later his chart was closed and he returned home. All that remained of the previous condition was some slight weakness in the two smallest fingers. The atrophy of thirteen months of disuse could not be denied—but Barkley was a happy lad. He was willing—yes, eager—to tell his story to all who asked about it.

No, not all conversion hysterias originate in early childish sexual maladjustment. Barkley was hospitalized August 26, 1944, with the clenched, spastic, paralyzed hand. Thirteen and a half months later, on October 8, 1945, he was assigned to the Special Treatment Company at Welch Convalescent Hospital. Four days later, October 12, 1945, hypnotherapy broke that thirteen months' paralysis—the hand opened.

PART IV

THE HYPNOANALYTIC TREATMENT OF AN ENTRENCHED PHOBIA

CHAPTER 20

MARGARET WAS AN OLD MAN

We fear thunder. We fear lightning. We fear earthquakes, water, snakes, other people, and death. But nothing can cause greater suffering than the fear of the enemy within—a man's fear of himself.

It was an early April morning. The topic in group therapy had been "Fears and How to Control Them." There was much heated discussion among the men about this subject. At the end of the hour a visitor approached the therapist.

"Could I have a few words with you in private, Lieutenant?"

"Certainly, let's go up to my office."

The young lieutenant who had requested the conference seated himself in the chair and then related the following:

"I was wounded and came here a few months ago as an orthopedic patient. Now, I am about to be released from the hospital and assigned on the staff as a duty officer. That's why I happened to drop in and listen to the discussion today. I wonder if you could help me with the fear that I've got. It's so strong at times that I simply can't sleep at all."

"Can you tell me more about it?"

"I don't know just when it started, but I guess it was back in Italy. I kept constantly having the feeling that somebody was trying to 'get me.' I simply had to have a light every night, or I couldn't sleep at all. It was about December, 1943, when this fear first began. It becomes less at times, but I never lose it. I'm worried now about my new job. They'll expect me to be duty officer on certain nights, and I don't know if I'll be able to go about alone in the dark."

"Do you remember anything before you came into the Army which might be related to this?"

"Yes, I remember an incident, which happened in 1939. I returned to my apartment and found that it had been ransacked by a robber. I was slightly uneasy in the dark at that time, but later it didn't bother me."

"Do you know who the burglar was?"

"No, but I thought at the time that it might have been a certain individual with whom I had gone to the races. He lost quite a lot of money betting. I never had any financial dealings with him. Later on this fellow left town—I just can't seem to recall his name. Do you think that you could help me get rid of this fear?"

"Let's see, I believe that you're on a duty status?"

"Yes, I'm going to be. Do I have to be a patient?"

"No, not for the time being. I can arrange to see you at various times while you are stationed here as duty personnel."

"I understand that you do work with hypnosis. Do you think that would help me?"

"I don't know, but we can see."

Lieutenant ———, let us call him Patient X, was given postural swaying suggestibility tests. He responded favorably to these. An appointment was made for two days later.

And so begins one of the most interesting cases that has ever come to the author's attention. Neither the patient nor the therapist on that early April morning had the slightest idea how many strange paths would be followed or how many dozens of hours would be required in the search for the cause of X's fear of the dark.

The sessions are presented in the order in which they occurred. The reader may find it interesting after he has the story of the treatment to review the entire case. He will find that much which at first is nonsensical assumes integrated meaning in the light of the final solution to the problem. Ideas, associations, wishes, dreams, and symbols which came out of the patient's "unconscious" during the sessions fit together like pieces in a jig-saw puzzle only when one knows the final pattern.

The entire treatment required a total of some sixty-five sessions over a period of a year. Five were held within the first two months and the other sixty during the last six months of the treatment period. During the initial stages of therapy the therapist had the active collaboration of a member of the American Psychoanalytic Association. In the latter part of the therapy consultations were held on the progress of the case with another psychoanalyst. His suggestions were of considerable assistance in planning the therapy.

This case is not presented as a complete "analysis," but it does represent a deeper and more intensive study than any previously described. In it, advanced techniques which had not been brought to bear in other cases were developed and utilized. Some of these methods have not been described in other publications on hypno-analysis and may prove to be useful extensions of hypnosis and projective methods in depth therapy. They are described here in the experimental form in which they were tried.

From this treatment did not emerge the completely adjusted individual. There was no loss of all neurotic personality traits. There were many questions yet unanswered, many motives still unexplored. Yet, without doubt, Patient X did undergo a major psychological operation.

Session of April 15, 1945; Interview Under Trance

Patient X was placed in a light hypnoidal trance and revealed the following:

He hated his father, because his father once hit his mother. He tried to attack his father but was too small to do so effectively. He was devoted to his mother. This was related with considerable emotion and anxiety. He stated afterwards that he didn't want to talk of it, as he never had before, but he felt "compelled" to do so. He was greatly disturbed over the fact that during trance he was unable to open his eyes although he had tried "with all my will." It was not fear, merely the phenomenon that amazed him.

He divulged more interesting facts after he came out of trance and stated that while in the Army he was terribly afraid of night patrols. His former wife gave birth to another man's child. It could not be ascertained whether his fears of the dark emerged prior to his wife's illegal pregnancy or afterward. After his divorce the patient was happily remarried.

He said that as a child he liked the dark because he and his best friend would go out in it together. However, he mentioned that now he must have the light on at night.

During this first hour the patient was able to enter only a very light trance. However, two days later more significant material was uncovered when he was interviewed under a deeper trance state.

Session of April 17, 1945

Patient X was placed in a medium trance.

"Can you tell more about your first marriage?"

"I was tricked into marriage by the girl. She claimed that she was pregnant, and that it was my fault." The patient elaborated this point in detail.

He was then regressed to age ten, where he indicated that he had a fear of rattlesnakes. He showed a great deal of disgust for "filthy" things.

When advanced to his present age once more, he mentioned that the Arabs in Africa were "filthy" and that so also were Italian women. Asked to discuss more about his first marriage, he said that when he left for overseas he was disgusted with his wife—but "resigned." He said that he knew she would play around and wouldn't be true to him; so her pregnancy was no surprise.

He was able to recall that the man whom he thought might have broken into his house was named Harry, but he could not remember the last name. He reported that this man was involved in shady deals. On emerging from trance, he opened up with the following interesting information.

"I guess I didn't tell you before, but my father was quite sick in the nineteen thirties, and he had to be hospitalized."

"What kind of sickness?"

"Well, I guess it was a kind of insanity. They sent him to a mental hospital. I've been wondering whether such things are hereditary."

"There is no direct evidence that insanity is inherited. I wouldn't let it worry you. Do you want to tell more about your parents?"

"I was always attached to Mother. I felt that Dad let her down. I just told him about my present marriage recently. This was the first contact that I have had with him for some time. You know, Mother died two years ago. Father was weak. People could push him around. He was a good money-maker, but he took flyers. I remember one time that a man wanted him to hide something—I don't know—some bootleg material. I know Father refused at first, and he was then bribed by this man through the use of his attractive thirty-year-old daughters."

"How did it make you feel when you learned this?"

"I felt very, very bitter about it. I remember that it was shortly after this that father took to brooding. He would keep looking out the windows. Then they took him away to the hospital."

"Weren't you rather young at the time?"

"Yes, I was in my early teens. I learned about Father and these other women only when Mother told me."

Session of April 23, 1945

Patient X came in today in an enthusiastic mood.

"I've got a couple of leads for you. I think they are important and worth investigating. The first one happened when I was around twelve years old. I saw two of my friends who had been drowned.

They were brothers. It was at night, and I was very much afraid. I could hardly go home. And the second one happened when I was around five years old. I remember that I was scared by an older girl. She was dressed up like an old man. It happened in late evening, and I remember that I was petrified. My aunt told me that it was a girl dressed up like a man. I think both of these things are important. I've been thinking of them since the last time we met. Incidentally, I felt quite a lot better since our last session and have been able to sleep well."

Patient X was placed in a trance by the waking method, and the right hand dissociated from the rest of the body. He was then regressed to age fourteen.

"Do you fear anything?"

Patient X replied, "No—No—No!" At the same time the hand wrote "YES."

"Whom do you fear?"

There was no answer. The patient pursed his lips as if to indicate that he wasn't going to speak. After a while the hand wrote, "MY FATHER."

"Why do you fear him?"

The hand wrote, "HE IS SICK."

"Tell me more about it."

The hand continued writing, "HE SITS AROUND AND STARES OUT THE WINDOWS." The patient was then induced to describe further his father's psychotic episode.

Next he was returned to various ages when he could not sleep because of a fear of the dark. In each case he said that he was afraid of a "man." But when asked to name the man or to write his name, he said that he didn't know. The hand always wrote, "I DON'T KNOW."

Next he was asked directly, "Is it your father that you fear in the dark?"

The hand answered, "NO."

After continued probing about his fears the hand finally wrote the word "MARGARET."

Patient X was now regressed back to various age levels. *He described how he once disliked a certain boy who was a bully.*[1]

"Now you're going to go back and be five years old. Something is happening which frightens you. What is it?"

---

[1] This seemingly innocent point takes on crucial significance ten and a half months later in the treatment.

Patient X froze in his chair. The color left his face. He became white and gripped the handles of the chair tightly.

"I'm walking down the fields. It's getting dark. Something jumps out at me. It's an old man. It's an old man in black. I'm scared to death. I start running. I'll never forget that man."

"Who was the old man?"

"My aunt said that it was Margaret. She's about sixteen years old. I never did quite believe her though."

"Now, X, you have just run home from being frightened. You're in the house—your aunt is in the house. You're in the front room. Look! Here comes somebody. Why, it's the old man—isn't it? See!"

Once more the patient stiffened in his chair. The therapist continued, "Look! The old man is taking off his clothes. Why, it isn't an old man at all. It's only a girl. It's Margaret, isn't it? Isn't that funny—it's just a funny joke. There's nothing to be afraid of. It's only Margaret."

Patient X relaxed in his chair, and a smile began to creep over his face. "Yes, it is Margaret, isn't it?"

"And now, X, you are going to grow older. You are going to grow up to be six, seven, eight—eight years old. X, do you remember about Margaret—the one dressed up as an old man who frightened you?"

The patient nodded—smiling.

"Do you remember afterwards she came into your aunt's parlor, and you saw her take off the old man's clothes? Then you knew that it was Margaret, and you weren't afraid any more, were you?"

Again the patient nodded.

"Just remember that you won't ever be afraid again. Now you're going to grow older—older—older. You are becoming nine, ten, eleven, twelve—twelve years old. Do you ever remember being frightened by an old man?"

Patient X laughed, "It's only Margaret."

He was reassured once more and told that he would no longer fear the dark. He was then awakened.

"You know, Doc, I feel grand. I feel wonderful. It's just like a great load has been lifted." He then described in detail his "memory" of the old man disrobing which proved to be "only Margaret." He displayed considerable amusement in relating the story.

On May 14, three weeks later, the "memory" of Patient X concerning the Margaret incident was tested by recall questions. It had continued as "adjusted."

CHAPTER 21

THE PROBLEM IS MUCH DEEPER

At the end of the previous session X had left feeling in fine fettle. Gone were his anxieties. Now he had "discovered" the cause for his fear of the dark. It was easy. As a five-year-old child he had been frightened by a little girl dressed up in an old man's clothes. This had happened at night. Something had now occurred which had brought back this memory. The source of the fear had been uncovered and now was resolved. The burden had left—the phobia was lost—or was it?

On the 23rd of May, a month after the session in which the "Margaret memory" was "adjusted," X came in and requested a resumption of treatment. The reassurance received from the last session had vanished. All the old anxieties and fears were now emerging once again, proving that more than "Margaret" lay at the base of this phobia.

He was placed in trance, and the right hand dissociated.

"Do you worry about your father?"

X replied, "No." The hand proceeded to write, "N—YES."

"Why do you fear your father?"

The hand traced the letters, "I DON'T KNOW."

"Can't you tell something about it?"

The hand wrote, "AGIVATE."

"'Agivate,' what's that?"

This time X replied, "It means 'aggravate.'"

"What about 'aggravate'?"

"I was afraid that Dad would have another one of his attacks. Perhaps he would interfere with my personal life, or become an added burden. He wouldn't care. He's not sensitive to the trouble that he causes others."

"Is there anything else about this situation that bothers you?"

"I wonder if I will become that way—like Dad, you know."

"Is there anything associated with your father that reminds you of a fear?"

"Yes, I recall once when I was a very little boy that Dad killed a bat. I was very much afraid of the bat. I didn't actually see him kill the creature, but I saw the dead animal afterwards."

No more could be disclosed under hypnotic trance, so the patient was awakened. When the incident involving the bat killing was called to his attention, he appeared greatly surprised.

"Why, that happened when I was only two or three years old—I wonder whether my troubles have anything to do with sex?"

"Do your parents have anything to do with this?"

"I only know that my father broke up my mother's home. Sometimes I'm afraid that he might act in the same way to my home. I'm also worried about whether maybe I may become like him."

"Can you tell me any more about yourself?"

"Suspicion. That's a word. You know, that's the way I feel lots of times about people. Sometimes I feel that people on the street are talking about me. I know it's ridiculous. I try to push it out of my mind, but it keeps cropping up just the same." This was the first evidence that the patient had given of paranoidal tendencies.

On May 31 another session was conducted with the dissociated hand under deep trance. Following are the important points which emerged.

W: Your hand is going to write now what it is that you fear in the dark, but the words will all be scrambled—the letters will be mixed.

The Hand: MESONE.

W: Can you tell me what that means?

X: It means "someone."

W: The Hand is going to write another important word.

The Hand: NOSREP.

W: What does that mean?

X: That means "person."

W: Can The Hand tell more about *what* person?

The Hand refused to write.

W: I think The Hand is going to write. It's going to write something important.

The Hand still refused to write.

W: Now it's beginning to move. Now letters are beginning to form. It has to write—it has to write.

The Hand: NO, NO, NOBODY. It paused a moment and then continued I DON'T KNOW. At this point it began to draw a picture—a rather weird little manikin. After two attempts at this picture it wrote underneath the word MYSTIC, and then MOVIES.

W: What about this? Where did you see it?

The Hand: PHANTOM OF THE OPERA.

W: What about 'Phantom of the Opera'?

The Hand: LON CHANEY.

W: Where did you see this show?

The Hand: DENVER.

Upon coming out of trance the patient mentioned that he remembered being frightened by seeing this motion picture when he was a small child. No other material could be elicited at this session.

.   .   .   .

It was four months later, October 3, and the therapist was seated in his office when there was a knock on the door.

"Come in."

The door opened. There stood Patient X, anxiety engraved on his face.

"Doc, it's getting bad again. It's getting terribly bad."

"Tell me about it."

"I've had a lot of responsibilities lately, and I'm getting more and more tense all the time. I can't sleep at night. Every time I go out in the dark there is that horrible clutching fear. I keep telling myself that it is going to go away. But it isn't. It's been getting worse. You're the only person that I know who can help me."

Patient X indeed showed his lack of sleep. His face was wan and haggard. There were tremors in his hands. His speech came haltingly. There were "jitters" over his whole body.

It was best to offer some palliative treatment at first. So he was placed in deep trance and given posthypnotic suggestions of relaxation and euphoria. He was also told that he would be able to sleep well the next few nights.

On October 8 he came in once more and reported that he had slept well the first night after the previous treatment. After that the fears had returned, and he could not sleep. It was decided that a longer-term, deeper treatment must be initiated. In order that he might have some insight into what we were trying to accomplish he was given an early manuscript draft of Part I of this book. This was in rough form at that time, and was designed to explain the structure of neuroses and their treatment to patients. The therapist and patient together went over the material concerning the causes of a neurosis and the theory of analytic-type therapy. At the end of this time, it was felt he had some insight into the nature of his condition, what analytic therapy would be like, and especially important, the factors of resistance and transference. Strongly emphasized was the point that emotional resistance is often a sign pointing to very significant material.

Session of October 15, 1945

X came in today in a worse state than ever before. His fears and "jittery" nerves were now seriously interfering with his Army work. He reported the last few nights as having been "very rough." He then described the following dream.

"Someone was chasing me. I was in a car. There was a girl beside me—I guess the girl was my wife. I don't seem to remember any more about it."

"What does it make you think of?"

"It doesn't make me think of anything else. That's all I can remember about it."

X was next placed in a deep trance and told that he could remember the dream more in detail. Whereupon he amplified it as follows:

"I'm driving along a highway. It's a big highway—four lanes. Someone is driving the car in the front seat. It looks like my wife is driving it. No, that's funny—my wife can't drive a car. Anyway, someone is chasing me. The car is chasing me. The person that I fear is in the car behind me. It has a big nickel-plated engine. That's funny—my wife can't drive this car. The man is getting closer and closer." Tremors appeared all over Patient X. He jumped about in his seat.

The therapist encouraged with, "Go on. You can finish the dream now. You are able to finish the dream."

But he replied, "Everything stopped—everything stopped. I can't see who is in the car. I can't see who it is that is chasing me. What is it that is chasing me? Everything is dark—everything is dark." No amount of probing could bring further description of the dream or associations to it.

Accordingly, he was given suggestions that he would sleep well tonight and would not remember anything that was discussed in trance—that he would have no headaches—that he would have euphoric feelings. On emerging from the trance state he mentioned that he had worried about his wife, because "she is alone." No further attempt was made to explore the point at this time.

On October 22 the patient reported that he had been able to have one good night's sleep immediately following the last treatment. After that he was again jittery and afraid that someone was going to enter his room. He slept very fitfully and could not go out in the dark.

At this session he was given the Thematic Apperception Test, previously described, in an attempt to uncover some possible dynamics. Some of the more interesting stories which he imagined are reported here.

PICTURE 3BM

(FIGURE OF INDEFINITE SEX SEATED ON FLOOR WITH FACE BURIED IN COT; REVOLVER-LIKE OBJECT ON FLOOR NEARBY)

"This is a girl—it must be a girl. Wonder what she is crying about? She is a very poor girl—a WAC. According to the surroundings it must be more or less like a barracks—a poor home, or it might be a jail. This girl probably committed a crime. She is in a detention home or a home for the wayward. She is crying."

PICTURE 4

(WOMAN RESTRAINING MAN WHO HAS ANXIETY ON HIS FEATURES)

"This man has just got married. He has lost his job and doesn't know what to do. He is disgusted with life. Hasn't got much confidence in his future. The woman beside him is his wife. He has already told her about leaving his job for no reason at all. The boss is mean and selfish. He wouldn't go back to that job if it was the last thing he had to do. The wife is pleading with him, calming him down. She is trying to tell him things will be all right—not to worry. He won't listen to her. He is very proud. He has got good features. Probably the reason he lost his job is no fault of his."

PICTURE 6BM

(YOUNG MAN IN DARK COAT HOLDING HAT AND STANDING BESIDE A MOTHER-FIGURE)

"I can really tell you something about this picture—but I won't, though. He has had incestuous relations with his sister—don't put that down. These people live in a small town, and this mother had only one child. It's this boy. The boy wants to leave home and go to the city and make his fortune. His mother argues back. His mother doesn't want him to go. The picture is on that moment when he leaves without the permission of his mother. Let's give him a name—Johnny. Johnny goes to a city, a big one. He doesn't get along very well. He doesn't make much money—no friends. He struggles and struggles. He makes no headway. Finally his money is all gone. Jobs he gets are left-overs—one-night work—dish-washer. Then one day in a room right next to him there moves a girl, a woman, and he makes her acquaintance, and from then on life is different. This girl probably comes to love Johnny, and he knows she is a prostitute. He loves her. She has a strong hold over him, so much so that he begins to pimp for her. She taught him every-thing she ever knew about people he is going to meet. And in due time Johnny becomes a racketeer, with girls all over the city and living the life of luxury happily ever after."

PICTURE 7BM

(OLDER MAN AND YOUNGER MAN)

"What in the hell would this be? Father and son—uncle and nephew? This young man has come to the office of this famous lawyer. His wife is giving him trouble, and he wants a divorce. He suspects her of intimacy with another man. They have two children. They have been very happy. Now all his dreams and his hopes, everything he has worked for, have gone to pot. He is drinking and staying out late at night. He becomes very seedy in his appearance and is gradually going to the dogs. The older man, knowing him as a boy—a small boy—tries to help him to get on his feet but with no success. The young man finally commits suicide."

PICTURE 8BM

(RECLINING FIGURE BEING OPERATED UPON; GUN ALONG ONE SIDE OF PICTURE; YOUNG BOY, APPARENTLY DREAMING, IN LOWER PART OF PICTURE)

"Now what the hell is this? I see a shotgun. I see a man with a knife cutting a man up. This young boy—what is he doing in the picture? I don't even want to talk about that." (The patient pushed the picture away, rejecting it.)

PICTURE 10

(TWO MIDDLE-AGED FACES, MAN AND WOMAN, AFFECTIONATELY NEAR EACH OTHER)

"Why in the hell don't they make these pictures so that you can see them? These are parents about fifty or fifty-five years of age who

have just received news that their son has just received an addition
to the family—first grandson that they have, and they are all very
happy." The patient put the picture away and said, "That's all. If
I say any more I'll probably say the baby swallowed a pin and died."

At this point the patient seemed to be tired of the test pictures; so
he was placed on the cot preparatory to entering trance.

He asked, "Doc, can I put myself to sleep?"

"Certainly," replied the therapist, "just look at the blue light.
Count up to fifty and imagine that you are going to go to sleep."
Patient X stared at the blue light. In about thirty seconds his eyes
closed, and he was in trance. He was given suggestion tests of hand
levitation and then asked, "Are you in a deep sleep?" He shook his
head, "No." Whereupon, he was given more suggestions of sleep.
A little later his hand automatically came up by itself and touched his
face, a signal which had been used in previous trance sessions to indicate that he had reached a stage of deep sleep.

He was now questioned again. "Are you in a deep sleep?"

This time he responded, "Yes."

"X, now you are going to see in front of your eyes a scroll of
paper. There will be words on this scroll. I would like to leave you
for a while. The scroll will revolve and unfold. You will be able
to read what is written on it. You do not need to talk about what
you see. There are things on that scroll which have to do with
your worries and with your fears. Can you see the scroll of paper?"

"Yes," replied Patient X.

The therapist then left the room for a period of ten minutes.
When he returned X was wide awake, his eyes staring, and fright
on his face.

He said, "I woke up—there was a thud. Something like a black
roll of paper went 'bang.'" He was given reassurance, placed back
again into a deep trance, and once more asked about the scroll.

"I can't see the scroll. The paper is all black."

"Now there is going to be a light behind the paper. You will be
able to see the words."

"I can't see the words—it's all black. The light is going out. The
light is going out—now it's all black again." The projective technique had failed. Nothing more could be uncovered.

During the first induction of trance he was told that he would
sleep "very well tonight and also tomorrow night." He was now
asked about this.

"What is going to happen tonight?"

He smiled and replied, "I will sleep well."

"And tomorrow night?"

"I will sleep well then too."

He was given further reassurance and posthypnotic suggestions on this point and then awakened. In the conscious state he seemed a little disturbed because he could remember the first break in trance. He also claimed that he remembered something about a black roll of paper which fell "down with a bang." He was given reassurance on this and did not exhibit any external signs of anxiety when he left.

Many possible leads can be deduced from the TAT stories. In picture 3BM the seated figure is interpreted as a girl although it is more commonly considered as a masculine figure. This may mean that unconsciously Patient X feels homoerotic drives and identifies with the feminine sex. These are not acceptable to his Super-Ego, since he concludes that, "This girl probably committed a crime. She is in a detention home or a home for the wayward." There is a bare further hint in picture 8BM where he exhibits such obvious resistance at the "man with a knife cutting a man up." Knives are often used as phallic symbols in dreams. We must assume by the remark, "This young boy—what is he doing in the picture? I don't even want to talk about that," that he has experienced an unpleasant association. As a perseverance of this we find the hostile resistance carrying over into the next picture, "Why in the hell don't they make these pictures so that you can see them?"

In picture 4 we see the hero as a very proud resistant figure who sees no good in father-figures, "the boss," who is depressed and subject to feminine influence, continued but ineffective.

In picture 6BM the hero is described as changing from a person of determination and highly ethical character to virtually a psychopath. The ending of the story "And in due time Johnny becomes a racketeer, with girls all over the city and living the life of luxury happily ever after," is typically psychopathic. This occurs after he leaves Mother. An association of sexual fixation toward sister intrudes itself at the first—the sister may actually be a symbol of Mother. He sees himself as loved but not loving.

In picture 7BM we find that father-figures (the "famous lawyer") are unable to restrain him from moral disintegration and finally self-destruction. This does not augur too well for his relation with the therapist. In this story also he hints at a rejection of the female, "he wants a divorce."

Picture 10 may indicate that he (or a part of him) actually wishes the approval of parents. However, in the end he cannot "stomach" the idea and comments, "If I say any more I'll probably say the baby swallowed a pin and died."

His resistance to the therapist and the conflictual nature of the material elicited by the stories is emphasized by his desire to be independent of the therapist and take his case in his own hands. ("Can I put myself to sleep?") This was further accented by his resistance to any projective suggestions such as the use of the roll of paper.

Session of October 26, 1945

On October 26 more Thematic Apperception Test pictures were administered. His responses were as follows:

PICTURE 11
(WEIRD PREHISTORIC SCENE)

"We have had an earthly disturbance—earthquakes and landslides. Can't make out this object in the extreme front. The object in the left is blended into the background. It could be an animal. I can see webbed feet. It could be a delusion. These are animals here. They are round. It may even be prehistoric times. It may be years ago. It looks like dinosaurs. I can't see much else in this picture."

PICTURE 12M
(YOUNG MAN RECLINING ON COUCH ASLEEP; OLDER MAN LEANING OVER HIM WITH HANDS IN FRONT OF YOUNG MAN'S FACE; SOMETIMES CALLED THE "HYPNOTIC" PICTURE AND USED TO TEST ATTITUDE FOR OR AGAINST HYPNOSIS)

"Well, we have here a boy. He is a young man. He is lying on his couch. He is the son of this man, the old man, and he has just come back home and has laid down to rest. He has slept too long, and his father is trying to wake him. The boy hasn't seen his father for many years, and this is his first trip away from his job. He wanted to come home to tell his father that he was going to get married and invite his father to go with him back home. The older man had lived in that community for years and years. He finally decided that the boy should go home alone, and at a later date return to pay a visit to his father—which he does. He gets married and has a little boy and is very happy. The father gets old and dies. The young man lives happily ever after."

PICTURE 13MF

(WOMAN COVERED WITH BLANKET, BUT WITH BREASTS BARE, LYING IN
BED; MAN STANDING IN FRONT OF BED, FACING AWAY, WITH ARM
OVER FACE)

"Boy, I could bring out a lot of ideas here. Must keep this clean,
though. Has he raped her or something? Well, he hasn't done anything—probably his wife. This man has led a very hard life. He
struggled and struggled. His wife has been a sickly woman. He
has nursed her for years—worked his fingers to the bone. She was
not getting any better—no money for medical support. He tried
many ways, many doctors, and the doctors said that his wife needed
fresh air, that she would die unless he took her away. One day he
comes home from work very tired and heartsick and ill at ease, and
rushes to the living room couch where he has made a place for her to
be on, and found that his wife is cold and dead. The man proceeds
to kill himself."

PICTURE 15

(WEIRD-LOOKING OLD MAN STANDING IN GRAVEYARD)

"This looks like something out of Cruikshank. This is a sort of
mystical cartoon of some time ago. It looks like a surrealist picture.
This is a sick old miser, and he hasn't any children. And because of
his miserliness and stinginess, and the way he has neglected his
family, the more he made, the more they died. Some of them grew
to manhood and had children, but they too passed away, and he
buries them all on his mansion—on his estate in a manner in which
no one knew except him. There are no names on the gravestones,
and he would go there and remember which one—and all about it.
At last he finally realized how wrong he had been. He wanted to
see his children alive and around him and happy. He was very
miserable in spite of his millions, and he realized what he had done
and suffered for his misdeeds."

PICTURE 16

(COMPLETELY BLANK WHITE CARD)

"Some one is kidding you, Watkins. I don't care what you say,
there is no picture here at all. I won't look at it." He stared at the
blank card for a little while and seemed very much amused. When

urged to continue and project something into it, he held the picture in front of him, shut his eyes, and said, "First thing that comes into my mind—very beautiful woman. But then again this is a picture of a lawn. It is a golf course. In the distance you can see the background of one tree. And half way between, a group of men is approaching. This is a happy domestic scene. These men are playing golf. The golf players have played for years and years together—getting neither better nor worse. They always remain on the same level. They are a group of tired old businessmen out there on daily excursions. Suddenly out of the sky storms a bunch of rocs. You know, a roc is a mythical giant bird. They come soaring down, and they see these golf players, and they fly upon them and crush them. There is big destruction over the whole earth, and nothing can stop them. After they have eaten everybody, as they can eat only humans for their diet, they eat all the animals, and then they eat themselves, until nothing is left. What is nothing? All is nothing, and if you think I'm going to sit here and tell you more about nothing you are crazy."

PICTURE 18BM

(APPARENTLY INEBRIATED MAN WITH TWO WHITE HANDS HOLDING HIM UP BY THE SHOULDER; THIRD WHITE PATCH ON SLEEVE WHICH MIGHT BE CALLED A HAND)

"How many hands has this guy got? Too many hands. That's a crazy picture. It looks like he is in ecstasy. Can't be a woman. This is a poor drunkard. He has gone on a drunk all his life. These are hands. He is dreaming. His hands are in front of his dream and are holding him back, and during the past years he has been becoming a chronic alcoholic. The hands are the product of his imagination. He struggles to get clear from them. He succumbs and passes a bar and saloon, but the hands are pulling him back. He goes into the saloon and starts drinking again. That's how he ends his life."

PICTURE 19

(RATHER IMPRESSIONISTIC PICTURE OF HOUSE)

"Now what in the hell is this? I see a chimney. If you think you're going to fool me this time, you're not. It reminds me of a dream I had once. It was about a house I had that was nestled on the sea, and to the rear there was a long stretch of open space. In front was the big ocean. I couldn't believe that there were animals running around the house, wild animals, and I couldn't get a boat to leave; so I just had to stay there—and I lived there for years and years—until the end of time." This is a rather interesting response when viewed in the light of the dream fantasies interpreted in Chapter 26.

In the second half of the TAT test we find even more significant material. In picture 11 the patient describes "an earthly disturbance"—his disturbance—but essentially rejects the picture. The lizard head in the foreground preoccupies him to some extent. Because of its shape it is sometimes made into a phallic symbol and precipitates anxieties related to the male genital.

In picture 12M we find that the hero wishes closer relations with his father even though "the father gets old and dies," and after that "the young man lives happily ever after." This must indicate his wish for the good father, since he did not feel consciously very close to his father.

In picture 13MF there is the same sexual slip at the beginning followed by the "cover-up." The "wife" or feminine figure dies and the man "proceeds to kill himself." We might infer guilt feelings about his relations to some feminine figure whom he considers he had neglected.

His guilty fears about his future are most exemplified in picture 15—the rejection of his relatives and the final need for them.

In picture 16 his associations start with sex, "very beautiful woman," proceed to a rather futile scene of middle age which is destroyed by overwhelming mythical monsters—perhaps his own "monstrous" impulses. It ends in oblivion.

The same theme of the hero who progressively disintegrates and reaches final destruction is portrayed in picture 18BM. Even here the homoerotic association reaches his mind, "Can't be a woman." One wonders about the great preoccupation with "hands."

Picture 19 reminds him of a dream which suggests his inability to escape from his "wild impulses."

A summary of themes drawn from all the stories reveals the following:

Forces in Hero

1. Struggle: hero rebels against mother and against wife
2. Fatalism: hero struggles with the environment—finally succumbs and ends life in resignation

3. Cynicism: apathy toward life; fatalism—resignation
4. Misdeeds: conscious guilt—need for introgression
5. Basic interests are lacking in heroes
6. No religion: heroes violate their own code of morals
7. Hero suspects wife of infidelity
8. Heroes desire to regress to childish days
9. Hero desires to tell father of marriage—expected rejection
10. Success does not bring happiness
11. Heroes do not appreciate the love of others—mother, wife
12. Heroes are slaves to bad habits (homosexual implications?)
13. Anal preoccupation (response to picture 20, not reported here)
14. Need for succorance
15. Heroes are in a state of conflict and indecision
16. Heroes are dejected and filled with gloom

Two very common themes seemed to be contradictory.

1. Hero is inadequate and feels much guilt
2. Hero is rejected by others because of events for which he is not responsible

Of the twenty stories, two had happy endings, nine had unhappy endings, and nine had neutral or indecisive endings.

Sessions of November 2 and 4, 1945

On the 2nd of November the patient reported that his fears and anxiety had now reached a point where they were seriously interfering with his Army work. He asked whether it would be possible to have his duties so arranged as to give him some freedom from stress and night work. This was arranged through the proper channels of authority.

He was placed in a deep trance and given suggestions of euphoria and ability to sleep. (Whenever sessions of this type were used— direct suggestive palliation—it was recognized that these were like giving headache powders or sedatives. They did, however, become necessary from time to time to keep the anxiety from reaching too acute a stage. Sessions of this type were interspersed between the meetings of more analytic type.)

The next day Patient X reported that he had slept well—that his anxiety was somewhat lower.

On November 4 some of the implications drawn from the Thematic Apperception Test were discussed with Patient X. It was suggested to him for the first time that he might have some repressed hostility toward his wife. He at first rejected this concept, but later admitted that there might be a great deal under the surface which he had not previously been willing to admit. He mentioned ways in which his wife would irritate him, and how he would retaliate by attempting to dominate her. He seemed to have a great need to dominate her and to win out in an argument.

The discussion then returned to his feelings of inadequacy. He emphasized the point that he had always wanted to be the "big shot." It was suggested to him that this was a neurotic wish and that, in wanting to dominate his wife, he was continuing this neurotic trend. The hint was then offered that he let her have her way a little oftener —that he find out the pleasure people get by being big enough to allow others to win in an argument occasionally. He seemed rather intrigued with the idea and said he was going to try it.

Session of November 5, 1945

Today the Oedipus complex was discussed with the patient. He was greatly interested and said he recognized many elements in it which applied to his own life. He then related an incident in which his father almost smothered his small sister. The child was crying, and the father attempted to stifle the cries by putting a pillow over the child's face. His aunt intervened in time. This sister, ultimately, was the one of whom the patient became quite fond.

He was next placed in trance and asked to discuss his inadequacies. An interesting point arose as follows:

"I was always afraid to go out and meet people directly."

"How do you mean, directly?"

"I mean I could never do house-to-house selling—as for example, going from door to door, selling Kotex."

"Kotex? Why does that idea come into your mind in connection with your inadequacies?"

"I don't know—I just said it is all."

"Yes, I know. But why did you say Kotex? Do people go from door to door selling Kotex?"

Patient X remained in deep trance but showed considerable irritation at this point. At first he refused to discuss it. Then he could not associate to it, but finally he began to admit that maybe there was a certain significance—that sex did arise in his mind in connection with his own Ego inadequacy. It is apparent that this slip might have been explored much further.

Sessions of November 6 and 8, 1945

Patient X first discussed the new changes in his assignment. These permitted him lighter duties and time during the day for his therapeutic session. He was placed in deep trance in fifteen minutes and given direct suggestions of euphoria, relaxation, freedom from worry, and ability to sleep. He awakened, stated that he was feeling "very grand," and left in a cheerful frame of mind.

Two days later on November 8 X reported that he was sore and stiff from "too much athletics." There had been no evidence of nervousness, fears, or inability to sleep for a week. He was given some reassurance, but no attempt was made to uncover any more material.

Sessions of November 14 and 16, 1945

On November 14 an interview was held in the conscious state in which the patient described details of his sex life.

"When I was seven or eight years old I had relations with two little girls. I guess it wasn't a real relation—just sort of play. But I remember I enjoyed it, particularly because there was an element of danger. One of them—*she had a big brother, and we were all scared of him.*[1] I remember a little later there were some five or six of us fellows, and we took a girl into a pup tent. One of the boys was the girl's brother. The boys all went in and had relations with her in turn. I know I was a stranger in the group at the time, but I had already had relations with her sometime before, and I didn't want to go in. Maybe it was because of the crowd.

"I guess the first time I had a real relation was when I was around twelve or thirteen years old. It was with the maid next door. She was about sixteen or seventeen, and I remember one evening after she had put the child to bed, and the parents had gone to the show that evening, two other boys and I took her out in the back yard, and while one of us would have sex relations with her, the other boys would guard the front and see if the parents were coming back. I was a little afraid of this because there was a boy that had been going out with her, who was a strong fighter, and he would have beat the hell out of me. He had been going fairly steady with her—and having relations with her.

"And then when I was about thirteen or fourteen I went with two other boys to a house of prostitution. And the other boys teased me

---

[1] Again a significant lead, but one not exploited at the time.

because I wasn't as big as they were. I wasn't particularly anxious to have relations, and I didn't have any money, but the other boys put up the two dollars, and I went ahead. I remember it made me quite proud. It was especially satisfying, 'cause I felt that I had arrived at manhood. Anyway, I bragged a good deal about this to the other boys in the neighborhood." Patient X paused a moment and frowned. "I regret this happened. I feel that I lost something there."

"How did your parents feel about sex? Did they ever talk to you about it?"

"Sex was never discussed in our home. I remember when I was twelve to fourteen years old, I went in for a lot of kissing parties— you know, petting and necking—but when I got older, in my early twenties, I slept with a lot of women, one after another. I remember one particular incident which certainly scared me, although I didn't seem to be frightened at the time. I was picked up by a married woman, and I went to her apartment. After we were through, and I was only partially dressed, she looked out of the window and said, 'Good Lord! My husband is coming.' So I went into the closet and hid, and she closed the door. Her husband came in, and I heard them talking for a while. I guess the husband was a much larger man than I was. Anyway, I planned if he opened the door to the closet I was going to sock him and run. However, she induced him to go away, and after they left I came out and put on the rest of my clothes and beat it." He repeated two or three times, "I can't understand why she took such a big chance."

Patient X then continued. "I remember once I was going steady with a girl about the same age as myself. She came from a very nice family. There were two living rooms in the house, and while the parents would stay in one living room, she and I would have an affair in the other one. The parents were always very considerate and knocked before they entered. I guess they didn't know what was going on."

"How long did this continue?" asked the therapist.

"Oh, it went on for about a year and a half."

"Didn't you ever fear that you would be caught?"

"No, I never seemed to worry much about it. However, one time I left my coat with a condom in it on the stairway, and when I came back, her mother had discovered it. The mother was mighty upset, but she didn't tell the father. She refused to believe me when I lied like hell and said there was nothing between us."

"What finally happened to you and this girl?"

"Well, after about a year and a half I drifted away, and I think I was really in love with her at the time, but I wasn't in any condition to get married, and I didn't even consider marriage."

Two days later, November 16, X reported a dream which had caused him to wake up. He could faintly remember something about a girl on a doorstep, but he insisted the dream was not significant. He was unable to remember the rest of the dream, although he felt he should try to do so. Some time was then spent in rehashing the material he had revealed about his sex life during the previous session.

It was obvious by this time that Patient X's sex life had been a most dramatic one. We now had innumerable pieces to the jig-saw puzzle. Yet the kind of pattern they would form—how they fitted together—was still completely unknown. However, it was increasingly evident that much more than Margaret was at the heart of his phobia.

CHAPTER 22

CONFLICT: ONE BODY—TWO PERSONALITIES

In the analysis of Patient X's stories, which he devised to explain the Thematic Apperception Test Pictures, many contradictory trends were evident. Variations of projective technique were used to study these.

Session of December 4, 1945

The patient was placed in a deep trance in a period of one minute by the eye-fixation method and regressed back to the age of six. He named most of the children in the first grade of school. He was then advanced to his present age and was told the following story:

"There are twin brothers by the name of Melvin and George Amberson.[1] These boys look so much alike that people often mistake them for the same person. They are now young men. Melvin represents everything that is good in a man. He does what is right. George signifies everything that is bad and evil. He does what is wrong. These boys have many bitter quarrels. George tries to get Melvin to do the things he shouldn't, and Melvin attempts to reform George. Do you understand?"

"Yes."

"Now I want you to tell me more about Melvin and George. Imagine the story the way you want and dramatize the lives of these two boys."

Patient X then carried on as follows: "I am Melvin. I went to school, then to high school, then to college. I became a chemist, worked very hard in my life to achieve what I wanted. I am a chemist. There is nothing to look forward to except hard work. All my life I have been good to my parents and good to my family. I have tried to do right with others. I have never been able to gain anything in life, such as important position, or good jobs, or money. I have nothing but hard work to show."

X paused a few moments and then said, "I am now George. I went to high school, although I didn't go to college. I started to go

---

[1] This name sufficiently resembled the patient's real name to permit a ready identification.

to work, although I never stuck at it long. I traveled for many years —traveled all over the world—and have seen everything in the way of life. I speak several languages. All my travels are due to a man who was a big money man in the States. He owned a big armament factory which made small armaments—caliber arms and small rifles. I talked my way into his good graces, and by stepping on other people I finally became a big success. I married his daughter. I'm satisfied. I have lots of money, but I got it at the expense of others. My brother Melvin is still struggling and getting nowhere."

The suggestion was now made to Patient X that he describe more fully the conflict between George and Melvin.

He replied, "George wants Melvin to accept his money so as to open up a bigger plant and make a lot in the armament business. Melvin won't accept. George thinks he's crazy. Melvin says that everything should be clean, open, and above-board. Melvin won't have any part of it, because of all the things George has done to his family."

"What has George done to his family?"

"George did petty things and hurt them in many ways which he shouldn't have."

The patient was then shown picture 4 of the Thematic Apperception Test.

"You may slowly open your eyes, but stay in your sleep. As you open your eyes you will look at this picture, and you will be Melvin. You will be able to tell me a story of what has happened in the picture and what is going to happen—the way Melvin would see it."

Patient X slowly opened his eyes and shook his head a number of times, twisting the picture back and forth.

"I don't think there is anything good in this picture. Both the man and the woman portray hardship. She is trying to hold him back by some method, but he doesn't want to be held. George will be able to tell you much more about this."

The patient was instantly told to close his eyes and go back into a deeper sleep. He was then instructed to open his eyes and see the picture the way George would look at it—he would be George.

Slowly he opened his eyes and said, "This boy and this girl—she forced this man to marry her. For a while things went all right, and they were happy—at least he thought it was, but it really wasn't. He was much too fickle. He wanted other women, until finally she caught up with him, and he finally told her he doesn't want her. He is telling her that in the picture. She begs him to stay. Finally one day he fails to return to her. He goes away and doesn't ever come back."

"And what happens to the girl?"

"The girl gets a divorce. She married somebody else and starts to play around with other men."

Patient X put the picture aside. The therapist started to reach over on his desk for the next picture. He had told X to return into the deep sleep and had informed him that he was no longer George.

In a moment of confusion the therapist said, "When you wake up this time you will play the part of Melvin, *the bad boy.*"

Patient X reacted immediately and vehemently. "Melvin is the good boy. George is the bad boy." This reaction was offered with considerable emotional expression and great disgust.

The therapist immediately corrected himself. "Now you will open your eyes and be Melvin, the good boy." The patient was then shown picture 11 and he replied as follows:

"These are prehistoric times. There is a giant lizard at the left. Right over here are some animals. Naturally, the giant lizard is trying to get at them. He isn't able to get the animals, however, because they run out over the road, and they escape."

"Now you are forgetting about being Melvin and going back into your deep sleep. This time when you wake up you will be George."

Patient X slowly opened his eyes, and in an angry voice said, "There's nothing in this picture. What do you want to show me something like this for? It is ridiculous. Any one who would draw pictures like this must have his head in the fog. What the hell! This looks like a lizard. It's a stupid picture. I can't see anything about it." And the George personality threw the picture down. This was a most interesting response and quite in contrast with the behavior of Melvin. It takes on considerable significance when reviewed in the final solution of Patient X's problem. As noted before, the lizard's head and neck, the most prominent feature in the picture, is often associated as a penis symbol.

Next, picture 12M was shown to the Melvin personality, which responded as follows: "This is a sickly boy. He has been supporting his father and working very hard. He comes home at night. The old man doesn't like it because he has to work so hard. He is sickly too. One day the boy flops on a couch. The old man walks over to him and tries to soothe him. He wants to help the boy along. This is an intelligent boy, but he's working at a job that he's not fitted for; so the old man gets dressed and goes to the factory to talk to the foreman. He then gives the boy the right kind of job. The boy is very happy and successful and gets promotions and raises in pay."

To this same picture 12M, the George personality responded with,

"This is in a club house. This boy is traveling across the country. He has a few hundred dollars sewed in his shirt, but he doesn't want to spend it. The damn fool ought to know not to keep it there. The old man sees the boy and figures he might keep it on him because he looks good. He goes over and takes the money out of the shirt. The old man beats it. The boy wakes up and is broke. He goes to the police, but the police don't believe his story. They won't back him up. Instead they throw him for three days in jail as a vagrant. He wants to get back at the police, but he can't do it, and when finally they take him off to the city limits he goes away beaten and broken. He wants to do to others what they did unto him."

The session was terminated at this point. He was made amnesic for all responses evoked under trance, and then awakened. He had no recollection of anything that was said while asleep.

The differences in the stories given by the two personalities to the same picture make clearer the conflicting trends indicated by the patient's reaction to these same pictures in the conscious state as described in the previous chapter.

To Melvin, father-figures are kindly and helpful; to George, they are menacing. To Melvin, stories have happy endings; to George, they end tragically. To Melvin, heroes are hard-working, honorable people; to George, they are bums or hoboes with a bitter, cynical view toward life. Much of X's past career had been like George, but obviously Melvin, the Super-Ego part of his personality, had been severely condemning. And so there was inner conflict.

The next day, December 5, an extremely long session was held in further studying the relationship of the George and Melvin personalities.

Session of December 5, 1945

Patient X was placed in deep trance by the eye-fixation and metronome method after a period of some ten minutes. (He stated afterwards that it was difficult to enter trance at this time. These new projective techniques were obviously meeting with considerable resistance.) The following dialogue ensued:

W: Tell me about your feelings.

X: I have a feeling way down so deep as if there is not a care in the world—no worries. I feel in a really deep sleep.

W: Do you remember about George and Melvin?

X: Yes, I remember them. George—he was cruel and mean.

W: Now you will become George. You are now George. Tell me, George, what do you fear?

George : I don't fear anything.

W : Are you afraid of the dark?

George : No.

W : You're going to forget all about being George. You're going down into a very deep sleep, and this time you are going to become Melvin. Do you understand? Melvin, what do you fear?

Melvin : I'm afraid of George. He is cruel. He does things people wouldn't do. He picks on me. He tries to get me to do things I shouldn't.

W : Like what?

Melvin : He tried to get me to steal my father's car one night.

W : Did George ever try to get you to leave your wife and go out with another woman?

Melvin : No, but George is a very fickle person. George is not afraid of anything.

W : Are you afraid of George in the dark?

Melvin : I'm not afraid of George in the dark because I can see him.

W : Now you're going down into a very, very deep sleep. You will still be Melvin. I'm going to show you a picture, and I want you to tell me a story all about it. [This was picture 15 in the TAT Series].

Melvin : I can't understand this picture. Nothing in here to talk about. Evidently a graveyard caretaker among his tombstones. He is a very sensitive and evil person. He just looks like it. He spends all his life in a graveyard. He has gotten like a tombstone— mysterious and ghoulish. He goes among the stones at night like a miser and gloats over them. A silly picture—wonder who ever painted it. [He tossed the picture aside].

W : Now you're going to go back into a very, very deep sleep, and this time when you open your eyes you will be George. [The George personality was now shown the same picture, No. 15.]

George : This old guy is probably among all his relatives. He has some big estate. He's been burying all these people—could be his wives, half of them. Maybe he's sorry about it, though probably not; he killed so many of his relatives directly or indirectly. Nothing is too good for him. He probably ends up by committing suicide.

W : Now, George, I'd like to show you another picture. Tell me a story about this one. [George was shown picture 18BM.]

George : The painter didn't draw this picture right. Three hands and two hands. That's five. Couldn't be six or four—but that's five. [George looked most perturbed and began to count the hands again in a puzzled fashion. Then he continued.] This is a drunk. He's been on a binge for two or three days. The burglars are following him, and they're rolling him now. The police will pick him up and put him in jail. He's been there before. Just another stumblebum— no good.

W: Now you're closing your eyes and going back into a very, very deep sleep. You're forgetting all about George. You're turning into Melvin. You will now open your eyes and be Melvin. [The Melvin personality was now shown the same picture, No. 18BM.]

Melvin: He looks like he's being robbed. Some one is trying to take his money away from him, if he has any. He may be a habitual drunkard, just beaten and robbed—is found by the police and thrown in jail. They don't believe his story. He's been there before. Anybody who drinks like that deserves to be rolled for all he's got. [The patient paused.] I can't figure this out. What's this extra hand? [Melvin stared at the picture for a while. As there was no further response, the therapist reached over and started to take the picture. Melvin refused to relinquish it, but finally put it aside by himself.]

W: What's the difference between you and George?

Melvin: Oh, George is a normal person, but he don't like me. He's no good. He's got some good traits, but some of them are bad.

W: What are George's good traits?

Melvin: He's kind to dumb animals, maybe, but he's bad because he doesn't care what he does to you in order to accomplish his own ends. [Next the Melvin personality was shown picture 16, the completely blank card, and told to visualize a picture on it.]

Melvin: I can't see a thing—can't imagine a thing.

W: Try real hard now. Try to see something on it.

Melvin: I see a lovely girl or scenery or something out in the distance. There in the foreground is a cloud, a slight wind. It would spoil a picture like that if people were in it. Looks like some place I've seen. Looks like it would be Pike's Peak.

W: Now you are closing your eyes and going back to sleep—a very deep sleep. When you open them again you will be George.

[The patient slowly opened his eyes. The therapist looked over and said, "Hello, Melvin."

X replied in a very disgusted voice. "I'm George. You know I'm George."]

W: What's wrong with Melvin?

George: He's just a baby and hasn't learned anything yet—too good for his own good. I tried to straighten him out, but I guess he's going to have to be all right as he is.

W : Here is a card. It's just blank, but I'd like to see if you can imagine a picture on it. What do you see there?

George : I can draw a picture for you—want me to draw one for you? I'd like to draw something. [George started taking out his fountain pen. The therapist, in his desire not to have the card spoiled, said, "You can draw something some other day, George. Right now I just want you to describe what you can see there," obviously passing up an opportunity from the therapeutic standpoint.]

George : This is Palmer Lake—Broadmoor. Gorgeous. I was there when I was a kid years ago. I was there with all the family— father, mother, sisters, and brothers. Picnicking grounds are here. We had a big car, and I would drive it up to Pike's Peak. [The patient then tossed the card aside.]

W : George, did you ever have any experiences with women?

George : Yes, I remember when I was thirteen years old. I had an affair with the girl next door.

W : Did Melvin ever do anything like that?

George : No, Melvin never had any time for that. He doesn't believe in it.

W : Did you ever have a quarrel with Melvin?

George : Yes, I remember once he ruined my crystal set. He hit me back, and then I knocked him out. I'm not sorry.

W : Now you are going down into a deep sleep and close your eyes. This time when you open your eyes you will be Melvin.

[When Patient X opened his eyes this time he looked somewhat dissociated—as if he was not quite sure who he was.]

W : Are you George?

X : Yes.

W : Well, then where's Melvin?

X : He's around somewhere—I guess.

[The patient wrinkled his brow, looked around in a rather befuddled manner, and then shook his head. "Now, I'm Melvin— yes, I'm Melvin." The George personality seemed to be much more stable than Melvin. It was always easier to turn the patient into George than it was to change him into Melvin. In later sessions, when he was given his choice of being either one, he usually chose to be George.]

W : Do you remember an incident about a crystal set and a fight with George?

Melvin : Yes. He's a better fighter than I am. I don't have any resentment toward him. I kind of stay out of his way most of the time. [Shaking his head.] George keeps bothering me—trying to push inside me. He tried to dominate me when I was a child. He could run better and fight better.

W : Melvin, tell me, do you fear the dark?

Melvin : Yes, I am afraid in the dark.

W : You are now going to go down into a very, very deep sleep. Your eyes are closing. This time when you open your eyes you will be George. Who are you now?

X : I'm George.

W : What is it that Melvin fears in the dark?

George : I don't know. Melvin's a sissy, but I don't know what it is that he fears.

W : George, I'm going to remove the feeling from your right hand. We are going to take it away from you; so it will no longer be under your control, and it will write by itself.

George : No, here! Do it with this one instead. [X withdrew his right hand and thrust out the left hand. Accordingly, his left hand was anesthetized and the hallucination given that it was disconnected from the wrist. The George personality then looked at the hand and burst out laughing.] Look! I don't have any control over it. It's just floating out in air—isn't even connected to my wrist.

W : I am going to count up to three, and when I finish the count of three, George, the hand over which you have no control will write what it is that Melvin fears. It will write the word scrambled or backwards. One, two, three.

George's Left Hand (dissociated) : NAM WONK TNOD I. [This was, of course, "I don't know man" written backwards.]

W : Tell me something about Melvin.

The Hand : MELVIN IS WEAK.

W : What does Melvin fear?

The Hand : LIFE—LIFE IN GENERAL. TOO MANY SETBACKS.

W : Does this mean failure?

The Hand : NO. NOT ENTIRELY. FRUSTRATION.

W : What does this mean?

The Hand : BECOMING SUCCESSFUL.

W : I think now you're going to be able to write more about the deeper meaning of Melvin's fear.

The Hand : I DON'T—

W : You do too know—quit writing 'I don't know.' You know a lot more than you've been writing. Now get busy and write something important. [Whereupon The Hand started scribbling again.]

The Hand : A TERRIBLE BEATING.

W : What about a terrible beating?

George: I don't want to write with this hand any more. I want to write with the other one—the right one. [The patient then took the pencil in the right hand and wrote in an entirely different script.]

George's Right (undissociated) Hand: MELVIN WAS BEATEN TERRIBLY BY A GANG OF BOYS WHEN HE WAS 7. HE PUT UP A GOOD FIGHT BUT LOST. HE WAS LAID UP FOR TWO WEEKS. IT COULD MEAN—

[At this point the patient stopped writing and said, "I can't write any more with this hand." The pencil was removed from his right hand and returned to the still dissociated left hand where it finished the sentence. (See Figure 6.)]

George's Left (dissociated) Hand: MANY TROUBLES COMBINED INTO ONE BEING.

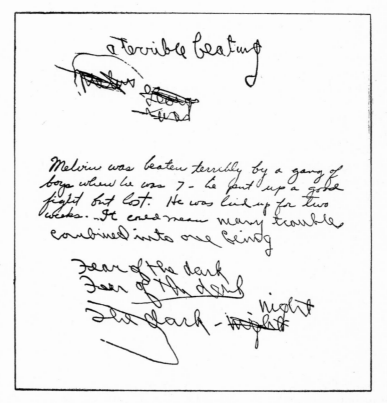

Figure 6. Handwriting Under Hypnotic Trance by George's Left Hand (Dissociated) and His Right Hand (Not Dissociated)

W : What are these troubles?

The Hand : FEAR OF THE DARK. THE DARK NIGHT. DEATH. A MAN DIED AND I SAW HIM BEING EMBALMED. DEATH. MELVIN AFR—DK.

W : Tell more about what Melvin fears in the dark.

The Hand : PROBABLY KILLED HIM.

W : What would probably kill him?

The Hand : I DON'T—

W : [breaking in again with simulated anger] Oh yes, you do too know. Quit writing 'I don't know.'

The Hand : NO. NO.

W : I'm going to hold this card in front of your eyes. You will open your eyes slowly, and you will see a dark grey field. Then something is going to emerge which is very significant in regard to Melvin's fear.

[George slowly opened his eyes and gazed at the card. The Hand started scribbling and scrawling all over the page. First it wrote out long lines of NONONONONONO, and then wrote, I DON'T KNOW. Next, the hand started to draw a picture twice, and then scratched it out. It had begun to sketch an evil-looking skull.]

W : What is this?

The Hand : [drawing an arrow pointing to the skull's mouth] A DEVIL.

W : Where did you see this devil?

The Hand : 8. [The Hand kept writing this figure 8 over and over again, tracing one eight over the other.]

W : Go on. That's fine. Tell me more about it.

[The Hand added a "1" in front of the "8" and a "4" after the "8," and then wrote a "7" after the "4." Then it changed the "7" into a "9." 1849.]

W : That's fine. Go on. Write some more.

The Hand : 1849 WINTER STREET, OMAHA. [City and street changed in reporting here to protect anonymity of the patient.]

W : What happened there?

The Hand : FUNERAL. DEAD.

W : Go on.

The Hand : A MAN DIED AND I SAW HIS BODY BEING EMBALMED. DEATH.

W : Were you afraid of it at this time?

The Hand : NO. I WASN'T AFRAID.

W : Can you tell more about it?

The Hand : I DON'T KNOW. I DON'T KNOW.

W : All right. Now you're going to go back into a very deep sleep. Feeling and movement are coming back into the hand. The hand is once more being connected to the wrist. You're going to forget all about being George or Melvin. Soon you'll wake up, and you'll feel very good. You will not remember anything that happened during this session. Now I am going to count up to five, and you will wake up and feel very good. 1, 2, 3, 4, 5.

X : My, I feel good. What time is it?

W : It's four o'clock.

X : Four o'clock. Ye gods! Where have I been the last hour and a half?

W : You've been asleep and resting.

X : Did I tell you about a lot of things?

W : Yes, you did, but it's getting late today. We'll talk about them some other time.

Patient X accepted this and departed in good spirits.

At the end of sessions like this one, the question often arose as to whether the material uncovered should be revealed to the patient and integrated into the conscious or used to provoke further associations at once, or whether it was better to keep the material from the patient for the time being until all ramifications in this area could be explored. This latter course was often taken on the theory that the revelation of the material already elicited would provoke anxiety and initiate greater resistance and blocking. The preferable course depends upon the patient, the session, etc. It is a matter of judgment each time— no one procedure is always best.

This session is an example of complex therapeutic technique. Combinations of projective methods were used simultaneously : dissociated personality, dissociated handwriting, scrambled words and card reading. Sometimes forcing methods were adopted to overpower minor resistances, with retreat into more nondirective tactics in the face of major resistance areas.

The next day, December 6, Patient X reported in an apparently happy frame of mind. The therapist looked over at him and casually remarked, "By the way, did you ever happen to know any boys by the name of Melvin and George Amberson?"

Patient X smiled. "Say, I know somebody by that name. It's been going through my mind for the last day. Did I dream them? Say, Watkins, have you been creating a new person? Huh! I know those names. They're related in some way."

The therapist asked, "Who would you think they were?"

X replied, "Taking a wild shot in the dark they might be brothers.

They're closely related, and they're related to me somehow. Maybe you've been planting those two people in my mind. They might even be me. In other words, you've been trying to give me a dual personality."

The previous session was now reviewed with the patient. He accepted the fact that, although the two personalities had been artificially created, there was inside of him a conflict, and that different parts of his own personality did identify with Melvin and with George. The implications of Melvin's and George's responses to the Thematic Apperception Test pictures were discussed, and also the relation these had to the stories given by X in the conscious state, as described in Chapter 21.

By the end of the hour the patient not only accepted but seemed quite willing to advance the concept that there had always been Melvin and George personalities within him and that the different desires and motives of these two were partially responsible for the conflict which he possessed. Only one other point emerged at this session. He admitted that in spite of his happy marriage he still had desires to "play around"—desires which he had made no attempt to carry out.

Session of December 10, 1945; Conscious Interview

"I had a dream. I was in some sort of school examination. We were getting our papers back with grades on them. I was sitting at a long table. All the papers were marked 'poor,' 'unsatisfactory,' 'bad,' 'no good.' My name was not on top of the paper. The name was blurred. I couldn't read it. I wonder if that name could have been George?

"By the way, did I ever tell you I had a brother by the name of Robert? He's a rather weak person. I beat him up once. I knocked him down."

No associations could be made to the dream, and no other important material emerged.

Session of December 12, 1945

"I had the same dream last night, only it wasn't in school. It was in some sort of a classroom, and I was sitting at a long table. We were getting the papers back from the test. They were all marked 'very poor,' 'no good,' down to the last paper. The name was blurred."

X was placed in deep trance and asked to visualize the dream once more.

This he did and added, "Here's a red check mark. It means 'very poor.' "

The therapist suggested, "Look up in the corner. See if you can see a name there."

"Yes, now I can see the name of George S——."

"Who is George S——?"

"He's a boy I knew when I was a kid. He was a mean bully. He's no good. He made us do what we shouldn't do." [2]

"What's that?"

"I don't remember exactly."

No other information could be elicited, so the session was concluded.

Session of December 14, 1945; Free Association Under Trance —Dissociated Personalities

Patient X was placed in a deep trance.

"Today you are free to talk about anything which comes to your mind. You may be either George or Melvin, and you can switch back from one to the other just as you wish."

"Oh well—how could I be Melvin at one time and George another? I think I'll be Melvin."

Patient X yawned for a while and then began, "I shouldn't have left the old Junior High School. I was cock of the walk there. I could have been student president. My name is Melvin Amberson. That's two names. I wish I was back in high school. Had the most fun. Used to be in charge of the school color-bearers. Had a lot of prestige in those days—captain of the athletic teams—fastest runner in school. They always chose me. What does it all mean after all? Doesn't mean a thing. What is there in life but a little bit of snatched happiness? Memories treasured—being carefree—doing what's right and not being overambitious. If I could only see and find pleasure in every little thing I would be happy—just little simple things of everyday living. Melvin wants more, not for himself so much, but to be able to walk the streets in dignity—people to look upon him as a good honest person—to consider him part of any community. George is too far away—out of sight and out of mind. I've got to face people—face myself."

---

2 Certain of the statements above have been italicized. These were points closely associated to the key to the entire problem. They show how often the heart of the conflict was touched upon—and then missed by both therapist and patient.

"What is it you can't face?"

"Lack of ability—no talent. I try to see how to live the simple life, and I can't see. I betcha down deep in George he's got a fear; that's why he puts on this terrific stunt. He knows that I know it. When he wants something real bad he gets it, but it's all front. My feet are on the ground—he's floating. I would like to have some of his skill about life sometimes, though. I don't have the knickknack. One must have the knickknack—even a child prodigy. I used to love the dark. There's a room in the cellar that was in the dark. Butch and his brother—I saw them drown. I saw their bodies. I ran home. Those bodies were awful. I don't want to go back. I can't go back."

"But you must go back. You must go back in your memory and see everything clearly."

"Their bodies are a big blot of green paint."

"Keep on looking down at them."

"There are flashing lights. I got sick that night. I ran home and threw up. I was afraid to go to the water."

"Was George around?"

"No, just Melvin. George was not around. Oh no, George wouldn't have stayed there, but he wouldn't have been afraid."

"You say George wouldn't have been afraid?"

"George. That's one of my names. He would kill me with a knife. I don't know. I can't stand knives. I feel fear when you mentioned this. I just came in the house. I saw my house had been ransacked. I wasn't scared until afterwards."

"All right. Now you're going to wake up. When you do you will remember distinctly everything which we talked about today. I am going to count up to five, and you will be wide awake and remembering everything clearly. One, two, three, four, five."

Patient X opened his eyes. All the material which had emerged was discussed with him. The George and Melvin personalities were brought somewhat more clearly in focus—especially the many fears held by Melvin.

Session of December 15, 1945; Free Association Under Trance-Dissociated Personalities

X was placed in deep trance again and told that he could talk about whatever entered his mind, and that he could be either Melvin or George, changing at will from one to the other. He clenched his hands, blinked his eyes, and then said, "I guess I'm going to be George. George has a sister—*George S*—has a sister too. He has two sisters. One is named Harriet, one my age and one much older. Harriet is about my age—eight years old. One day George S—and two or three other boys, whom I don't know, and Harriet went down to the railroad track. We were pulling a cart with an animal in it. We also had with us a small pup tent. We went down to the railroad track underneath a tunnel or bridge and set up the tent. Harriet got in it, and all the boys took turns going into the tent with her. I used to meet Harriet before at times and tried to have sex relations with her. I was the last one in the tent. I didn't do anything. I was afraid her mother would find out and hurt me. Even the crippled boy was carried into the pup tent. When he came out he said he couldn't do anything—that he was too big for her. George S— is certainly a dumb cluck about his sister. Anyway, it's none of my business."

"Are you still George?"

"Yes, I'm George, and I'm about fourteen years of age. I remember this happened in Omaha. Harriet was in Philadelphia. This little girl's name was Amy — Amy —."

"Do you think Melvin would know the last name?"

"I don't think so. Does a name mean anything anyway? I hate to tell you—I wasn't going to tell you this. My buddy and I, Jack Carr, we took that girl and had sex relations with her. She was only a kid not very bright, but was she stupid. She told her mother, and her mother went to the juvenile authorities. We were taken down and talked to by the judge. He gave us the devil. The man told us we've got to be good boys and that we had clean records at school. I certainly felt scared. I remember the day that trouble ended. It was such a relief—just like losing a load off my shoulders. I walked out of the court room into the sunlight."

"Did you feel guilty?"

"Oh, yes."

"Are you still George?"

"Yes, I don't feel like talking any more. What was that girl's name? Oh yes, it wasn't Amy, it was Marsha. I don't care now. What a funny person. Oh well, so it goes." And the patient laughed quite heartily.

"Suppose you turn into Melvin now and talk the way Melvin would."

"I don't want to be Melvin. I'd rather be George."

No other new ideas emerged. Accordingly, the patient was awakened and there was some discussion about how much more dominant the George personality appeared to be.

Session of December 17, 1945; Conscious Interview

"I had a screwy dream about a car. I was driving in my car at night. All of a sudden I came to a big hill. I couldn't stop. I looked over the steering wheel. I went rolling through the night. It was black, and then I woke up. I had that dream during an afternoon nap." No associations could be given to the dream. The patient began to describe another incident.

"The time that I was robbed, my mother was in the hospital, and I was going with a married woman. I took this woman home by myself. We went to bed. One time her husband wanted to fight. I calmed him down. He knew I was seeing her but didn't know I had sex relations with her. I had been gambling a lot with her at that time. I lost a lot of money—practically everything. Then this woman, she became pregnant, and she wanted to have an abortion. She told me about it and made an appointment with the abortionist. She had had one before, but that time by her husband. I felt real guilty. I was supposed to pay the $150 for the doctor, but I didn't have the money and couldn't get it. I had lost the money at the races gambling. I came home one night and told her that I would get the money the next day, but I never did."

"You say all this happened about the time your mother died?"

"Yes, Mother died about a month after I had the trouble with this woman. We had been together New Year's Eve—trying to knock it out. Mother died a month later, and three months after that I was inducted into the Army. When Mother became ill she had a malignant cancer. First it was a black growth on her toe. They took her toe off and put her in a home. She got along fine, and then it came into her leg, and they amputated the leg. I didn't know at the time that she had a cancer. When I found out I didn't tell my brothers or sisters. I felt guilty afterwards, because I had a car, and I didn't go to see her much. I didn't realize that she was sick (or I didn't want to). The day she died I went out that afternoon. She was unconscious. They called me. My cousin picked me up, and when I got there it was all over. I had to drive it out of my mind. I feel very guilty about it."

"Do you feel guilty about it because you had been spending time having an affair with the other woman—time which you might have spent with your mother?"

"No, I don't think that's the reason I felt guilty." There seemed to be considerable doubt about this point.

"Is there anything else that happened about that time?"

"Yes, that was the time my room was ransacked—I guess it was about the first time I was afraid of the dark."

Sessions of December 18 and 20, 1945

When Patient X reported today, he claimed that he felt somewhat better than usual. He had not been conscious of his fear. He then discussed his parents more in detail.

"I remember father was taken to the — Mental Institute in 1932; but he seemed to improve, and they took him home. While he was at home, I would always think about it before I went to sleep. I was afraid father would come in and kill Mother and me with a knife. The fear left me after he was taken to the hospital. You know, I thought about this the other night, and a nice glow came over me. It was a relief. I thought I must tell you, and then I forgot. This is probably the most important thing that I've told you. That feeling came back right now. I feel much better after telling you."

"Did you ever worry about becoming like your father? Did you ever think that you were the same kind of person as your father?"

At first the patient denied this but later admitted the possibility. His reaction to father images on the TAT test was called to his attention—Melvin's response to the picture of the old man bending over the young man.

("This is the young man—he is sickly—this is his father—*he is sickly too.*")

Since the reaction to this picture was a Melvin projection, the possibility was discussed that Melvin identified with the father even though George, the dominant personality, did not.

It was obvious that something significant had been dislodged during the session of December 18. On December 20 X reported that the night following the preceding treatment he had become terror-stricken and was unable to sleep until morning. He had a constant fear that there was a man with a knife who would stab him. He claimed that he had tried to bring out the idea that it was only his father, as suggested at one of the previous meetings, but it was with difficulty that he could associate this, and when he did, relief was only momentary. An uncovering session was then held.

"X, today you are going to be able to write automatically without being in trance at all. You're going to write while you are awake and out of trance. I shall hypnotize you first and dissociate your hand. When you are wide awake we will continue the session, but you will not have any control over your hand. It will write by itself. Do you understand?"

"Do you think I can do that, Doc?"

"Let's try."

The patient was then placed in deep trance, and the left hand was dissociated. When given permission to write, the hand wrote, "IS IT DARK?" and when asked what it was that X was afraid of, the hand wrote "SOMEONE." Next it started to write, "I DON'T," then it stopped and wrote, "A MAN." Without further prodding it proceeded to put down, "WHO IS IT? WHO IS IT?"

The patient was now told that he would be awakened and that he would have no feeling or control over his hand, which would write automatically. The hand answered, "OK." Patient X was awakened from trance.

"Gee, Doc, my hand feels very funny."

"Can you move it?"

The patient looked at it, seemed to try, then gave up. "No, it's all numb."

"Let's see what it will write."

X stared at the Hand in a fascinated manner while it drew a picture of a man on paper. After this the Hand wrote, "WHAT CAN I DO TO HELP X?" and a line was drawn over pointing to the figure. (See Figure 7.) Next the Hand wrote, "X NEEDS HELP," followed by "I WILL HELP." The Hand now proceeded to draw another figure of a man with a slanting forehead. After it the Hand wrote, "CAN THIS BE FATHER?"

Patient X looked at the picture and smiled. "That reminds me of a man I once worked for, who was unscrupulous. He ran a grocery warehouse. I didn't like him. I didn't approve of him or his wife, but I couldn't quit because jobs were hard to get. That was way back in the middle thirties. I had been working for around sixteen dollars a week—even though I was with him for two years. Sometime later this man wanted me to come back because help was scarce for that kind of work, which he said needed training, and he offered me thirty-two dollars a week, and then forty dollars. I turned him down. The more he offered, the madder I got. Finally I exploded and cussed him out and asked him where he got all his money, and whether he could face his children."

"Do you think this picture of a man is really that of the employer?"

At this question the Hand wrote, "YES, A PART."

Patient X commented, "It reminds me of me, and also of my father, and a lot of other people too."

The patient and therapist then discussed Melvin's and George's struggle. The point was brought up that the employer at the grocery warehouse was another individual who was unscrupulous, but who made a lot of money. Patient X emphasized how many shady deals this employer had pulled and remarked, "They call it business."

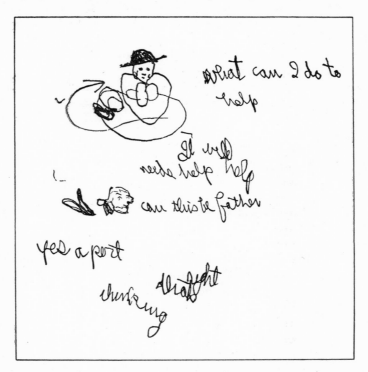

Figure 7. Automatic (Dissociated) Handwriting by Patient X When Not in Hypnotic Trance

"What did you do during these days—after you left that business?"

"Well, I worked for a taxicab company. I remember riding one day in a cab, and the driver told me, 'People look down on us for being cab drivers, but I like it because I am completely free. I have my car, and I can go where I want to.' This appealed to me, so I went down to the company immediately and applied for a job, and I finally became a cab driver. They gave me a cab for beginners first—to use in the daytime. I didn't make very much money. I tried very, very hard. I was conscientious. Then I noted that a lot of the other cab drivers would make money chiseling. They would overcharge the patrons—steal them out of house and home. I remember one man who charged a patron three dollars and a half to take him over a thirty-five cent route. Then I was transferred to the night run. I learned how to chisel too, and how to judge whether a patron would pay a lot and charge everything I could get out of him—especially out-of-town travelers." [3]

Some discussion followed about the relation of Melvin to George, and how, apparently, Melvin had charge of Patient X during the early period as a cab driver. George took over later and began to make a great deal of money in more unscrupulous ways. He was asked what attitude this symbolized in him.

He responded with, "I don't know quite what you mean."

"Well," continued the therapist, "let's let the Hand write."

Whereupon the Hand wrote, "DON'T DO UNTO OTHERS WHAT YOU'D WANT THEM TO DO YOU." The Hand then underlined the word "DON'T."

Patient X continued his associations. "I remember once I picked up a young woman. She was a prostitute, but I didn't know at the time. However, later I took her to a house, then I brought her some business. I was pimp for her. I know it's lowdown, only I did it just a few times. Then I decided it was rotten business, and I wouldn't do it any more; so I quit, and it didn't bother me any more."

"Are you sure that you really put it out of mind, and that it really didn't bother you any more?"

"Of course, I did. I quit it—didn't I?"

"Let's ask The Hand whether it's really out of your mind or not."

"If The Hand says I haven't forgotten it, The Hand is a damn liar, because I know it doesn't bother me any more."

The Hand began to move and form the following letters: "THOSE LYING IN MUD MUST CLEANSE THEMSELVES."

Patient X studied the writing of The Hand for a while and then cursed, "I'll be damned." Next he remarked, "Say, could you leave The Hand that way. It would be a handy fellow to have around with me all the time." Then he took his right hand over, affectionately patted the left hand, and said, "Nice work there, boy." The questioning was continued.

W: Do you have feelings of guilt bothering you?

The Hand: NO EFFECT ON MIND BUT HOW ABOUT THE HEART?

W: Explain this statement more.

---

[3] This incident in his life closely resembles the theme of the story he told to picture 6BM of the TAT pictures in the previous chapter. The hero struggles to succeed along approved lines and then turns to unethical behavior in order to achieve success.

The Hand: THE BEST THINGS IN LIFE ARE RESPECT, DIGNITY AND TO BE ABLE TO LIVE WITH ONESELF.

W: Who do you suppose wrote this—George, Melvin or X?

The Hand: GEORGE.

[It appeared rather astounding to both the patient and therapist that this one of his double personalities would be writing statements of this type.]

W: Tell me more about it.

The Hand: GEORGE NEEDS THIS. CAN GEORGE BE HAPPY? After a moment's pause The Hand answered its own question. NO.

W: Is this associated with the fear of the dark? Is it George's guilt feelings that perhaps are condemned by a punishing Melvin?

The Hand: YES, YES.

W: Can you associate any further to your fear of the dark?

The Hand: I WALK INTO A BLACK PIT BUT MY EYES CANNOT SEE.

W: Is this feeling of guilt and the punishment which might come from it the real reason for your fear of the dark?

The Hand: AMONG MANY, ONE. YES, ONE. IT IS A STRING ATTACHED TO A PUPPET—ME, GEORGE, MELVIN.

W: Do your many different personalities pull the string?

The Hand: YES, YES.

W: Can you expand this further and tell what else goes into your guilty fears—what other things are part of the phobia?

The Hand: FATHER, PREVIOUS JOB, NO HAPPY MEDIUM.

W: What do you mean by 'no happy medium'?

At this point Patient X broke in and began to talk. "You know —happy medium. That means ups and down—feeling of being highly adequate and at other times greatly inadequate." He paused a moment, and the Hand again started writing.

The Hand: LIFE IN THE FUTURE NOW THAT I HAVE RESPONSIBILITIES AND INADEQUATE ABILITIES.

W: Were you afraid that because you think you have inadequate abilities you may not be able to meet life squarely? Do you feel that you might resort to criminal or unethical methods in earning the things you want in life—and that if you do, you would be punished for this? Can this be what you fear?

The Hand: IT CAN.

W: What would happen to you if you did unethical things?

The Hand: I HOPE NOTHING.

W: What would your unconscious do to you?

The Hand: I HOPE MY UNCONSCIOUS MIND NEVER FINDS OUT.

W: What would happen if it did find out?

The Hand: AN UNHAPPY LIFE. It then underlined the phrase several times.

W: How many different things go into your fear of the dark?

The Hand scribbled a line up and down the page much like a bracket, apparently indicating all that had been written.

W: Can you tell me more about this?

The Hand: I DON'T KNOW HOW TO ANSWER YOU.

W: Do you think that because you feel inadequate you might do unethical things to get what you want?

The Hand: I CAN'T PREDICT SUCH THINGS. THE DARK IS AL-WAYS THERE. ONE CAN'T WALK WHERE ONE CAN'T SEE. IN THE SAME LANE AS WITH LIFE.

W: Why is it you can't identify the man in the dark who symbolizes your fears?

The Hand: RETRIBUTION IS UNKNOWN UNLESS IT HAPPENS.

W: What do you mean by that?

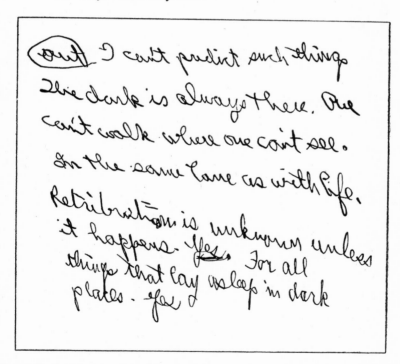

Figure 8. Automatic (Dissociated) Handwriting by Patient X When Not in Hypnotic Trance

The Hand: FOR ALL THINGS THAT LAY ASLEEP IN DARK PLACES. (See Figure 8.)

W : Is the man with a knife in the dark a symbol of retribution because retribution is unknown?

The Hand: YES.

Patient X was now placed in a deep trance. All this material was discussed with him—the feelings of inadequacy, the guilt associated with his life as a cab driver, the guilt for his many sex experiences, his failure to pay enough attention to his mother just prior to her death. All these matters were discussed under deep trance, and he seemed for the first time to accept the point that *he feared because he felt guilty.*

At this point X began to smile. He remarked, "I am very anxious to have you wake me up. I feel as if a great burden has been lifted." He was awakened and departed in a smiling, jocular mood.

In airing his guilt feelings and recognizing their connection to his fear of the dark, Patient X had pierced a significant point of resistance. He had taken a definite step forward—but stormy weather still lay ahead.

CHAPTER 23

THE KNIFE OF MR. Y

The day following the previous session, Patient X was supposed to have reported for another treatment. He did not show up. Later in the afternoon he telephoned and gave an unconvincing excuse. Another session was scheduled for December 23. Again he failed to appear—this time he had overslept. Another appointment was set the day after Christmas, but still another reason arose why the patient could not come.

Whenever a patient fails to report following a deep uncovering session, the following can often be inferred:

1. Something very significant was touched upon during the previous session.
2. This has initiated a great deal of anxiety.
3. This in turn has caused resentment to arise toward the therapist and has mobilized the patient's resistance. This resistance now manifests itself by causing him to avoid treatment.

Indeed it was the 28th of December before X was able to keep an appointment and return for treatment. The resistance was entirely obvious, and attempts to hypnotize him were unsuccessful. He entered only a light hypnoidal state and emerged from it within a minute or two. His actions of the previous week were reviewed with him, and it was pointed out that apparently something he wished to conceal was being threatened. The nature of resistance and negative transference was discussed. He seemed to be greatly interested. Toward the end of the hour there was an apparent change in the transference back to the positive state.

Just before the session was finished the therapist asked, "By the way, have you had any interesting dreams lately?"

"I believe I've had a few," returned the patient, "but I can't seem to remember any of them."

The therapist slowly closed the patient's chart, and without looking at him remarked, "I believe you're going to have a dream within the next day or so which will have considerable significance."

"What makes you think so?" asked Patient X in a rather startled manner.

"Oh—I just think so." (Here is an attempt to initiate a dream through suggestion in the waking state.) The next session was scheduled for December 31.

This meeting was not held. A dark cloak of resistance descended over X, and for nearly two weeks he became completely inaccessible. A session attempted during the first week of January proved to be entirely nonproductive. He bristled with antagonism. His anxiety was such as to prevent him from being hypnotized at all—and no attempt was made.

Since the patient's anxieties had become so strong, it was decided at this time that he should be relieved from the pressure of duty and be hospitalized as a patient. Accordingly, this change in his status was arranged.

On the 7th of January the next development occurred. X called the therapist that morning and requested an afternoon interview. His face was eager and smiling when he entered the office.

"Doc, I've gotta tell you about a dream I had. It happened five days ago—but I had to test it out myself. That's why I didn't show up."

Then X, with considerable gesturing, related the following:

"I dreamed that you were arguing with an unknown person. This individual was the man that I fear. I couldn't see his face—let's call him Mr. Y. Mr. Y kept saying, 'Give me a chance to prove that you do not need Lieutenant W. You should not go back to see him any more.' And while he would say that to me you didn't speak. You just stood there shaking your head rather slowly. This went on for quite a while, and finally I thought, 'I won't go back for treatment for a few days.' I was going to see what happened. Nothing seemed to happen—I didn't get any better—I didn't get any worse. I still had that same fear of the dark. Then last night I had almost the same dream again. You and Mr. Y were arguing, but this time you dominated him. I remember that you told me to return, and as you said this, Mr. Y faded away completely. This Mr. Y, this person I fear in the dark, he must represent my whole complex. I wish we could find out who he is."

"We've associated to your dreams before. What do you think this one meant?"

"I remember you said that a neurosis tries to direct the patient's attention away from the real trouble—you know, that mother-bird-and-nest example, which was in one of the first chapters of your book.

I bet whatever it is that makes me fear the dark is also afraid of you, and it is trying to get me to give up treatment."

"I think you have made a rather good interpretation. Why do you think that Mr. Y made such strenuous efforts to persuade you not to continue treatment?"

"It must be that we have got him cornered—that we are stepping on his tail. Maybe we are getting close to his hiding place, and that's why he is putting up so much resistance."

This was a good bit of insight. A patient is indeed much easier to treat when he has sufficient intelligence to recognize the significance of resistance and negative transference. The discussion of these phenomena held during the previous period of resistance was bearing fruit.

The notes of the previous sessions were then reviewed, and he was asked, "What seems to be the most important point that runs through all we had just uncovered prior to this period of resistance?"

"I guess it is that *my fear is a projection of guilt feelings.*" Patient X himself first mentioned this idea, but almost immediately afterwards retreated from it. However, by the end of the hour, after considerable more discussion, he again accepted this point and stated that he felt this to be a very significant advance.

The acceptance of this point, following the extended period of negative transference, was undoubtedly one of the most significant moments in the entire treatment. One important layer of resistance had been penetrated, and one very important piece of insight had emerged—*"My fear is a projection of my own feelings of guilt."*

Patient X felt guilty about many things, about his mother, his many sex affairs, and his unscrupulous treatment of some of the women involved, his rather shady record as a taxi driver. He was not proud of any of these parts of his life, and he felt guilty concerning them. These guilt feelings were projected into his fear of the dark. This much he knew—but the phobia continued. Something else, something deeper, lay at the basis of this fear, some guilt that he had not yet mentioned. The rest of the hour was spent largely in the conscious state discussing the significance of his dreams concerning Mr. Y.

"Do you think that Mr. Y is the man you have always feared in the dark?"

"I don't know. He could be or he could not be—but Mr. Y is sinister, he is the symbol of fear."

"What does fear make you think of?"

"I fear a knife from a man in the dark. Maybe it's something to be inserted into me—not a knife—but a part of action to guilt."

"Guilt for what?"

"I don't know—I wish I knew."

"X, do you remember the other day when we were discussing symbols in psychoanalysis—dream symbols? What did objects like a knife usually stand for?"

"You said that people commonly dream them to represent a penis."

"That's right. Now concerning this knife, you just made a very interesting remark. You said, 'maybe it is something to be inserted into me, not a knife, but a part of action to guilt.' Did you ever think that perhaps this could have some homosexual implications?"

Patient X frowned—there was just a trace of anxiety which swept across his face. He bit his lip rather promptly, and then remarked, "I never thought of it that way. I'll think of it." He did not seem to want to continue this discussion; so he was shown the picture that he had drawn under trance during the session of June 20th.

"What does this make you think of?"

"It looks like an animal with a wolfish look." Patient X turned the picture about, studying it carefully. "I used to have a childish fear of dogs. The whole key may lie in a dog. I used to have a dog called Buster. He was a mean devil. He fought with other dogs. I sicked him on some kittens, and he killed them. I got sick afterwards. It made me feel funny. I don't seem to feel any resistance to telling about this. It comes so easily. I wonder whether there is any significance to it?"

"Do you remember writing, 'I walk in a black pit'? What does that make you think of?"

"The black pit may mean my inadequacy—something I can't see— I walk in it alone. I guess the pit is life. Perhaps I can't see in life because of my own inadequacy. I'm unable to see life itself—that black is just a symbol of helplessness. Huh, isn't it funny that the hand writes scripture? I know that I don't normally talk that way."

X sat rather quiet, engrossed in thought. Casually he remarked, *"Wouldn't it be funny if Mr. Y turned up as a woman?"*

"You keep talking about your inadequacy. What do you mean by inadequacy?"

"I mean that I can't do things—you know—with my hands. I'm not skilled. I can't repair or make things like other people can." There was considerable hand contortion as a demonstration.

"X, did you ever notice that sometimes, while you talk to me, you seem to be washing your hands? Why do you do that?"

"I don't know—why is that important? I just seem to do it, that is all."

"A man moves his hands around like that when he is trying to wash something off them—perhaps something filthy?"

Patient X frowned. "That seems rather silly to me."

This line of questioning was now discontinued, and the patient was placed in a deep trance in a period of three minutes—there was now a period of increased rapport. The therapist said:

"Tonight you will have a most significant dream. It will relate to your attitude concerning the treatment and will also point toward your main problem. You will not remember my talking to you. You will not remember my having suggested this dream to you, but you will have the dream tonight and be able to report it tomorrow. You will also feel very good and have no sense of pain or headache when you wake up."

Patient X opened his eyes and sat up on the cot. "How long have I been asleep? Say, I feel pretty good." He looked over at his shoulder and rubbed it. "How did you know that I had a pain in my shoulder?"

"I didn't."

"Well anyway, you took it away, because it was there when I went to sleep."

Session of January 10, 1946

The state of high positive transference continued, and Patient X was rather enthusiastic upon reporting for this meeting.

"I had two dreams last night. They happened just before I woke up. I want to tell you about them. This was the second one. I was in a white room, and a lot of people were walking back and forth, passing my bed. I was in the bed. Then you came along and looked down and said, 'I'm going to make you go to sleep. You haven't slept well lately.' Then you started counting. You kept counting for a long time, and then you went away, and immediately came back, and you were dressed differently. The first time you were in a white suit, and the second time, in a dark suit; and then I remember I said, 'I can still recognize you.' Whereupon, you said, 'I want you to dream, and tomorrow when you come back to see me I want you to tell me all about it'; and then I answered you by saying, 'I'm going to dream something important.' At that point I couldn't dream any longer, but I woke up."

"What ideas come to your mind in connection with this dream?"

"Well, it signifies hospitals. They have white rooms. Oh, yes, I remember another dream I had. This was a battle dream. I was riding in a jeep with my sergeant, taking up some ammunition to a distributing point. We had not had good instructions from the advance party as to where we were. We were on a road in Italy, and there was an Army tank with a man standing up in it. He came by, and I asked him by waving my hand if it was all right to go on, and he waved me on by him. We skirted the tank, and it was a narrow road. Then we went on ahead until I suddenly realized we were in enemy territory. They started firing at our jeep. We jumped out on the side of the road. We were five or ten yards from the jeep, and there was a brick house there, a two-story house to my left. Half the roof was gone—half of one side was gone. Coming around the corner I saw a Jerry, and he didn't see me. He was crouching by the side of the building. Suddenly he turned and saw me and stood there frozen. In an instant I had my carbine on my hip pocket pointed right at him. I pulled the trigger—it wouldn't go off. He stood there, arms out, and then with a sudden motion he ran into the house quickly. Then my sergeant and I got up and came running back. We heard rifle and machine gun fire all around us, and we were running. I got hit, and then I woke up."

"Do you have any associations to this?"

"This is a true story. There was the tank driver. I feel a little hostile at him yet because he caused me to get shot up. He should have warned me. There were mines on the shoulders of the road, and it was dangerous. The sergeant was shot in both legs and the testicles. I always felt it was my fault. I got one letter from him that he couldn't use his legs. When I think of him I feel funny. Shucks, I don't know how I could get in touch with him—better write the War Department. I would sure like to know how he is getting along. This was a true dream all except in one respect. I actually shot the Jerry." Pointing with his fingers, Patient X said, "Ping, right through the forehead—it was sure a beauty shot. The sergeant and I were lying on the road. Two Jerries came up. One stooped down and asked me if I were Polish. I said 'No.' He asked me if I were American. He spoke in German. And when I said 'yes,' he didn't bother me. It was a miserable night. It happened on May 13, and on May 14 was Mother's Day. They picked us up at seven or eight o'clock next morning when our bunch advanced and pushed the Jerries out." Patient X stopped for a moment and appeared to be thinking rather quietly. Then he remarked, "Do I feel so guilty about this boy? You are the only person I have ever told this to. I shouldn't have let this happen if I had used my head. My chain of thoughts just don't seem to be right." He could not explain the dream further.

The patient was now placed in a deep trance.

"Can you tell more about what your dream in the hospital means?"

"Yes, the white rooms mean that I am sick. I am ill. I am in a hospital—it refers to my phobias."

"And what about the people walking in front of your bed?"

"Oh, yes, I remember now—they mean all my troubles. That's what they are. They're walking by. They want to help me. Huh, funny thing—troubles don't want to help you. Somebody is making them help me."

"Who?"

"You."

"What kind of troubles?"

"My whole life of troubles. Everything connected to me. They are on a string. They are connected into one cog, and you are in white and trying to help—to drive these people away. They disappear when you come along, and then when you put on a black suit, that means that some one is trying to drive you out. The black suit wasn't you, because I said, 'Oh yes, I can still recognize you.' But the black suit indicates to me that you are not so good. I can see evil in the color. It seems that you are not trying to help me at all. You have dark, black aspects. Dark means somebody is trying to dress you up as evil. But there is white underneath. I beat them to it. He can't dress you up."

Without stopping, the patient suddenly launched into the battle dream. "Why do I have to go forward? Why? Why? That's the second time I came close to death. Three times and you're out. I wonder why I was spared?"

"Does your being hurt symbolize anything?"

"It symbolized the fact that I was punished for my inadequacy. I have normal abilities, normal brain power—why does it fail me?"

"What do you mean by inadequacy? Do you get any associations in connection with it?"

"I can only see trees, tops of trees. It's a mountain in Colorado. It's up at Grant Lake. I went there on a camping trip. It was very nice." He then rambled on at length about his picnic in the mountains.

The therapist next prepared to continue the session as an "in-and-out" interview.

"Whenever I count up to five you will wake up; but any time that I tap twice with my black pen on the table you will immediately and instantly go back into a deep sleep. Do you understand?"

"Yes."

"One, two, three, four, five." Patient X opened his eyes. He was removed from the cot and seated in a chair beside the therapist's desk. The session was continued.

W: In the dream about the hospital—do you recognize any of the people who went by you as symbolizing any particular troubles?

X: I don't think I can. [The therapist lifted his pen—tap, tap. Instantly Patient X closed his eyes and entered a deep trance.]

W: Do you recognize any of the people who went by you as symbolizing particular troubles? [X could not associate in any way. Accordingly, the therapist counted, "one, two, three, four, five." Patient X opened his eyes and blinked. He looked a little bit surprised but didn't say anything.]

W: How did you feel when you lay out on that battlefield wounded?

X: Very peaceful, as if I wanted to accept my fate within. [The therapist again lifted his pen—tap, tap. Patient X's eyes closed once more, and he entered a deep trance again.]

W: Why did you feel so peaceful on the battlefield?

X: Oh, it's because until that morning I didn't seem to have any hope. It was very easy though. It wasn't as tough as I thought it was going to be—to die. I felt calm and resigned.

W: When did guilt about the sergeant first strike you?

X: It was about a week later—in the hospital.

W: Did anybody say anything?

X: A couple of officers came by and asked me how it came about that I was up so far. It made me feel bad because they were calling attention to my inadequacy.

W: One, two, three, four, five. [X opened his eyes.] Can you tell me more about shooting the German?

X: The carbine didn't jam. I actually hit the German—right between the eyes. [The therapist lifted his black pen—tap, tap. X instantly closed his eyes.]

W: Why did you dream that you didn't kill the Jerry?

X: Maybe I didn't want to kill him—still I didn't have any guilt.

W: What did this German look like?

X: He had a mustache—silly to dream about it—there is no remorse.

W : Is there anybody whom you know that has a mustache—somebody in the family?

X : No, but I had an uncle and cousin who had a mustache—but it didn't mean anything.

The session was concluded at this point, and the patient awakened.

"Say, Doc, have I been doing anything funny this hour?"

"Why?"

"I think I've been going into trance some."

"What do you think made you go into trance?"

"It had something to do with that black pen of yours. I know I would feel a little uneasy when I saw you pick it up—I didn't want you to pick it up."

X was told about being linked to the black pen and reassured concerning it. He was placed back again in deep trance, and the black pen suggestion was removed. He exhibited no anxiety when he departed.

Session of January 14, 1946; George, Melvin, and X Hold a Conference

The first thing X reported at this meeting was the reappearance of a fear the previous night. He was unable to open his eyes. He knew he was not asleep. He was awake, but his eyes were closed, and they kept sticking together. He said that he had previously experienced this same fear last September. Last night, however, it had returned in a most acute form. He had been unable to sleep throughout the entire night. He also mentioned that he had experienced several dreams during the few periods he could doze fitfully. He was unable to recall any of them. He was placed in a deep trance after considerable resistance. Under trance, he could easily recall the dreams which he could not remember in the conscious state.

"Would you tell me what it was you dreamed last night?"

"I dreamed I was talking to a man who was eating peaches."

"Peaches—what about peaches?"

"Wheelbarrow—the man was eating peaches out of a wheelbarrow, and he had eaten all of them."

"What associations come to your mind in connection with this dream?"

Patient X refused to associate but immediately launched into a description of another dream. Quite often he would do this. He would not associate to any one dream until after he had first related several—apparently all that had occurred the previous night.

"There was a big black bird flying through the air. I tried to catch the bird, but I couldn't."

"Who did this bird represent?"

"He was Mr. Y—some kind of enveloping power."

No other associations could be secured at this time; so a complicated projective technique was tried.

"Your right hand is losing all sense of feeling and movement. It is no longer under your control. Now it is under the control of George—the George personality. It will write whatever George wants to say." This was accompanied by rubbing the hand and the usual suggestions hallucinating the hand away from the wrist. The same suggestions were then repeated with the left hand. He was told, "Your left hand is now no longer under your control. It will write only for Melvin."

The patient was next told, "In a minute I shall wake you up. You and I will continue our discussion, but you will not have control over either of your hands. George will write with the right hand, and Melvin will write with the left hand. They will make their own comments independently of you or of each other, and can do so whenever they wish."

The patient was then seated at a desk, pencils placed in each hand, and sheets of paper conveniently arranged. He was then awakened. He seemed a bit surprised and stared in a puzzled manner at the two hands over which he had no control.

The George Hand: WHERE IS X?

W: X can speak with his mouth. You are not in trance now. You're wide awake. You and I can talk as usual. Only your hands are not under your control. The two hands will write for George and for Melvin. Do you think maybe George might be able to interpret some of your dreams further?

The George Hand: THE MAN IS EATING ALL THE GOOD THINGS THAT BELONG TO X. X HAS MANY ABILITIES BUT CAN'T BRING THEM TO LIGHT. [There was a close natural association between "peaches" and the true name of Patient X.]

W: What about the man in the dream?

The George Hand: THE MAN IS [The hand filled in a small space with black pencil lines and then continued writing.] DARKNESS, BLACK, BLACK.

The Melvin Hand: [This hand drew a picture of a peach and labeled it. Then it wrote.] WHY DOES X FEAR?

The George Hand: BECAUSE HE IS AFRAID OF HIMSELF.

The Melvin Hand: DOESN'T HE HAVE WHAT EVERYBODY ELSE HAS?

The George Hand: X IS A NORMAL SENSIBLE MAN WITH NATURAL INCLINATIONS FOR THE PROPER METHODS OF LIFE. FRUSTRATION AND INFERIORITY COMPLEX WILL NOT HELP HIM.

W: Do you notice the significance, X, of the dream choosing peaches to symbolize your various abilities and possibilities? It's associated to your name, isn't it? What relation do you think all this has with your feelings of guilt?

The George Hand: IF A MAN DOESN'T TAKE ADVANTAGE OF OPPORTUNITIES GIVEN HIM HE DESERVES NOTHING. LET THOSE WHO FEEL GUILT SWIM IN THAT GUILT.

The Melvin Hand: WHAT ARE THE OPPORTUNITIES?

The George Hand: WHAT DIFFERENCE DOES IT MAKE AS LONG AS HE GETS WHAT HE GOES AFTER? KILL OR BE KILLED—MELVIN WOULD SAY THAT WAS WRONG. HE'S NUTS! IT'S JUST A PHRASE LIKE EAT OR BE EATEN. THE STRONGEST SURVIVE.

X: The numbness is going away out of the Melvin hand. I think it's gone entirely now. It feels perfectly normal. [X lifted his left hand, opening and closing the fingers.]

W: Is the George hand still numb?

X: Yes, it is.

W: I think it will go on writing significant material then. [The patient and the therapist held their breath, and both looked at the George Hand. Nothing happened.]

W: I think maybe George might tell us more about the guilt feelings.

The George Hand: YES, OF COURSE—WHY CAN'T YOU SEE THAT YOURSELF. CAN'T YOU UNDERSTAND. WHY GO ON WITH THIS NONSENSE? [Both X and W stared at the hand in astonishment.]

W: Is George angry?

The George Hand: YES.

The George Hand was then reassociated by merely rubbing it until feeling and movement were restored. After the hand had been connected again to X, the therapist and the patient began discussing some news events of the day. While this was going on the George Hand started "doodling" on the top of the sheet of paper. X seemed to be paying no attention to it. The Hand first made an 8 and two zeros, then a picture of a house, an odd pattern, some circular scribbling, a picture of a funny old man, and a circle. (See Figure 9.)

"X, look what your hand is doing."

X glanced over and remarked, "What about it?"

"Doesn't it seem a bit odd that it is making all that doodling on the paper? Does that mean anything? Can you think of anything in association to those figures?" X tried but could not associate in any way to them.

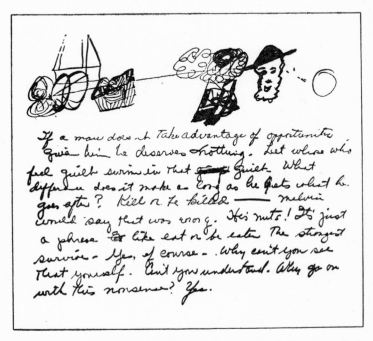

Figure 9. Dissociated Handwriting and "Doodling" Performed by the "George Hand," Patient X Being Out of Trance at the Time

The patient was now placed back on the cot, and a deep trance induced. "You will open your eyes while staying asleep and look at these funny pictures that you drew. What do they make you think of?"

Patient X opened his eyes and gazed at them. "Nothing—I can't think of anything."

To be certain there was no trace left of the dissociated hands, these were now specifically removed by direct suggestion.

"Tonight you will have another dream. This will indicate still further the nature of your guilt feelings."

"I think it's a good idea. I don't want to forget the dream. I'm going to take a paper and pencil to bed with me."

"Do you think you could associate any more ideas in connection with the two dreams you told me? What about the bird—you said something about an enveloping power?"

"I don't see anything about the bird now. I remember something, though, that happened the other day. I was out walking in the dark, and suddenly I had the feeling that Mr. Y was there, but Mr. Y no longer had his knife."

The therapist repeated this in a nondirective manner. "Mr. Y has lost his knife?"

At this moment the patient became very excited. With raised pitch and a voice filled with emotion he repeated, "Mr. Y has lost his knife. Why didn't you tell me this before? Mr. Y has lost his knife."

The therapist asked, "Why has Mr. Y lost his knife?"

Patient X merely continued to repeat, "Mr. Y has lost his knife— Mr. Y has lost his knife." Suddenly he sat up on the cot with his eyes wide open, emerging instantly from a deep trance.

"I've got the most wonderful feeling, the most wonderful feeling I've had for a long time. *Mr. Y has lost his knife.* Now I can handle that guy. I feel as if a great weight has been lifted from my shoulders. I'd like to find a dark place right now. I want to try it out. I'm sure I'm not going to have any more fears."

The therapist tried to quiet his enthusiasm. "Better not be too optimistic. You've had feelings something like this before."

"Never like this before. This is important. Mr. Y has lost his knife."

"Do you think perhaps this means that part of your fear is gone? Maybe it represents a partial gain in insight because you now realize that guilt feelings are at the basis of your fear. Recognition of this point may have reduced the fear symbolically by causing Mr. Y to lose his knife—thus making him a less fearsome creature."

"Yes, maybe that's true. Maybe that's what caused it. I only know that I'm happy—that I'm not afraid. I can handle that guy. This is the most important thing that has happened in the whole analysis. *Mr. Y has lost his knife.*"

CHAPTER 24

DREAMS OF FEAR

Mr. Y had lost his knife, but he had not yet disappeared. When Patient X reported for treatment again ten days later, his anxieties and fears, though greatly improved, continued to exist. However, instead of a severe manifest reaction, he now began to exhibit his difficulty symbolically through dreams.[1]

Sessions of January 16, 17, and 21, 1946

The patient was placed in a deep trance. He then related the following:

"I had a dream last night. I saw what appeared to be a horse. Sitting on the horse was a man. When I got closer, I saw he was made of wood—but he functioned as a person. I was trying to get over a fence when I woke up. The horse galloped off. I'm hazy about whether the horse was made of wood or not. Then I also dreamed that there was a live horse, this time a very huge one. I tried to get on him, but I couldn't. I forgot to tell you I've been feeling a lot better since the last time."

"What ideas do you associate to this dream?"

"The thing I've been worried about—I saw it—it's not real—it's not a live animal. He had a black face and a long stick for a head. Huh, sticks don't mean anything."

"What does the fact that he was made of wood, sticks of wood, symbolize to you?"

"Sticks don't mean anything—I've been looking at the wrong side of the picture. That was Mr. Y, and I don't have to be afraid of him."

"What do you think Mr. Y's knife stood for?"

"I don't know, but he's lost it anyway. You made him lose it. You hit a certain valve, and the guilt is gone. I'm not trying to hold that back any longer. These guilts are hidden now, and I won't be able to see them any longer. We can keep them down."

---

[1] This phenomenon often appears in the late stages of depth therapy, especially in obsessive cases.

"Perhaps it would be better to release them and bring them out in the open rather than keep them down."

X then associated to the second dream as follows:

"The horse seemed disgusted with me. I couldn't get on it. Maybe this means I haven't completely cleared up my problems. Yes, that's what it means."

At this particular moment a knock sounded on the door. It was the company clerk with the information that the therapist was wanted on the phone.

"X, I shall be gone for five minutes. While I'm away you can have another very important dream. You can tell me about it when I return."

Five minutes later, Patient X related the following dream:

"I was in a drugstore—people all sitting at the counter ordering things. One person behind the counter is a girl. She is redheaded and very busy. She is by herself. She reminds me of my first wife."

"What do you mean 'she is very busy'?"

"She needs help."

"Who should help her?"

"Not me."

"Do you have any guilt about not helping her?"

"Only that I ever undertook such a marriage. It hurt too many people."

"What else do you see in this dream?"

"That's all there is. I'm not afraid any more, though, because people are not standing behind my back. They're not talking about me any more."

"Why do you feel this way?"

"I don't know. I just don't feel suspicious of others. Maybe it has something to do with Mr. Y losing his knife."

"You will wake up and feel very good. You will remember everything which we have discussed today."

The next day, January 17, the session was spent in a conscious review of all the various incidents about which the patient felt guilt. There seemed to be a certain gain in insight. A new motive had recently entered his life. He had become increasingly interested in taking advantage of the "G.I. Bill of Rights," returning to college, and becoming an athletic teacher. He exhibited considerable confidence in his ability to achieve this goal. This new motive was encouraged, and he was directed to sources of information. This constructive drive, coming when it did, was evidence of increased strength.

When the patient came in on the 21st of January he complained of back pains. He had wrenched his back the previous day while engaged in sports. These pains were apparently organic in nature. He stated that he had been meeting Mr. Y some in his dreams, but Mr. Y was not a threatening creature now. He was unable to remember specific dreams. When placed in a deep trance he still reported no dreams. The session was spent by the patient under trance, integrating past material without assistance. It was handled as follows:

"X, you are completely free to review the entire treatment up to this point. You can flit back through your mind and pick up the significant matters. You can then summarize to yourself the progress that we have made. I shall let you sleep a long time. At the end of this period, you will understand what areas need further exploration."

X was then permitted to sleep for forty-five minutes. At the end of this time he was questioned concerning his conclusions.

This session may have brought about better integration through a review of previously uncovered material, but nothing new emerged. He said that the most important point was Mr. Y losing his knife and indicated that this symbolized the loss of guilt feelings to him. He claimed that he could now understand himself better. He then suggested that we explore further:

1. The area of guilt and feelings of inadequacy still remaining
2. Mr. Y

When asked about sex, he said he did not believe it to be an important factor. It was suggested to him that he would have another dream which would point to a significant area needing exploration. Following this, he was given suggestive treatment for the pains in his back. When he awoke, he said that his back pains were gone.

Session of January 22, 1946

X could report no dream in the conscious state, but when placed in deep trance he described one as follows:

"I was running through doors chasing somebody—I don't know who it was. They were running ahead of me. We came to one door. He was holding the door on the other side. I looked through the keyhole and saw an outline. I gave one big pull, and the handle came off. I heard some one laughing and yelling. Then I woke up. I wasn't afraid of him, though."

In his associations it was obvious that this was Mr. Y whom he was chasing. Attention was called to the point that now he was chasing Mr. Y, whereas six months ago Mr. Y was chasing him with a knife.

He then said, "I think that's the key to the whole situation, and the door represents something that is closed." He further added that, "The handle represents something that is holding out."

He was now questioned about other dreams. At first he claimed that there were no others and then said, "Yes, I do remember one now. I dreamed of a tiger."

"What about the tiger?"

"Oh, there's nothing to it. You wouldn't care to hear it. It's a silly dream." (Obvious resistance.)

"I don't mind listening to a silly dream. Let's hear it."

"Well, OK. There was a tiger driving a taxicab. I got into the cab. He wouldn't let me go where I wanted to go. He jumped in back. He was biting me and clawing me. I woke up. I wanted to go some place. I don't know where."

"What does 'tiger' make you think of?"

"Maybe the tiger could mean another part of me—jumping on me to tell me to stop. I was fighting myself."

"What part of you could the tiger be?"

"It might be George."

"Do you think maybe this also indicated that the time in your life when you were a taxicab driver needs further exploration?"

"It might be. Oh yes, now I remember another dream. I was walking along a bridge. Suddenly I fell. I was falling—falling—falling. Then I woke up."

"What do you think of in connection with this dream?"

"I can't think of anything in connection with it—oh, but I remember another dream now. I was running along the street—along the car tracks. I couldn't move, and a street car was coming."

"What do these dreams of falling and of being chained to street car tracks symbolize?"

"I guess they mean fear—I fear something."

"What parts of your life do you think we should explore next?"

"I would go back to Margaret. I would also go back to the time of my father. I was always afraid that he would do something drastic when I was asleep at night. I can control a taxicab, but I can't control my father—I don't know what he would do with a knife."

"Do you think that your father might be Mr. Y?"

"It can't be one person. We have already established that it is many—or are we wrong?"

There was then some discussion concerning the symbolism of knives—because they could be inserted into a person—like an erect penis. He agreed that this was possible, and then said, "I have always been afraid of knives." Further discussion followed about how "we have now (emasculated) Mr. Y by removing his knife from him."

Patient X was now regressed back to the time of Margaret, and he said, "She came out of the corn patch all dressed up. She had a beard, black hat, and cane [Note "doodling" of the George Hand in Figure 9, page 308], and I didn't know until later that it was really Margaret."

"When did you know?"

"After they told me."

"Who?"

"Everybody. I was afraid though, and I wouldn't go out. I wouldn't believe them."

"Did you actually see her removing the clothes, so that you would know that it was Margaret and not an old man?"

"No." (Apparently the memory as adjusted last April had not continued in the recall form—under trance.)

"You said that Margaret was dressed in black. Is Mr. Y dressed in black too?"

"Yes, but Margaret had a cane, no knife—huh, a cane could be a knife. There is a certain fear of it just the same."

"Isn't it possible that a cane could symbolize a penis as well as a knife? Did you ever see Margaret undress in front of the group and remove the old man's clothes?"

"Oh yes, I remember now. It was Margaret and not an old man. I remember distinctly. I saw her take the clothes off in the parlor." (The "adjusted" memory now asserts itself.)

"What else do you think we should discuss?"

"I think we should talk about the time of the taxicab driving, about Father and his knife, and about the Margaret situation."

It was now time to end the hour; so the patient was given a post-hypnotic suggestion that he would remember everything that had been discussed. Just before he left he made the following comment: "I never told you this before, but a few houses from me there lived a beautiful woman. She had two children. She tried to seduce me. I resisted her. I was very interested and did some sleuthing. To my knowledge I was the only person to whom she had made advances. I resisted her—now, I wouldn't resist. She had poise, character. Men were 'nuts' about her. For some reason or other she was attracted to me. She was very beautiful. I always thought of her in a kindly light."

"When did this happen?"

"Oh, this happened a long time before I was a taxicab driver."

Session of January 23, 1946

X claimed today that he had not been sleeping well. He had suffered for three nights with the back pains. The pains seemed "to be going down into the left testicle," and he felt they were getting worse and not better. He then revealed another dream.

"I was going to some type of school. My brother also was attending this school. Mother came to see us. She wanted to leave us. I told her that a place was hard to find, and I gave her the best possible directions. She left. I received a call from the principal of this school, who wanted me to take charge of a parade. While going downstairs I met my brother, who was on the steps. We exchanged greetings. He was in the line with a number of students. He had books under his arm. I went to the principal's office. He told me I was to take charge of a company. I then found myself in military clothing, all dressed, but the other companies and students were dressed in civilian clothes.

"Suddenly the parade leader, who was dressed in a pair of slacks and sport shirt, ran out in front of his company and started to form all the groups of companies. Mine was at the extreme end. The man who was assisting me started to run toward them. My legs couldn't move. I got tired and couldn't run. I told him to go and form the parade. Then I heard a voice off to my left, coming from a very old house, calling my name. The house was so dilapidated that it had very little sides or front. All you could see was shingles tacked together like a car shed. It happened to be my mother who was calling me. She was walking toward me saying that she couldn't find our house, and she was sorry that she had ever left home. They were calling me back to the parade. I didn't know which way to turn. I told her to wait, and I would come back to her after the parade."

"Can you interpret your dream?"

"I don't know. My brother was a grade below me in school. I was the captain of the color guard. The main fact is that I was in military clothes, and I didn't want to be."

No important associations could be secured. However, concerning his mother, he mentioned that she was "a guiding hand." The next day, January 24, he was able to associate more to the dream, and he said regarding the principal, "He knew I could do it. He wanted me to try out leading the companies."

"Who is the principal?"

"Maybe it's you—I remember my brother on the stairs with the students. He wanted to say hello. I'm proud of the fact. I always wanted his approval. He respected anybody in a position of leadership." (Notice the close identification of the Melvin (Super-Ego) personality within the patient to his brother, who was a weaker person physically but whose approval the patient wanted.) "I think the people on the stairs symbolize my admirers and the folks who would think I was a big shot. My brother, he probably thinks I'm a sucker—I didn't really mean that. You know, my brother can run real fast. I remember I chased him once, and I caught up with him, because I could run faster. Everybody said, 'whew, look at him run,' and they admired my ability to run fast. I think seeing my brother on the stairs symbolized to me the admiration of other people. It meant that I was a great man walking down the stairs. I remember one time when I chased my brother. He hid in the dark—in the evening—behind the fence; so that I wouldn't find him. I stumbled over him though. I didn't hurt him. I just let him go."

"What does the idea of the civilian costume mean to you?"

"I guess it's that I want to get out of the Army. I think leading the parade means my life work. I knew I could do it if I could only get to it."

"What do you associate to the old house?"

"That seems to be my mother."

"Do you think it could mean your mother's body?" (She was very sick and died of cancer.)

"Yes I guess that's what it means. You know, you ought to be a dentist. You have the ability to pull things out of people. I remember I felt pretty guilty about leaving mother—going back to the parade."

"Do you think this meant deserting your mother? In real life you planned to go back to her, but she died in the meantime?"

"Yes, that's what it means. That old house is the symbol of our home, very dilapidated and broken. I didn't get to leave the parade of life and return to her."

The symbolic representation of a person by a house is common in dream work. The individual is then characterized by the house's condition.

Session of January 24, 1946

The day was spent in a conscious review of the last five sessions, especially the preceding one concerning the matter of guilt for having neglected his mother. The patient had mentioned the need to sell his car. It was a rather flashy, big car. There was some discussion today concerning the fact that the car was a "front"—it was George —"trying to be somebody I'm not." The therapist suggested to him that the car served as a crutch, a crutch for his feelings of inadequacy, and that it was interesting that now he was beginning to feel strong enough to do without it. In his desire to go to school, the patient felt that he needed the money rather than the prestige of the car.

Another session was held on January 25, giving reassurance and integrating on the conscious level material uncovered in the last few hours.

Session of January 28, 1946

Patient X could recall no dreams and reported no anxieties or fears over the weekend. He was placed in deep trance and told that he would dream for five minutes. He was informed that he would dream something about the present progress of the treatment and where Mr. Y was now. After five minutes he was asked whether he had finished his dream. After replying in the affirmative he described it as follows:

"I was walking down a straight road as far as the eye could see. Suddenly it became very dark. I couldn't see a thing. For a moment nothing affected me, and I suddenly began to feel a change of thoughts. I became hysterical, fought myself to gain control. I knew that I couldn't go back—had to go ahead. I was afraid to go on—almost became panicky. Then it suddenly became light, and I walked along. I walked along this road. It was a beautiful road with flowers on the side. The air was fresh and clear, and I came to a house. It seemed as though it were suspended in midair. I couldn't resist entering. When I went in there was nothing there—no foundation and no furniture. It was a desolate hall, but I found a staircase, and I climbed it. On the second floor I came to a door. It was the only door upstairs. I opened it and went in and saw a beautiful room, gorgeously furnished, sofas and furniture. There was a fireplace in it, flowers around it, and big rugs on the floor. Over in one corner was a desk. In another was a typewriter. I went over and sat down and looked out the window, and I could see the ocean, a beautiful body of water. I sat down to typewrite. I typed continuously for a long period of time, and the words kept pouring out on the sheet of paper. Suddenly I stopped and took the paper out of the machine; and when I looked at it there was nothing on it, and then I knew I'd forgotten something. There was no ribbon on the typewriter."

"What do you associate to this dream?"

"Well, the road is a path that I am to follow. It's straight. It's got a definite aim. It's a definite purpose, like becoming a teacher. The dark—that's the trouble that is going to beset me. I will have to fight it, overcome it—like these fears. The light means successful handling of these fears. That's the beautiful day. The house is a structure, my own structure because it doesn't have any foundation to it. It's suspended in the air and shaky. The first floor is pretty vacant. I must build my house from the ground up. The first floor is empty and doesn't have any furniture in it. That means my background."

"What about the stairs?"

"I can't think anything about them, but the typewriter is a symbol of my ability, and the work will disappear because of my own negligence. I failed to foresee and provide for this."

"Did you have any fear in the dream?"

"Only when my feet were chained."

"I'm now going to count up to ten. When I do you will dream again about Mr. Y. One, two, three, . . . ten."

Patient X began to twitch all over. He started with anxiety. He exhibited tremors, and his breathing came in a labored manner. This continued for a minute. Then he would relax; then it began again and would disappear once more after a minute or two. Finally he began to talk.

"I was standing in a big place or field—like a desert. In front of me were a dozen different lanes or roads. I wanted to go on one of them and get some drinking water, because I was getting right thirsty. I started down the one on the extreme left and had gone about ten paces when suddenly a fierce animal appeared in front of me. He had bared his teeth and grimaced at me. I ran back. Then I tried each one of the roads, and each time there was the animal, and he showed his fangs and wouldn't let me go through; so I came back and lay down on the ground. I was very, very thirsty, but I didn't really care. I couldn't go on. That was all."

"I think maybe you can add more to this dream. Do you want to go back and finish it? You can describe it as it is happening."

"I'm very thirsty, but there is a little girl coming toward me. She's taking me by the hand. She is taking me out of the woods, but I can't stop her. Nothing can stop her; but there is no animal, and we come to a light spring, and I kneel down to drink. I look in, and I see the face of the animal. I look in again, and only the little girl looks down. The animal is gone. I drink, and the little girl is gone now, but I don't care because I can go on by myself, and the water is so very, very good."

"What does the little girl make you think of?"

"She is the helping hand."

"What do you mean by the helping hand?" (X had previously referred to his Mother as "the guiding hand.")

"It's you—and others. Some one to guide me. She's just a little baby. What a little girl should do, I should be able to do. She needs to be led herself."

"Can you think of anything else about her?"

"No, she just means the helping hand—oh, but I see a beautiful horse, a beautiful animal. He's that big black horse again, isn't he?"

"Yes, he is. All right, you're going to catch him and ride him. He is coal black. There is nobody on him."

"I don't think I can catch him. I'm trying to catch him. I've got hold of his nose, but he keeps moving away and in a circle—running away. Now he's gone. I would just rather watch a horse like that. I knew I shouldn't try to ride that horse. He was very beautiful." Patient X turned his head reproachfully toward the therapist, "You said to ride him."

"Why don't you try to ride him again?"

"I wouldn't hurt him, but I can't see him any more."

"I'm going to count up to ten once more, and then you'll have another dream regarding Mr. Y. one, two three, . . . ten."

After X had dreamed for five minutes, he began to relate the following: "I was in a party, a Hallowe'en party. Everybody was there. I knew them even though they had their faces covered with masks. A girl came up to me and took me by the hand. She was in a mask, and she said, 'Follow me,' and then led me downstairs off into a little wood. Then she said, 'Do you know who I am?' and I said, 'I don't know.' She said, 'Don't you want to find out?' Then she said, 'Catch me.' And she ran into the woods. She was quick, and I couldn't catch her. I heard her laughing and laughing. I wanted to stop her, but I couldn't catch her. You were driving me on to catch her. Something tells me I can't catch her. I wish that I could. I could hold her hand. She's playing tag with me."

"Are you afraid of her?"

"No, she isn't sinister, but she makes me very nervous and excited by her actions. I wasn't afraid of her. I could leave her alone if I wanted to. I didn't even have to follow her down. She is only toying with me now—because you are here to help me."

Patient X was now awakened from trance. He could add nothing more to his description of the dreams.

Sessions of January 30 and February 1, 1946

On January 30 X reported that he had not noticed any sign of his fears lately. He was given the poem "If" by Rudyard Kipling. The therapist and the patient read it together. He was very much impressed by the inspirational possibilities in it. He was then placed in a light trance. He related the following dream:

"I saw Mr. Y in a dream. I was in a house. Mr. Y was waiting for me to come out. He was playing with a lasso. Then you were with me, and he went away."

No associations could be evoked to this. He was then told, "During the next two weeks you will have a very significant insight into Mr. Y."

While this suggestion was being given, there was a change of expression over the patient's face, and he suddenly blurted out, "I see sort of a cloud formation. There's a face in it. All I can see is his face. Nobody else can see it. I'm looking at the face. It's distorted—now it fades away—but I can see something just the same. I think this means that I'm really going to uncover Mr. Y after all. You know, I had this dream once before. I remember I couldn't open my eyes. It was the other night. I felt very helpless, and then when I got out of bed—that is in my dream—I became the size of a pigmy, and I couldn't get back in again. I couldn't open my eyes. I finally did so only with a great deal of effort."

"Were you afraid of this?"

"I guess I wasn't too much afraid at the time."

On February 1 Patient X reported some anxiety symptoms. There was obvious resistance at this time. He related the following dream:

"I saw a man's face. It was not clear. It was hideous. I couldn't describe it. His lips were red, and the gums were outstanding. He had black gray hair, and he was getting very hideous, but I wasn't afraid of him. He faded away, and I woke up." No other associations could be evoked except that this symbolized Mr. Y in another one of his many forms.

There was further discussion about the poem "If" by Rudyard Kipling, which the patient had now memorized. He was then shown diagrams in which the Ego was pictured as relatively weak and being pressed by the hostile forces of the Super-Ego, the Id, and the Environment. His attention was called to the purpose of therapy, namely, to strengthen the Ego and weaken the Super-Ego and Id drives so that he could successfully handle the pressures from within and the stresses from without.

When asked what part of him the Id represented he immediately said, "George," and when asked what the Super-Ego was he replied, "Melvin," and followed with, "I guess the Ego part is the real me." Our objective was then described as to strengthen X (the Ego) so that he could "keep George and Melvin in their place" and adequately cope with the problems of everyday life, the Environment.

The writer feels that therapy of analytic type is better if the patient has some understanding about the purposes of the treatment and how it operates. Patients get well through insight. Insight involves understanding, and progress is made much faster when the patient understands what are the therapist's objectives, and how he intends to accomplish them.

The treatment up to this point had been a series of uncovering sessions followed by integration and review. Review is very important, and insights must be restudied many times before the patient has learned them so thoroughly that he does not forget, repress, and slip back into his earlier neurotic patterns. Patient X was learning much about himself, and learning fast, but he had still not reached the heart of his difficulty.

CHAPTER 25

X APPROACHES Y

Three days later Patient X reported for treatment filled with great anxiety. Considerable resistance had again become manifest. He mentioned that he had not slept well—that he would lie awake and imagine the shadow on the ceiling was much more prominent and was coming toward him in a threatening way.

Almost as a side remark, he said, "I don't think this has anything to do with my problem. It's just a normal dream, but I dreamed I had an appointment with you. I rushed there, and when I got there it wasn't my time. It was scheduled for another day, so I went away." He was able to interpret this himself as a resistance dream showing that he did not want to come for his treatment and that he was afraid to come. He also told the therapist that he didn't think he should be hypnotized at this time because he felt so negativistic. He had the feeling that something very significant was going to come up in the future.

Next, he seemed most eager to discuss the layout of his apartment. Each night before retiring he would put out the light in the front room, pull the window down, and then, as he approached the bedroom, he began to experience a fear. It was suggested to him that perhaps this fear corresponded with his approaching his wife in the dark, and he seemed very surprised at this idea. He then mentioned that he also greatly feared to open the pantry door at night. He was asked if this had any relation to the time that he, himself, hid behind the closet door when the husband of the woman whom he was with came home unexpectedly. Concerning that incident he had said, "If he discovered me, I was going to slug him and run." He was asked whether his fear of opening the pantry door might be a projection of this same fear, with himself in the role of the husband. He seemed greatly interested in this idea but did not either accept or reject it for the time being. He did mention, however, that he had a great many fears for his wife's safety—fears that somebody might hurt her. There followed some discussion about how fears for the safety of others sometimes represented the conscious resolution of repressed wishes for their harm. He agreed to consider this point but could not

322

discover any reason why he might wish harm to his wife. His attention was called to his previously expressed desires toward other women—"window-shopping." Then he brought up an interesting point.

"She's been having some dreams in which she thinks I've been stepping out on her. Whenever she has mentioned them it has always made me angry."

"Why do you think it should make you angry?"

"I don't know. I don't want her to think that."

"Have you ever noticed how people bristle at criticism if there is some truth to it? Maybe you do have desires to step out on her. You realize that she senses these, and that is what makes you angry."

"Well, maybe I think that way at times, but I know that neither of us would really step out on each other."

The patient then brought up one other association. "The other night I became quite frightened at a slight sound. I asked my wife what it was. She said it was nothing. Then I looked in the mirror and noticed that I was white. I had white lips." Nothing else emerged at this session. The resistance was very obvious.

Eight days later, on February 12, the patient again reported. He had experienced a week of resistance and had failed to show up for his appointments. Now again, there was a change of the transference relationship in the positive direction. The session was spent in re-assurance and in strengthening his motivation toward his academic goal.

Session of February 14, 1946; Auditory Projective Technique

X was in a relaxed mood today. The period of resistance had gone. He reported no fears. Except for some difficulty in sleeping he had suffered no anxiety. It required about fifteen minutes to place him in a deep trance. When questioned about dreams he could relate none under trance. He was then prepared for a projective technique as follows: First, his right hand was dissociated in the usual manner. Second, he was told that he would hear whispered voices—that they would say something very important to him, and that his hand could write out all that he had heard. Then there was played into his ear a tautophone (Dictaphone) record. This had been previously prepared by the therapist and consisted only of an indefinite mass of whispering talk in which no clear words could be heard.[1]

---

[1] Although the jumbled whispering voices used as a projective technique did initiate a session which proved fruitful, the present example of this technique is not representative

X would not write at first and insisted that he heard only jumbled material. The dissociated hand displayed a lot of negativism, making wavy motions up and down. It then started to write.

The Hand: I DO - - - - - [I DON'T KNOW.]

W : Of course you know.

The Hand: JUMBLE. JUMBLE.

W : That's right. But what do these jumble voices say? They say something.

The Hand: THE HAND CAN'T TELL. X WILL TELL.

X : [speaking] It sounded pretty badly jumbled, but I do have a dream which the voice has made me think of. There is a horse. It is that same horse again, and he has a beautiful saddle and bridle. Everybody is trying to get on it, and the horse wouldn't let anybody get on. They asked me to try. I was afraid. The horse didn't move. He just stood there. I got one foot up on the saddle, but I couldn't get up. The reason I couldn't get up was because I had roots in the ground.

W : Do you think maybe the Hand could explain better your inability to mount the horse?

X : What do you want to let the Hand write for? I don't want the Hand to write. Why can't I say it myself? [Hostile remarks like this continued for some time. Finally the Hand began to write.]

The Hand: RESULTS ARE MEASURED BY DEEDS.

W : How do you mean that?

The Hand: HE WHO STEALS MY PURSE STEALS TRASH BUT HE WHO STEALS FROM ME MY GOOD NAME LEAVES NOTHING.

W : Who has stolen X's good name?

The Hand: YOU—WHAT? WHAT?

X : [covering his head with his hands] I'm not going to talk any more.

The Hand: LET HIM. I HAVE NO MORE TO ADD.

W : What do you mean by "let him"?

The Hand: WHAT?

W : Can you tell me more about what you mean?

The Hand: LA CASA ES NEGRA Y MUCHO SENORS. [At this point the Hand became quite rebellious and refused to write for some time. Eventually it was induced to hold the pencil again.]

W : I think the Hand can reveal more.

The Hand: NO. THE HAND IS OUT.

In other cases, not mentioned in this book, the writer has used this method with interesting results. Patients will often read into "the voices" words of guilt and condemnation stemming from deep-seated paranoidal tendencies within themselves.

W: You mean that the feeling has returned to the hand?

The Hand: YES NO.

W: What do you mean by that?

The Hand: NO ORGANS TO FORM WORDS.

W: Do you mean that The Hand is incapable of further writing?

[The Hand first wrote "NO" and then "YES," finally scratching it out. Then the patient became very angry. He started pouting like a small boy. He threw the pencil away. He threw the Hand away. The therapist put the pencil some six times in the fingers of the Hand before the Hand would grip and continue writing.]

The Hand: I HELP X TO RECOVER. MR. Y SAYS YOU ARE BAD FOR HIM. [A feeling of relief and a loss of tension seemed to come over the patient. Then he continued writing.]

The Hand: HE HAD CONTROL FOR A MINUTE.

W: Can you tell me more about Mr. Y?

The Hand: HE IS A NO GOOD LOUSE DRESSED IN CAMPHOR AND SMELLING OF EVIL.

W: Can the Hand write more about Mr. Y?

The Hand: HE IS ME. MY DARK PAST.

W: Can you explain more about this?

The Hand: NOT ENOUGH CONFIDENCE IN ME, X.

W: What do you mean by this? [The patient once more became very irritable, but the Hand finally started scribbling again.]

The Hand: YOU KNOW HOW HE HAS FALSE TEETH. HE IS A COWARD.

W: Does that mean that Mr. Y represents that part of you which is cowardly?

The Hand: YES.

W: In what way are you cowardly? What are you afraid of?

The Hand: NO MAN BUT VARIOUS DAILY ENCOUNTERS.

W: Do you think that the fear of Mr. Y has anything to do with your wife or marital difficulties?

[At this point Patient X became very anxious and tense. The Hand did not want to write. It threw the pencil away a number of times. Finally, the patient was induced to hold the pencil again, but the Hand would not write.

W: I am going to count up to five. When I say "five" you will have to write. One, two, three, four, five.

The Hand: SEX MUST BE CONTROLLED.

W: Can you explain further what this means?

The Hand: NO, MR. Y PLANTS EVIL THOUGHTS IN CONNECTION WITH SEX. [After a pause it continued writing:] X IS SATISFIED.

At this point feeling and movement began to return to the Hand, whereupon it was reassociated to the body and Patient X was placed back on the cot. The session was now continued on a more non-directive basis.

"You can discuss matters now without using your hand. The Hand wrote something about sex. What does this mean?"

"This means desires for other women." Then he added concerning Mr. Y, "He's the guy that put the bug where it shouldn't be—X is afraid of losing his potency."

"Why do you think that you're losing your potency?"

"Well, look at the life I've lived—continuous sex relations with women. Don't you think it would take away some from my strength —from my ability?"

"Did you ever try to have a child?"

"Yes, I think my wife has one now."

"What's your reaction to this?"

"I'm very pleased—if it's true." Patient X paused a moment thoughtfully, and then made the following interesting comment. "You know, last night I put the car away, and for the first time I didn't use a flashlight—didn't have any fear of the dark. In fact, I didn't even think of it. I didn't think of Mr. Y. I suppose you know that Mr. Y is my guilty fear of my past life—I haven't had such a bad life, haven't broken into any houses or stolen any money. I had a damn good life at times." Then he commented once more about Mr. Y. "I didn't even think of him."

The therapist next asked him if he would like to talk more about Mr. Y and also to tell why he had two weeks of resistance.

He replied, "You know why—you know why. I didn't want to talk about it."

The therapist kept pressing. "Why?"

"You know, Mr. Y was cornered. We were so close to his home. He was flanked on all sides. If he went forward, he ran into you. If he went to the right, he ran into you. If he went to the left, he ran into you; so he didn't have any place to go except to come back on me, and that is what made me all excited, anxious and tense.[2] He's right over the crest of the next hill. He hasn't got much ammunition left. I'm going to send out a scouting party. I'm going to lead that scouting party. I'm going to get hold of him and drag him out."

"X, in the next few days you're going to have a very significant dream, something to do with Mr. Y."

---

[2] One of the most interesting and valid explanations from the patient's viewpoint of just what happens when interpretation mobilizes anxiety and threatens neurotic repressions.

"If I have a dream that's significant, I'm going to come and see you if it's time for our meeting or not—even if you're at a dance. I'm going to come right over and tell you."

Patient X then began to ramble about a number of interesting but apparently inconsequential matters.

"You know, I saw a kid the other day with a broken arm and a lot of blood—didn't even affect me. That's the first time it never did." At this point X started joking. He wanted to talk about the recent fire department handling of the Auditorium fire. "It was badly snafued." Then he commented about Mr. Byrnes's talk on the English loan. He didn't think it should be granted. For about fifteen minutes he continued in this jocular manner.

Then the therapist suggested, "Let's play a new game."

Patient X picked it up instantly. "That's a good idea. It'll break the monotony."

Accordingly, the therapist said, "When I count up to thirteen, there will suddenly pop into your mind the number of days it will take until we finally uncover the last of Mr. Y and get him out of his lair."

Patient X smiled. "Make it fourteen."

"All right. One, two, three, . . . thirteen, fourteen."

Instantly X remarked, "Twenty-one." While the therapist was counting, X was making a number of rather odd-looking passes with his hands in the air. He seemed much interested at the number which had emerged.

"That's a lot of fun. Let's play that game again."

The therapist replied, "All right. I'm now going to count up to eleven, and some important word about what will happen to Mr. Y will emerge—only the word will be in scrambled form. Here we go. One, two, three, . . . nine, ten, eleven."

Patient X started reeling off the following letters: "R-E-M-B-A-E-C-O-G-Y. I know what the word is. It's 'remember.' I'm going to remember something which is significant and will have something to do with Mr. Y."

There was only a light trance remaining. Patient X was awakened. He said he felt very, very good. He was most happy—laughing and joking. While he was sitting there chatting, the therapist opened his appointment book, which had a page for each day, and started slowly counting pages, "One, two, three, four, . . ." At first Patient X didn't understand. Then he opened his eyes in amazement and smiled finally when number twenty-one was reached. The therapist drew a large circle around March 7.

"So that's the day we're going to beat Mr. Y. I remember now. I told you it would be twenty-one days, didn't I?"

About ten more minutes were now spent in discussing affairs of the day, and Patient X started to leave the treatment office. When he reached the door he turned around and looked back. "By the way, how are you coming with your book?"

"Oh, I get to do a little work on it from time to time."

"How many chapters are in it?"

"There will be thirty-three" [the number planned at that time].

"I thought you said there were twenty-one."

The therapist laughed. "There aren't twenty-one chapters in *my* book. There are twenty-one chapters in *your* book—and remember, the last one is twenty-one. Isn't that right?"

Patient X laughingly agreed.

Session of February 18, 1946

"I've been real anxious to tell you a dream that I had last night. I had an empty milk bottle in my hand, and Captain S— came to me and told me to go to his home to get a bottle of milk. It was night and dark. He said, 'Go over and get it.' I had a sudden wave of nervousness—a great wave of fear. I danced up and down and started yelling, 'No! No! I'm not going in there.' He then took hold of me and started walking me back to my house. After we got to the corner he said, 'Go home.' I ran all the way. When I got home I found myself in a high degree of sweat.

"I had another dream also. It went like this. I'm still trying to get on a big black horse who runs, biting at me. That's all."

"What ideas do you have in connection with the milk bottle?"

"Somehow it makes me think of my wife—maybe the milk symbolizes the pregnancy that she has. Do you know Captain S—'s wife is going to have a baby, and I think my wife is going to have a baby too."

In his other associations it was drawn out that he obviously had both a fear of pregnancy and a fear that his wife was not pregnant. From the immediate standpoint, if his wife was pregnant it would interfere seriously with his plans for schooling; on the other hand, if she was not, it would tend to emphasize his feeling that he had become impotent. There was some discussion about the fact that his first wife did not become pregnant when he was with her, but that she did become so when he went overseas—the basis on which a divorce was granted.

He then continued to describe the following material, associating rather freely. "I remember at the age of ten or eleven I slept in the same room with my parents. I heard father come into the room. My mother and I were in the room. I heard him and mother moving around. They were having sex relations—didn't use any contraceptives. It was when I was seven or eight years old that—"

At this point the patient started and said, "Say, do you know what? I don't know if this is the truth, or whether I'm making it up, but I just suddenly remember something. I had a very lovely aunt. She was beautiful. She stayed in the same house with us. I admired her very much. I had great sex desires for her. I tried to fulfil these, but I wasn't permitted to for some reason."

Then he stopped, thought a bit, and said, "You know, my father was in the same room with my mother, and I wanted to sleep with her. I knew that my father had been sleeping with her, and I wanted the same kind of relations. I made so much of a fuss that I finally got to sleep with my mother. I must have been a very small child, and while there I remember wondering whether I should do something with her—I was very passionate. This happened when I was around seven or eight."

"Did you have any guilt feelings about this?"

"Yes, I did. I felt very guilty—why didn't I tell you this before? You know, once I had the same desire with my sister. She was four or five years younger than I was. I was ten or eleven. I tried to have sexual relations with her. She objected strenuously, and I stopped. She told mother, who gave me holy hell. There was a woman, too, who lived nearby, and I had desires for her. She was sure built right. She was over at my home visiting, and so while she and mother were talking I brought in a rubber and asked mother in front of her what it was. I knew what it was all the time."

Patient X then started talking about his aunt. "I was sixteen or seventeen. I made advances toward her. She knew it, too, and she didn't stop me. We were bathing one time, and the waves were coming in from the sea, and I was standing right behind her with my arms around her on her breast and pubic region. She seemed to like it. I felt very guilty about wanting relations with my mother, but I didn't feel that way about my aunt."

Patient X then jumped back in his memory to the age of three or four and said, "It was about that time when I was taken off nursing from mother because the new younger brother came. I resented him a great deal at first because she let him nurse. I remember, though, they gave me a bottle to suck on until I was six or eight years of age. I was that old before I stopped taking the bottle to bed."

This concluded the session. The most interesting point about it was that, even though it was held in the conscious state, a great amount of very significant material had emerged. Whether X had actually experienced these incidents he had described or whether they were only part of his fantasy life was not too important. Either way they emphasized the underlying Oedipus complex which laid the basis for future guilt reactions. It was also interesting that this material appeared immediately after the session in which the patient had stated that Mr. Y would be uncovered within twenty-one days.

What had been disclosed had indeed been significant and anxiety-provoking. The patient did not show up again for two weeks, and when he did return his old uneasiness was quite evident. He was unable to give an adequate reason for failing to come in for treatment. He mentioned that he had experienced a number of dreams, but he seemed unable to remember them.

Session of February 28, 1946

X was placed in a light hypnoidal trance after considerable resistance.

"Would you care to talk some more about the sexual ideas you mentioned last time concerning your mother?"

There was no response—only blocking.

"All right. So you can't think of anything. Now I'm going to count up to nine and something will pop up in your mind that is significant. One, two, three, . . . nine."

"Barnyard fowl."

"What do you mean 'barnyard fowl'?"

"Well, this means chickens, pigs, hogs, etc." He was unable to associate further, but after some time he said, "There was a turkey which got the idea in my mind—a relatively large turkey."

He was unable to name any particular farms but when asked to associate the idea of a turkey on a farm he digressed as follows:

"I see a small store, just the corner of it. It is the site of a bakery. The back door is open at night. I went in, and I got some cookies. I was a little boy—only seven years old. There was another little boy who lived next door. He was a sneak. We only took a few cookies. I told the proprietor that her back door was open. I felt a lot better because I told her, but I beat the boy up because he told her that I went in. His father chased me. He was a tall man and caught me around the neck and squeezed me. I soiled my pants that time—the only time I ever did. It was at night, and it was dark then."

"What about the turkey?"

"Well, the turkey has got big feathers like a peacock or somebody who is strutting."

"Who is it that struts?"

"Well, that's myself. I put on a big front."

"Now, X, I want you to make the fingertips of your two hands touch each other. That's fine. Now each one of those fingers represents a root of Mr. Y. Pretty soon you're going to have a tingling feeling at the tips of one of those pairs of fingers."

X lay quietly on the cot. After a while he said, "It's in the third finger."

"All right. Remove all the fingers except the third fingers. Keep the tips of them together. Now right between those two finger tips a word is going to form. It will have raised letters on it, like the kind the blind feel. This word will slowly emerge, and you're going to be able to spell it out."

Patient X started spelling, "P-R-O-A-N-T-I-R-A-N-S-U-B-S-T-A-N-C-H-I-I-O-N-I S T."

The therapist was greatly surprised. "Do you think you could spell it again?"

Patient X spelled it again exactly the same way—even with the double "i"—then he added, "I read it years ago. Proantiransubstanchiionist. It was way back in the Civil War, and it was about a man who had a certain kind of social standing. They gave that name to him. He was a man that had a pro and con against certain elements. He had two different kinds of standing at the same time."

"What do you think the word means?"

"It means absolutely nothing—maybe it might apply to me, because it goes two ways at the same time."

"Maybe another word will come between your fingers."

"No, I can't feel anything."

"You concentrate real hard on those two fingers. Let's see if another word doesn't begin to squeeze in between them."

In a minute X spelled out the word "A-L-L-E-V-I-A-T-E," and then added, "You know what 'alleviate' means? It means to alleviate my symptoms."

No more words seemed to emerge automatically between the fingers, so another variation of this projective technique was tried. "Right between your two fingers will run a ticker tape. You know what a ticker tape is like? It will have raised words on it. You will be able to spell those words."

Patient X began spelling, "H-O-M-O-B-I-O-L-O-G-I-C-A-L-H-O-M-O." [3] He then spelled "P-R-E-S-S-I-V-E." "There's no word 'pressive.'"

"Maybe you mean 'oppressive'?"

"I'm a radio station—tick, tick, tick." Then he started spelling some more. "P-R-O-C-L-I-V-I-T-E."

"Proclivity? What's that mean?"

"I don't know. I'm going to count up to seven. When I say 'seven' an idea telling you what 'proclivity' means will pop into your mind. One, two, three, . . . seven."

"Of all things in the world. Proclivity is you—Proclivity Watkins. You have a proclivity for pulling things out of me." Then he added, "Do I have to hold these fingers together any more? You know, I can't open my eyes. I've been trying to."

At this time the patient began to associate again. "I was once run over by a sled. That was a long time ago. I fell off, and the one behind me ran over me." No further associations could be determined for this incident; so another projective technique was tried.

"In front of you there is a great fire. You can see it. It is a great picture in fire."

Patient X immediately seized on this unstructured stimulus and started fashioning a concept with it. "Yes, I see this fire very, very clear. It stands out like the wings of a bird—an eagle. The eagle is getting larger and larger. He is just standing there like a statue."

"What's the eagle mean?"

"I don't know what it is."

"I'm going to count up to five, and when I say 'five' an association will come to your mind which will tell you something about what the eagle means. One, two, three, four, five."

"Huh, when you said 'five' the bird disappeared."

"All right. Let's try another angle on this. I'm going to ask you some questions, and I want you to respond instantly. Do you understand me—instantly. Answer yes or no just as soon as I finish the question. Now regarding this bird, is it—you?"

"No."

"Is it—Melvin?"

"No."

"Is it—George?"

---

[3] This word is most interesting when compared with the final solution of the case.

"No."

"Is it—Mr. Y?"

"No."

"Is it—me?"

"No."

"Is it—your father?"

"No."

"This time I'm going to count up to seven, and when I say 'seven' a scrambled word will come to your mind. It will tell you something about what the bird stands for. One, two, three, four, five, six, seven."

Patient X started spelling, "H-E-R-A-E-T-C," then he added, "but I can't interpret it."

"All right. I'm going to count up to seven once more. This time you will be able to spell the word in a little better form. One, two, three, four, five, six, seven."

"I knew you were going to analyze it. I told you so. Well, here goes. C-H-E-R-T-E-A."

"Does it mean 'cheater'?"

"No, It means 'teacher.' "

"Tell me what the word 'teacher' brings to your mind."

"Well, the teacher struck me—Miss Jordon was her name. It wasn't my fault. The boy in front of me was a pet of hers and was jealous of me because I was the second highest in the class, and he turned around and whispered something. She came over and slapped me because he was a pet of hers. I then threw a bottle of ink all over her—all over her white blouse. She took me up immediately to the principal, and the principal, after finding out what was wrong, censured her instead of me."

"Yes, but I don't exactly see what all this has to do with 'eagle.' "

"Don't you see? An eagle is a leader—a teacher. You know, I'm going to be a teacher. I want to be an eagle that can fly and not have a broken leg. That means I need education and support because my own wings, my own education, are broken. It means that a lot of background must be required. It will take an awful strain."

"What about that long word, 'proantiransubstanchiionist'? [proantitransubstantiationalist?] What's that got to do with it?"

"Don't you see that it is a big long word? That is the front that I have to have. I always put up a big *impressive* front. [The reader will recall that X had spelled out the word 'pressive.' At the time the therapist had suggested this meant 'oppressive,' and X had not challenged this suggestion.] That's the kind of a guy I am."

He further integrated these concepts by pointing out that he wanted to be an eagle—a leader, but he felt he was more of a turkey, a show-off. He then discussed his wife's pregnancy and indicated that he was very pleased with the matter—said he wanted to become a father.

The thought was suggested to him, "See, you haven't lost your potency and power?"

"Well, that's right. I feel pretty good about it."

He had recently sold his car and accepted an older model. He seemed quite pleased that he did not feel as inferior about it as he thought he would. This was called to his attention, and he said, "Say, I've made a lot of progress. I feel better. I'm glad that you mentioned this to me. It means that I'm stronger and that I can take a lot more."

At this point he was awakened from his trance. He left the session feeling somewhat relieved and mentioned that he was anxious to report more dreams—for the final uncovering of Mr. Y.

A Period of Resistance

During the next week a tremendous period of resistance began. As the last of the twenty-one days began to pass and the significant date of March 7 began to approach, Patient X became more tense, more nervous, more jittery. His fears at night became stronger. Following the session of February 28 he did not report for some time. He conjured up one excuse and rationalization after another not to come in. It was obvious that a terrific battle was going on within him. He, himself, had set the date of March 7 for the final uncovering; yet down deep inside, Mr. Y was waging a tremendous conflict to remain hidden in his unconscious stronghold.

On March 6 Patient X came to the office, looking wan, tired, and haggard. His eyes showed the lack of sleep. He was nervous, tense, and jittery, and his face was covered with the deepest depression.

"We've been on the wrong track. I know there's no use of us going any further. We're never going to find the solution to my problem. I'm just going to have to live with it, I guess, for the rest of my life."

Mr. Y was obviously pleading to have the treatment called off at this point.

No attempt was made to do anything but to give X some mild reassurance. In his present state of agitation nothing more could be

done. However, his tension was lowered somewhat by the reassurance. Both in Patient X's mind and in the mind of the therapist
the next day loomed like a major ordeal—a psychological operation—
and as to the outcome there was only a question mark. Mr. Y had
been cornered. He was putting up a furious battle for his existence.

CHAPTER 26

THE MASQUERADE IS ENDED

For two weeks a decisive battle had been going on within Patient X. His nights were spent in helplessly tossing around the bed. The few moments of sleep were filled with vague forms of fear—dreams, fantasies. Headaches appeared often. At times tremors shook his body. Like poison he had avoided the therapist. March 7 was approaching, and Mr. Y, cornered, was fighting like a wild beast.

Session of March 7, 1946

Patient X opened the door. He came in and sat down, and for a few moments he did not say anything. The expression on his face was a mixture of anguished apprehension and stoical fortitude. After a while he spoke.

"There are dreams I meant to tell you about, but I can't think of them."

X was placed on the cot, and suggestions to induce hypnotic trance were started. In view of his state of agitation, the therapist had felt severe misgivings as to the possibility of actually inducing trance at this time. These were not groundless. Indeed, after the session was finished Patient X himself said, "When I came in I didn't think you'd be able to hypnotize me today."

However, after a period of fifteen minutes of sleep suggestions the patient's right hand slowly rose into the air and touched his head— the prearranged signal which had been used in each trance session to indicate to the therapist and to the patient himself that a deep degree of trance had finally been reached.

"X, you are in a cave, a dark cave, and there are steps leading down the cave, not into darkness, but into a light which is ahead. You are going to go out into this very bright light." The therapist counted steps.

The patient began to describe his dream. "It is all shining. There is a big, open, hollow tunnel. Light is in one section—there is nothing in the tunnel. There is only an old tunnel." X growled rather belligerently, "You got me to come down here."

"Maybe there are some pictures on the walls of this tunnel. Look around and see."

"Yes, it has markings. Some one has chiseled them on the stone. I am trying to see what they say. These markings were written years and years ago. Oh, the light is going out."

"You're very strong now, much stronger than you used to be. You can put the light on again. You can *will* the light on. I'm going to count up to ten, and as I do, you will be able to will the light back on. One, two, three, . . . ten."

Patient X smiled. "Yes, the light is back on again. Let me turn it on and off again. I want to see if it will work. I wonder if I could make colored lights too." A few moments elapsed while X "turned the light on and off again." After his smile indicated satisfaction, he was prodded again to describe what he saw.

"It is so light now the wall is turning all white. There are nurses and doctors around me. I see myself as a boy. It is at Saint A——'s Hospital. I had my tonsils taken out. There's nothing to it, but across from me is a boy who's blind. I wonder where he is now. My mother just brought me some ice cream. This throat feeling is hard to go down, but it does in time." X cleared his throat and began to speak in a hoarse, whispering voice, describing his feelings.

It was suggested to him that he look once more at the message on the wall, but he ignored this and continued, "I see myself being taken out of the hospital. I sit around the house. The boy friends come in to see me now. Naturally, they think I'm brave—the only time I've ever been in the hospital for an operation." [1]

"How old are you?"

"Ten years old."

"I'm going to count up to ten, and something will come to your mind that is very important—very, very important. One, two, three, four, ——."

X broke in. "You don't have to make it jell. I see now. There's a bully. His name was George S——. Huh! Did I ever tell you about him before? He was much older. Oh, I remember. He was the boy with the sister I told you about. I used to go out to the railroad yards and jump to the sand trestle. I was the only one who was brave enough to do it. If I had missed, there would be no telling where I would have fallen to. This boy said he wanted me to come up there with him, and I went up, and we were in a box car. He took

---

[1] The session today is in the nature of a major operation. It reminds him of the tonsil operation of his childhood and, as at that earlier time, he indicates his need for bravery and control.

his peter out. He wanted me to do something—to kiss him. Then
he said, 'Do it, or I'll beat you up,' and he rushed at me. It was a
railroad car filled with sawdust, and I got terribly mad and beat him
and beat him—kicked him until he cried and hollered, and then I
came to my senses, and I left. He got out, 'cause I saw him later. I
whipped him terribly. He was much bigger than I was. How could
I do it? There was some kind of a revulsion in me—something
terrible. I felt a lot better afterwards. Imagine me beating George.
It would be like beating Joe Louis today. I was still afraid of him,
though—even afterwards."

Here was the missing link, the handle on the last door, the fear of
Mr. Y with his knife, the great emphasis on athletic prowess, manhood, and leadership, the explanation of his many sexual affairs with
women—and now finally, the tremendous, blinding fear of this childhood incident. They all added up to what Patient X was afraid to
face within himself, the existence of which his whole life had been one
constant striving to deny. Almost instantly innumerable pieces of
jig-saw puzzle fitted together, and the pattern they made was—
latent homosexuality.

But insight to be helpful must reach down deep within the patient
himself. Could this understanding be initiated into X without creating a panic? Could this concept, obviously so terrible to X as to have
warped his whole life, be integrated into his understanding? The
session continued.

"This older boy—you said you felt fear toward him."

"Yes, it was intense."

"What kind of a feeling was it?"

"I never knew what it meant—it just came from within. Since
that time I've thought a lot about that boy. I wanted to tell you about
him, but somehow I forgot to."

"Did you ever have any other experiences involving homosexuals?"

"I've seen so many men approach me. I can tell them when I first
see them. I know them right and left. I know what they eat, drink,
and sleep. I've had enough of them as friends, but my relations for
them have always been platonic. I can spot them a million miles
away." X mused a bit to himself. "How do you think I can tell
them? My brother is the same way. Isn't it funny that I can spot
them? Doesn't affect me, though. Don't get angry at them any
more. I just believe they are sort of sick. I knew a girl, and she was
a lesbian—a very good friend of mine; only she got angry at me when

I started to go with a girl she had a crush on. We had *that kind* of a relation. I wouldn't let a man do that to me—but a woman, yes.[2] I got to enjoy it quite a lot."

At this point the therapist took the lead. "You know, X, something most people do not realize is that we were not constructed just man or woman. All men have a certain F or feminine component within them, and all women have a certain M or masculine component. Ordinarily, this doesn't cause much trouble, but sometimes people refuse to face or accept the fact that they have this in them. They feel drives in the direction of those which would be experienced by the opposite sex. They have been taught to be ashamed of this, so they refuse to accept the fact that they have these urges; instead, they repress them—they push them down into their unconscious, and a great conflict occurs—one in which the person tries to keep these urges hidden from himself, to deny their very existence.

"Let us suppose that a man has an F component within him—just an ordinary good man like other people, but for some reason he has been taught to reject this F component within him, and the F component is strong enough that, even though repressed into the unconscious and unrecognized, it exerts a considerable amount of control over his behavior. This man will do a number of things to deny the existence of his own F component. For example, if approached by a homosexual, he will become very, very angry. Have you ever heard some soldiers tell how they enjoyed beating up a homosexual who approached them? Why do you think they got such pleasure at mistreating the man? It was because in so doing they were able to deny the existence of feelings which they themselves had down deep inside. The reason they became so angry at his advances was because he was touching off some inner drive in them, which they instinctively sensed, but whose existence they did not want to admit. We call this *latent* homosexuality, because people who are like this don't actually engage in homosexual practices or behavior. They are people like this," and the therapist drew a square on a sheet of scratch paper, broken into two rectangles, the larger occupying about four fifths of the square. This section was labeled M, and the smaller called F, masculine—feminine.

"You see, men of this type, and that includes many persons, are very anxious to prove to themselves that they are one hundred per

---

[2] Homoerotic impulses can be gratified without anxiety when disguised as an oral heterosexual experience.

cent M. This man will engage in a lot of athletic sports—you know, chest-beating. He will aim to be a leader of men in physical activities. Perhaps he will exhibit a drive to have many sexual affairs with women. Why does he do all this? Why? He is trying to prove his masculinity to himself. Down deep inside, he suspects that there is this small F component. He is afraid of it. He refuses to admit its being there, and his whole life is spent in trying to deny its existence.

"Now there's nothing wrong in having this F component within us. We all have it more or less. If we are affectionate toward our fathers and our brothers, it receives partial development. These latent homosexual components are far more widespread than most persons are willing to admit."

Patient X broke in. "Yes, I've seen a lot of boys like that—one in the YMCA. A boy came in to urinate. I saw another boy watching him—with that look in his eyes, and I was shocked." Then he added, "Why do all these homosexuals have money? I never met one who didn't have money." (It will be noted that one of the patient's drives in the past had been to acquire money; this was especially true of the George component.) ·

The therapist further explained that there was a certain amount of homosexuality in a latent form in all of us—that there was nothing wrong about having a small F component—that it does not take the form of actual homosexual relations in most cases, but that many persons are afraid to face it in themselves. At one point when the discussion centered about homosexual relations, Patient X remarked, "I wonder what it would feel like to do it." ·

The discussion now returned to the great waves of anger which overcome many men on being approached by a homosexual—the great desire they have to strike or injure the homosexual. X remarked, "You know, that's me." Then he began to smile all over. The attention of the patient was then called to the fact that overt or actual expression of homosexual tendencies was regarded in the old Greek society as an accepted form of sexual expression, even though it is not approved in our present culture. He was reassured that it was not going to manifest itself in him by bringing about homosexual relations. He was told that all he needed to do was to frankly recognize that he, like a lot of other men in this world, had this F component within him, and that once he recognized it and ceased fighting it, he would no longer fear it.

Then the therapist asked, "How did this manifest itself in you?"

Patient X replied, "You know, Mr. Y—Mr. Y with his big knife, the knife which stands for the penis." At this point the tenseness began to disappear in his body. He remarked, "The darkness has faded away. Everything is becoming light."

"By the way, X, do you know what day today is?"

"Oh yes, it's March 7, isn't it? That's the day you said Mr. Y would be uncovered."

"I didn't say it. You said it. Now, I'm going to describe a dream to you, and you're going to finish the dream. You see yourself out in a field, and there is a big black horse in this field."

Immediately X said, "Like a flash I'm on top of that horse. I'm galloping off—I'm galloping off. I can ride it—I can handle it." [3]

The therapist continued, "Now I want you to see another dream. You are at a masquerade. Everyone has on masks. You know them all except one young woman. She runs downstairs with a mask on. You chase after, and she says, 'If you want to see who I am, catch me first.' Now go ahead and finish the dream." (The unresolved dream of Chapter 24.)

Patient X jumped. He writhed—he fidgeted—he wrinkled his face. Finally he replied, "I've caught her. I'm removing the mask. Huh—that's me. That's who it is. I'm the woman." (The F component finally unmasked.)

Once more the therapist suggested a dream. "You're on a desert again. There are many roads leading out in all directions. You are very thirsty. What happens?"

"I am walking down the road. There is no wolf any more. He is gone. Now all the many roads merge into one, and there is a clear straight road. Everything is fine. There are roses around it."

"You can walk down this road. Tell me what you see. Is there a house?"

"Yes. Only now the house has changed. It has been painted white. Now it has solid brick foundations under it. It is well built. It is now changed from the shaky foundations to the solid foundations."

"You know what the house means, don't you?"

"Yes, it means me."

"That's right. And now that you can be a real man, you'll no longer fear the old traces of homosexuality because you understand them. You don't repress them any longer. So Mr. Y is gone. You realize you have a small F component within you, like many others, only you're not afraid of it any more. You admit it, and then forget

---

[3] Contrast this with the repeated attempts made earlier to suggest to the patient that he could ride the horse, suggestions which had always failed previously.

it. That makes you a bigger man—*a more real man* than you were before. You have nothing more to hide from yourself. Mr. Y is gone. Melvin and George are gone now too. They merged into one person. That's you. They will not need to fight each other any more. I am going to count up to five, and when I do you will wake up. You will feel good, and you will remember distinctly everything we have discussed. You will understand and accept it. One, two, three, four, five."

Patient X opened his eyes and smiled. "Isn't it funny. I don't feel wild exhilaration. I just feel a calm sense of satisfaction—a feeling of relief, as if a burden has gone."

The material was now rediscussed with him in the conscious state, and it was planned to go over his entire treatment with him, word for word. Then his chart could be closed, and he could be returned to civilian life.

A Flare-up of Anxiety Following Insight

Moses and Aaron once looked over a hill and saw the Promised Land of Canaan, but it was only a glimpse. The Children of Israel wandered in the wilderness for years before they were permitted to enjoy that promised land. Sometimes insight is like that. The cause is resolved—the patient sees—he understands. It looks all too clear. Then the fog of resistance closes down—the clouds congeal—the light is obscured. The explanations are rejected—Mr. Y still had one round of ammunition.

Beginning that night, March 7, all the anxieties and fears returned to Patient X—returned in the most acute form he had ever experienced. For four nights he went through a virtual hell. He spent his nights again rising and tossing, and his days gritting his teeth, trying to swallow his anxiety. That which his whole life had been trying to deny had now finally emerged to the surface. He had now been made to look directly into the mirror at himself, and what he saw was not pleasing.

It was March 11 before he again reported in to see the therapist and describe the tortures through which he had been going. This time the therapist gave him some reassurance and once more pointed out the necessity of understanding and accepting, not rejecting. He left slightly reassured, but the death agonies of Mr. Y continued for seven more days.

Finally, on March 18, 1946, his anxieties and resistances had subsided somewhat, and he returned. Reassurance was given, including further discussion as to the meaning behind the material uncovered. At the end of this session he left feeling much better.

The next day, March 19, the hour was spent beginning a thorough, exhaustive review of the entire treatment. Line by line, word by word, event by event, the material was reviewed, placing the pieces in the pattern where they made sense as interpreted in the light of the uncovered key—the latent homosexual component which X had been desperately trying to conceal from himself throughout his entire life.[4]

On March 21 his anxiety had largely subsided. There were still some slight fears, but these were not incapacitating. The entire story of his life as uncovered was again reviewed and interpreted in terms of the denial of the repressed F component. Patient X began to accept more and to understand—began to fight less. Although the therapist did not let up for an instant in trying to make X face the true issue, the patient's Ego was constantly given support and reassurance—reassurance that there was nothing fundamentally wrong with him—that he was a real man—that he would become more of a real man by accepting instead of rejecting the uncovering of his F component.

Session of March 26, 1946

Patient X reported today that he had been sleeping well for five days. There had been some slight uneasiness once or twice, but he said that it was "not much." He had experienced no frightening dreams. He was not awakened in the middle of the night, and there had been no fear of turning out the lights in his house and moving about as previously. Concerning his fear of the dark at home he said, "I just forgot about it." There was no evidence of fear toward the dark closet, which once had caused him such severe anxiety. He mentioned that he had recently seen the picture "Lost Weekend," a story of the struggles of an alcoholic. This movie included some

---

[4] Much material elicited earlier in the treatment becomes logical as viewed in the light of latent homosexuality. The reader will recall the session of February 28 when the patient's dissociated hand wrote, "H-O-M-O-B-I-O-L-O-G-I-C-A-L-H-O-M-O." Or again the early session of October 15 and his dream of being pursued along the highway. We might interpret some of the elements as follows: "Some one is driving the car in the front seat. It looks like my wife is driving it." (My wife is more dominating, and hence more masculine, than I. She is in the driver's seat.) "No, that's funny—my wife can't drive a car." (She's a woman. She's not supposed to play the male role.) "The car is chasing me. The person that I fear is in the car behind me. It has a big nickel-plated engine." (I fear homosexual attack from the rear. The car with the "big nickel-plated engine" is a penis symbol.)

rather terrifying scenes. He felt pleased with himself that there were no jitters or fears of the dark after having observed the picture. His entire manner and attitude had changed to one of calmness and confidence toward the reorganizing of his life and his future.

Obviously no complete analysis had been accomplished nor had all the questions been answered. Certain strata of the unconscious mind had been penetrated. The existence of homosexual impulses had been uncovered, and his symptoms relieved. This material had been considerably "worked through."

We might ask such questions as why these homosexual fears first originated. What were the childhood fantasies that occurred in the sex development of Patient X which brought about the strong need to deny his F component? Why was the F component so strong as to exert such a traumatic effect on his life? Yes, there were many unanswered questions. Perhaps months or years of probing might be necessary to uncover them all, but we had reached a point where the analysis could be stabilized. It was time now for X to go home— for him to leave the military environment and return to civilian life, testing out his newly found confidence. There was time for only one more session—an hour designed to make a final check on his condition of insight.

Session of March 28, 1946

"You know I had a dream recently. I saw a baby. It was dying. It did die. Its heart protruded, making the skin extend. I saw it suffering, and then it was dead."

X was placed in deep trance in a period of fifteen minutes and was asked to associate and interpret his dream. He said immediately, "The baby is Mr. Y. He died. The heart showed that he was dying."

Next he was taken back to the field and shown the black horse again. He said, "It is very wild. It is running away from me. He comes back—he runs away—he comes back—he circles me—he stops. Now I walk over to him—I get in the saddle—I put one foot in the stirrup. He moved away again—he is moving away, and I can't get the foot in. I try to put it in. Now I'm on top of him. He is a wild animal—he throws me off. I'm getting on again. I'm riding some more. He jumps over fences and then throws me off again. I get on again. Now we are running. We are running down the road. He takes off into the air. I can ride him. And now he disappears. He is just a flash in the distance."

The therapist then suggested, "You will have a dream now which will indicate to you what your future is going to be in terms of your present adjustment. Will you be riding the horse in the future?"

Patient X was quiet for about five minutes. At times he would twiddle with his fingers, moving them around as he folded his hands.

At the end of this period he was asked, "Have you finished your dream?"

"Yes, first I saw a barracks, Army barracks like we have here. Suddenly, one of them began to change into a house. It was a nice house. It had a small fence around it. Outside the house was the horse. I started to go to the field, playing polo. I can't imagine why —riding him. Ha—you know I can't ride."

The therapist reassured, "You can ride *your* horse."

Patient X continued, "Anyway, we played polo. He was a nice horse to handle. Rather funny, though, he went over the fence fine when we were going out there, but he didn't seem to want to come back."

"What might that mean?"

"I guess that means that I'm going out of the Army into civilian life from the barracks to the house. It's a one-way trip. I'm not coming back."

"But you can ride the horse all right in civilian life?"

"Oh yes, I can handle him fine."

"All right, you are now at a masquerade ball. There is a girl there who has a mask on."

"She probably needs to keep her face covered because her face is horrible—my face." Then he laughed, "That's a good joke."

The therapist inquired, "Who is this girl?"

Immediately the patient said, "I don't want to chase her. Why should I chase her? I know who she is."

"Are you afraid of her?"

"No, of course not. I'm not afraid of her." He then began to rub his eyes. "I'm getting awake. I'm awake, but I can't open my eyes."

The therapist then checked on a minor point. "I would like to ask you something for curiosity's sake. You once said that Mr. Y was covered with camphor. What do you mean by 'camphor'?"

"When I was a boy I used to dislike the smell of camphor. They would put it to my nose when I had a cold. That is why I said that." (Homosexuality is a smelly business.)

"What has happened to George and Melvin?"

"Oh," replied the patient, "they have taken long trips—gone away, and they are not coming back. Poor Melvin." He mused a moment. "If they had combined their best traits in one person—what a person."

"Maybe they have. Is there any other point that you would care to bring up or interpret before I awaken you?"

"No, I guess not."

"Are you sure you know what it is that you've been fighting? Are you sure you know now, and that you will never forget it?"

"Of course, I know. I know it now. I want to get back to civilian life and start driving—the old push—the old force, like I used to have. If I were cleaning streets, I'd have the cleanest streets in the block. All I need now is to get back and get that old drive going. Mr. Y will be just a bad memory."

Patient X opened his eyes and smiled.

Summary of the Case

Just before leaving the hospital Patient X was given a Rorschach analysis. It was not secured under optimum conditions as he was somewhat impatient and uncooperative at the time; hence, the total number of responses was low. However, the results were indicative of normal personality functioning, with little evidence of neurotic maladjustment. Ego strength was good and regard for reality high. His intellectual approach to problems was along more general and obvious lines. Mild anxiety and depressive features were noted, but were much less intense than those which characterize a severe obsessive neurosis such as this patient had at the beginning of treatment.[5] Although he exhibited sensitivity to emotional stimuli from his environment, his capacity for emotional identification with others was still not fully mature and stabilized. The general Rorschach pattern was that of a normal and not neurotic personality.

For the benefit of those Rorschach specialists who would like to interpret it more in detail, the scoring is presented on page 347.

It is quite difficult to assess just what has been accomplished in this case. A patient may lose symptoms merely because of transference reactions or because of suggestion or motivational changes, in which case there is no real character alteration. However, Patient X shows not only loss of symptoms, but he also resolves all of his neurotic dreams, another test for successful insight. His Rorschach is indicative of nearly normal personality functioning. We have no

---

5 Unfortunately an initial Rorschach had not been administered at the beginning of therapy.

initial Rorschach with which to compare, but his symptoms and the material that emerged during the extended therapy could hardly have been manifested in a well-adjusted individual. The original diagnosis of a severe obsessive neurosis seems well substantiated.

		Main		*Add*		*Content*				
W	9	M	2	M	1	H	1	F plus	80%
D	13	FM	1			Hd	2		
d	1	Fk	1			A	6	P	7
	—	F	10			Ad	3		
	23	Fc	2			A obj	4	O	1
		FC'	1			At	1		
		FC	2			Obj	1	T/R	32"
		CF	3			N	1		
		C	1			Geo	1	Reaction time:	
			—			Art	1	Color	15"
			23			Emb	1	Achromatic	14"
						Cg	1		
							—		
							23		

RORSCHACH SCORES

(There was no shock on Card VI.)
Exp. Bal. M :C = 2 :5.5

The relief from symptoms proceeded by two steps. First, the fear lessened, and the phobia of the dark changed to anxiety dreams after the patient had come to accept that his fear was the projected manifestation of personal guilt feelings. These phobic dreams then resolved and left him apparently symptom-free after he had worked through his Oedipal feelings toward his mother and had disclosed his latent homoeroticism or fears of passivity. The entire pattern of his previous behavior becomes quite logical in the light of this need to flee from passivity (the F component).

In discussing "Failures with Psychoanalytic Therapy," Oberndorf (1948) states that, "Freud refers again to Ferenczi's article in which the latter emphasizes the paramount importance of two themes: 'the wish for a penis in women, and *in men, the struggle with passivity.*' [Italics ours.] Ferenczi in 1927 'laid it down as a principle that in every successful analysis these two complexes must have been resolved. Whether and when we have succeeded in mastering this factor in analysis is hard to determine. We console ourselves with the certainty that everything possible has been done to rouse the analysand to examine and change his attitude in this respect.' "

If by this criterion of "successful analysis" it would appear that Patient X has adequately worked through and resolved his "struggle with passivity" we might then consider his treatment to have wrought a genuine change in his basic personality. Time alone can provide the really final and valid test—continued freedom from symptoms and mature adjustment to life.

PART V
EVALUATION

CHAPTER 27

SUMMARY

This book has attempted a great deal. Yet the experiences in working with these severe psychoneurotics in the Special Treatment Company seemed to offer much of value which should be shared with other clinicians.

Only a representative fraction of all the patients treated in Company F could be described. Those selected give examples of treatment ranging from the simplest motivational to the more complex analytic types, from those which were reasonably successful to those in which there was only limited improvement.

From a number of these cases we can conclude that the enucleation of a few of the most severe conflicts, accompanied by an adjustment of environmental factors, may bring considerable relief. This "limited-help therapy" can through the medium of hypnosis be more widely employed to assist those neurotics who could never afford a complete psychoanalysis.

Undoubtedly some of the patients who appeared to be greatly relieved on leaving the hospital suffered relapses later. Their neurotic predispositions—plus the strong secondary gain of soldier disability pensions—were too strong to enable them to meet the stress of civilian life and its problems.

Attempts are being made by the author to contact the patients after they have had sufficient time to become "acclimated" to civilian life. From the few follow-up reports now available, we must conclude that the purely motivational "cure" in a strongly predisposed individual, accompanied by little insight, is at best a precarious one. These cases cannot be "cured" and then forgotten. Often the patients will require rather continuous attention throughout the rest of their lives to keep them in a state of health and adjustment. On the other hand, letters have already been received from some who claimed to be greatly improved after they had returned to civilian life. In one case the patient was discharged in a very poor condition. An unsolicited communication from him later reported a considerable improvement and credited the gain to the hypnoanalytic treatment. Of course, his recovery may have been the result of stabilizing environmental factors outside the Army. Still, it may have resulted from a "delayed" effect of the therapy, such as has been described by Yaskin (1945).

Government, education, and psychotherapy have all undergone in recent years a struggle between two fundamentally different approaches. In the political life of nations some have adopted the authoritarian or "ruler-centered" trend. In general these have developed into ruthless totalitarian states. A few, however, with more benevolent dictators, have achieved a greater degree of human happiness, even though it was based on paternalism. Other nations, notably our own, of course, have rejected the authoritarian concept of government and have developed along "citizen-centered" lines in which control inheres in the governed.

In education this same cleavage has been brought to the foreground through the rise of "progressive education." This approach is "pupil-centered" and is in contrast to the older authoritarian methods of pedagogy which were "teacher-centered."

The rise of psychoanalysts in the practice of psychiatry and of the school of nondirective therapists (Rogers 1942) in clinical psychology occupies a corresponding position in the field of psychotherapy. By being "patient-centered," these two approaches have developed the democratic concept into a therapeutic method. They evolved out of the failure of the techniques of reassurance, exhortation, and suggestion, with or without hypnosis, so widely and futilely practiced by the earlier treaters of mental maladjustment. As such they were in tune with the reforms in political and educational thinking sweeping the world.

Furthermore, these patient-centered methods achieved results. Many cases completely unresponsive to directive attacks dissolved under the patient probing of the psychoanalytic and nondirective therapies.

In spite of their ultimate success, these methods have one severe limitation. The large amount of time required means that only a few of our maladjusted people can be treated. If the neurotic must spend several thousands of dollars and devote an hour a day for one or two years to sessions with his analyst, only a few wealthy and highly motivated sufferers can be helped. These therapeutic approaches may offer a method of resolving neuroses; they do not solve the neurotic problem of our time.

Under nondirective or psychoanalytic methods, the inner conflicts may eventually emerge and be resolved, but in the process literally hundreds of blind alleys must first be explored. We have seen in the case of Patient X many of the false leads which were followed at the expense of considerable time.

However, it does not appear necessary that all the minor resistances, the fringe problems, must be worked through before the heart of a conflict can be attacked. Psychotherapy is basically a kind of education or re-education. In the schools the teachers have often found that it is better to point out the correct approach to an algebra problem than to permit the student to flounder for hours in nonproductive and frustrating effort. Likewise, there comes a time during the treatment of neuroses when directed guidance may bring greater return than the continued reflection of the client's feelings or the patient listening to his endless chains of associations.

The corrective emotional experience is especially speeded through the interpretive skill of the therapist. We have seen in the case of Harry Weber (Chapter 15) that failure to interpret properly when the opportunity was offered delayed the successful resolution of the conflict—a situation which was later remedied by interpretation. The results from these cases tend to confirm the affirmation of Alexander and French (1946) that recovery is not directly related to time spent in therapy, but rather is most dependent on correct and timely interpretations. It is in the development of greater interpretive skill that the psychotherapist can most improve the efficiency of his treatment. Interpretations fail to bring about an acceptance and emotional insight in the patient if they are not planted in the fertile soil of a high rapport and sound patient-therapist relationship. Success in developing this relationship, sensing the dynamic heart of the conflict, and skillfully timing and presenting his interpretations shows the true mettle of a psychotherapist.

Our nondirective therapists rightfully emphasize the individual's need for expressive freedom. They and the psychoanalysts have stressed the close relationship of adjustive maturity and independence. But there are other requirements that also must be considered. An individual may have an equal need for reassurance, for interpretation, for clarification, even for contradiction—and all these may not be unhealthy. In this interdependent social culture of ours a give-and-take quality in emotional ties both to the therapist and to others may be productive of better adjustment than the therapeutic goal of complete independence. It is not the lack of dependent relationships but rather the resolution of unhealthy ones which should be our aim. Therapists should not fear the establishment of necessary, helpful, temporary transferences as a support to the patient during therapy. The psychologically bankrupt person may sometimes need a short-term emotional loan to help him acquire Ego-solvency.

When enough has emerged that the therapist senses the heart of the trouble, a direct "incision" under protected conditions may afford more and quicker relief than gradual development of insight. Witness the case of John Hilton (Chapter 13). Many therapists warn that this will bring on greater anxiety than the patient's Ego can stand and may precipitate an acute breakdown—that too much insight too soon is dangerous. Yes, an acute reaction often occurs, but seldom one which cannot be handled by the neurotic patient with proper guidance and reassurance. Moreover, little progress ever occurs without accompanying anxiety.

On the other hand, there can be an equally great danger in procrastination while a storm is developing. True, if the patient is fed more than he can take, he will block and develop strong anxiety. He needs careful watching at this time. But a high positive relationship to the therapist can be used to strengthen him and give needed reassurance while he is assimilating the new insight.

It appears that if suggestion and persuasion are *strong enough* and are *skillfully presented,* with a good knowledge of the patient's motivational structure, insight can be "forced" *at certain stages* in spite of active resistances—the resistances are overwhelmed. This, of course, assumes that the patient is not psychotic, with a definite delusional system to fall back upon. Failures in early persuasive methods can perhaps be traced to lack of skill in their employment— attempts to force through concepts without the full utilization of *a great preponderance of motivational allies.*

Sometimes actual demonstrations of psychological mechanisms through experimentally induced neuroses under hypnotic trance may be effective in changing a patient's attitude. Wolberg (1945) and Watkins (1947a) have found this device useful in breaking key resistances.

This book has emphasized the values of hypnotherapy. It has been stressed that hypnosis does not supplant other methods of treatment. Rather, it gives them an opportunity for greater effectiveness in shorter periods of time by offering access to deeper levels of personality structure. This applies to all methods of psychotherapy, superficial or deep. With hypnosis a condition of insight can be achieved more rapidly. It enables the therapist to unearth and work through large quantities of significant material in a much shorter period of time than is possible in the conscious state. In this way he can make his knowledge and skill available to larger numbers of needy persons. However, it has definite limitations and is no substitute for therapeutic skill. It is hoped that the discussion of hypnosis in this volume will stimulate psychotherapists of various schools to experiment further along the lines of adapting it to their own techniques.

But the progress in this promising area will be seriously impeded unless both professional and lay prejudices against hypnosis are reduced. A first step in building more confidence and in opening research laboratories to the serious study of this instrument should be its elimination from the field of showmanship. Unprofessional stage demonstrations have served to bring the practice of hypnosis, and hence hypnotherapy, into popular and professional disrepute. Many patients who otherwise could be helped by hypnotic procedures cannot be treated by these methods because of the resistance created by their own prejudices—prejudices originally formed by witnessing ridiculous or alarming shows in which hypnosis was utilized for idle amusement.

The popular illusion that no one can be harmed by hypnosis regardless of its unskillful use should be corrected. Any psychotherapeutic method which can constructively alter personality structure is strong enough to do harm. The hypnotic blunderer can precipitate severe problems in the delicate or predisposed individual.

Those who go about startling the uninitiated with ludicrous suggestions on the stage insist that "you can't be hypnotized against your will," and "nobody can be forced under hypnosis to violate his moral code." These statements are often used to justify the continued performance of hypnosis for profit by entertainers. They are not scientifically established. In fact, as previously indicated, there are published studies which throw serious doubt on their validity. At least the matter today is controversial. Professional people could greatly improve the possibility of using hypnosis therapeutically by lending their efforts to the legal restriction of hypnosis to professional and scientific purposes and the exclusion of it from the entertainment field.

There has been much hypnotizing but not enough controlled research. The correction of this condition must come in our great research institutions. Our major universities, instead of looking askance at any psychologist who wishes to do research in hypnosis, might better provide funds, laboratories, and equipment for its study, just as they do in the fields of psychological testing or physiology. We greatly need more study of hypnotic phenomena under experimentally controlled conditions.

The problem presented by the neurotic disorders in our culture today is indeed a staggering one. Whether these adjustment problems were precipitated by military service or interpersonal stresses in civilian life, the essential features in their etiology and treatment are similar. They require a unified attack by all psychological disciplines. No one of us has the entire solution. Each, like the blind men and the elephant, has grasped a part of the truth and feels tempted to generalize from it. The challenge today can be met if all the related professions work together in mutual respect and collaboration: the psychologist, the psychiatrist, the psychiatric social worker, the psychoanalyst, those representing each "school" of psychotherapy, as well as colleagues from related disciplines such as the sociologist, the anthropologist, and the educator. Only by a pooling of our experience can we build the sound scientific structure of theory and practice which must underlie our mutual efforts to lessen the ravages of neurotic misery, so pandemic to our present culture.

GLOSSARY

ā = *a* as in *came* ō = *o* as in *pole*
ă = *a* as in *cat* ŏ = *o* as in *not*
ä = *a* as in *card* ô = *o* as in *orb*
a = *a* as in *alone* ö = *o* as in *obey*

ē = *e* as in *legal* ū = *u* as in *cube*
ĕ = *e* as in *end* ŭ = *u* as in *nut*
ë = *e* as in first syllable of *event* ü = *u* as in *unite*
e = *e* as in *maker*

ī = *i* as in *ice* ōō = *oo* as in *pool*
ĭ = *i* as in *bit* N = *n* as in French *bon*
 tü = *tu* as in *nature*

1. Military Terms

BAR (B-A-R) *n.* Abbreviation for "Browning automatic rifle."

CDD (C-D-D) *n.* Abbreviation for "certificate of disability for discharge."

Goldbrick *n.* Soldier who shirks his duties; *v.* To shirk.

NP (N-P) *a., n.* Abbreviation for "neuropsychiatric" (q.v.); neuropsychiatric patient.

OCS (O-C-S) *n.* Abbreviation for "officer candidate school."

Psycho (sī'kō) *n.* Slang term used by servicemen to refer to all patients with neuropsychiatric illnesses.

Retreat *n.* Official end of formal military duties of the day, symbolized by ceremony and lowering of the flag.

Snafu (snă'fōō) *n., a.* Army slang term composed of first letters of the "situation normal, all fouled up"; a mess or tangle; tangled or mixed up.

Zone of the Interior *n. phr.* The United States proper as opposed to the overseas theaters.

2. Professional Terms

Abreaction (ăb"rë-ăk'shŭn) *n.* The act of reviving the memory of a repressed disagreeable experience and giving expression in speech and action to the emotions related to it, thereby relieving the personality of its influence.

Affective (ăf-fĕk'tĭv) *adj.* Referring to excitations arising in connection with emotion; emotional.

Ambivalence (ăm-bĭv'a-lĕns) *n.* Contrasting emotions such as love and hatred, either or both of which may be unconscious, experienced at the same time for the same person.

Amnesia (ăm-nē'zhĭ-*a*) *n.* Loss of memory either physically or psychologically caused.

Analysand (a-năl'ĭ-sănd) *n.* Term used by psychoanalysts to refer to the patient under analysis.

Analysis (See "Psychoanalysis")

Analytic-type therapy *n. phr.* Referring to an eclectic depth therapy utilizing psychoanalytic principles.

Animal magnetism *n. phr.* Theory advanced by Franz Anton Mesmer to account for hypnotic phenomena. It held that these were explicable in terms of a magnetic fluid or force which flowed from a magnetized object or person to the hypnotic subject.

Anorexia (ăn-ö-rĕk'sĭ-*a*) *n.* Inability to eat, organically or psychologically caused.

Anxiety reaction *n. phr.* Neurosis characterized by anxiety, sleeplessness, anorexia, tremulousness, and miscellaneous pains. During the second World War it was commonly called battle fatigue, combat fatigue, operational fatigue, etc.

Aphonia (ă-fō'nĭ-*a*) *n.* Loss of voice, organically or psychologically caused.

Astasia abasia (ă-stā'zë-*a* ă-bā'zë-*a*) *n. phr.* Irregularity in standing erect or walking due to psychological conflict.

Asthenic (ăs-thĕn'ĭk) *adj.* Characterized by loss of muscular energy.

Belongingness, principle of *n. phr.* Principle of learning which holds that material is more easily learned and retained if it is presented in a logical, meaningful context.

Bender Gestalt (bĕnd'er gĕ-shtält') *n. phr.* Psychological projective test which uses a subject's drawn reproductions of a set of standardized configurational designs as a method of diagnosing personality functioning.

Camptocormia (kămp"tö-kŏr'më-*a*) *n.* Hysterical deformity consisting of forward flexion of the trunk.

Catalepsy (căt′a-lĕp-sĭ) *n.* Condition of muscular rigidity in which the body and limbs may be moved but keep any position in which they are placed.

Catatonic (kăt-a-tŏn′ĭc) *adj.* Of the nature of catatonia, a form of schizophrenia characterized by withdrawn manner, muscular rigidity, and general irritability.

Catharsis (ka-thär′sĭs) *n.* Unburdening the personality of disturbing complexes through verbal or postural expression.

Clinical psychologist *n. phr.* Psychologist who diagnoses and treats psychologically caused disorders.

Combat fatigue *n. phr.* Loose general term applied to war neuroses; specifically, anxiety reactions precipitated by battle.

Complex *n.* Group of concepts and memories related to each other which have an emotional basis and have been repressed into the unconscious.

Compulsion *n.* Uncontrollable urge toward an irrational act or speech.

Conversion hysteria *n. phr.* Neurosis in which anxiety is manifested by or "converted" into specific symptoms, often involving the loss of some bodily function.

Conversion reaction *n. phr.* Term used in Army neuropsychiatric classification to refer to those hysterical neuroses in which the symptom is specific and physical. (See also "Dissociative reaction.")

Defense mechanism *n. phr.* Device whereby the individual avoids anxiety by dodging a direct solution of his problems.

Delusion *n.* False belief not founded upon logical inference and which cannot be corrected by adequate proof of its falsity.

Depth therapy *n. phr.* Treatment which has as its objective the gaining of insight into unconscious motivations.

Direct suggestion *n. phr.* Suggestion given to a patient while he is under hypnotic trance.

Dissociative reaction *n. phr.* Term used in Army neuropsychiatric classification to refer to those hysterical neuroses in which the symptom is specific and psychological, such as somnambulism, amnesia, or fugue. (See also "Conversion reaction.")

Dynamics (See "Psychodynamics")

Eclectic (ĕk-lĕk′tĭk) *adj.* Selecting methods from various sources; used here as pertaining to a therapy which does not rely exclusively on one theoretical system of psychology.

Ego (ē′gō) *n.* The conscious self that is aware of personal experiences and in touch with reality; ability of the organism to achieve its objectives and goals.

Electra complex (ě-lĕk'tra kŏm'plĕks) *n. phr.* Complex developed in the female child; corresponding to the Oedipus complex (q.v.).

Enuresis (ĕn-ü-rē'sĭs) *n.* Involuntary discharge of the urine.

Epigastric (ĕp"ĭ-găs'trĭk) *adj.* Pertaining to the region over the stomach.

Euphoria (ü-fō'rĭ-a) *n.* Sense of well-being and buoyancy.

Free association *n. phr.* Analytic technique of therapy in which the patient is permitted unrestricted mental activity; it is assumed that his chains of associations tend to lead toward areas of mental conflict.

Fugue (fūg) *n.* Disturbance of consciousness in which the patient performs purposeful acts of flight from familiar surroundings without later recollection of the acts.

Functional *adj.* Affecting the action of any organ (or of the mind), but without physiological change of structure; sometimes used as the equivalent of "psychogenic."

Gestalt (gě-shtält') *n.* Mental pattern or configuration.

Grand mal (grän mal) *n. phr.* Epileptic fit in which there are severe convulsions and loss of consciousness. It is controversial whether the disease is functional or organic or both.

Hallucination (hăl-lū"sĭ-nā'shŭn) *n.* Perception of objects with no reality, or experience of sensations with no external cause.

Horizontal exploration *n. phr.* Term used in this book to refer to the study of incidents, experiences, emotions, feelings, and ideas of the patient when regressed to a former age-level under hypnotic trance.

Hyperesthesia (hī"per-ĕs-thē'zhĭ-a) *n.* State of heightened sensibility to touch.

Hypermnesia (hī"perm-nē'zhĭ-a) *n.* Superior memory; unusual recall or retentiveness.

Hypnoanalytic (hĭp"nö-ăn-a-lĭt'ĭk) *adj.* Characterized by the use of psychoanalytic techniques in conjunction with hypnosis.

Hypnoidal state (hīp-noid'ăl stāt) *n. phr.* Light degree of narcosis resembling hypnosis.

Hypnosis (hĭp-nō'sĭs) *n.* Sleep-like state induced by the hypnotist in a subject. It is characterized by heightened suggestibility.

Hypnotherapy (hĭp"nö-thěr'apĭ) *n.* Treatment of an illness under hypnosis.

Hysteria (hĭs-těr'ĭ-a) *n.* Neurosis characterized by emotional excitability and various specific symptoms. It is explained psychoanalytically as the result or conversion of unconscious conflicts into physical or psychological symptoms. (See also "Conversion reaction" and "Dissociative reaction.")

Id (ĭd) *n.* Unorganized region of the unconscious. It is considered to be a reservoir of primitive and unsocialized impulses.

"In-and-out" *adj.* Characterized by repeatedly placing the patient into hypnotic trance and taking him out in order to ascertain both his conscious and unconscious reactions to questions.

Innate *adj.* Inborn, inherited, not acquired.

Insane *adj.* Legal term inferring lack of mental competency to undertake contracts and assume obligations. "Psychotic" is the psychiatric term which is roughly its equivalent.

Insight *n.* Understanding; appreciation of deeper significance of behavior.

Levitation, hand (lĕv-ĭ-tā′shŭn) *n. phr.* Raising of the hand. When unconsciously executed by a hypnotized subject in response to a suggestion, it becomes a test of the depth of trance.

Libido (lĭ-bē′dō) *n.* Basic psychosexual energy. As invested in objects or people it constitutes the expression of all love impulses.

Malingerer (ma-lĭng′ger-er) *n.* One who feigns illness or disability in order to avoid duty.

Mesmerism (mĕz′mer-ĭzm) *n.* Hypnotism as practiced by Franz Anton Mesmer and his followers.

Minnesota Multiphasic Personality Inventory (mŭl-tĭ-fāz′ĭk) *n. phr.* Objective psychological test designed to evaluate types of personality disorders.

Narcosis (när-kō′sĭs) *n.* Stuporous or sleeplike state produced by a narcotic drug.

Narcosynthesis (när″kö-sĭn′thĕ-sĭs) *n.* Therapeutic technique in which traumatic memories are reconstructed under a narcosis induced by barbiturate drugs.

Neurological (nū″rö-lŏj′ĭ-kăl) *adj.* Pertaining to neurology, the science dealing with the nervous system and its diseases.

Neuropathic traits (nū″rö-păth′ĭk trāts) *n. phr.* Traits pertaining to, or similar to, functional nervous disease; childhood nervous traits such as nail-biting, stuttering, and enuresis.

Neuropsychiatric (nū″rö-sī″kĭ-ăt′rĭk) *adj.* Pertaining to that division of medical science which includes neurology and psychiatry.

Neurosis (nū-rō′sĭs) *n.* Functional nervous disorder, without demonstrable physical lesion. It is marked by the presence of physical or mental symptoms and an impairment of living efficiency or adjustment but not by a disturbance in the perception of reality as occurs in the psychoses.

Normal distribution *n. phr.* Usual distribution of scores in psychological measurement of a group of individuals. When represented graphically, these tend to approach the form of a bell-shaped curve known as the "normal" or "Gaussian" curve.

Obsession *n.* Uncontrollable urge to dwell upon some thought or perform some unnecessary action.

Obsessive-compulsive reaction *n. phr.* Diagnostic term used in Army classification of psychiatric disorders to refer to a type of neurosis marked by obsessive thoughts and compulsive, repetitive actions.

Oedipus complex (ĕd'ĭ-pŭs kŏm'plĕks) *n. phr.* Psychoanalytic theory, named after a character in an ancient Greek legend, which holds that the young child in a family tends to develop a sexual fixation on the parent of the opposite sex and a hostility toward the parent of the same sex; normally used with reference to the male child.

Operational fatigue *n. phr.* Term used by Army Air Forces during second World War to refer to war neuroses largely of the anxiety-reaction type; combat or battle fatigue.

Organic *adj.* Pertaining to the physical structure of the individual; structural rather than psychological.

Parkinson syndrome (pärk'ĭn-sŭn sĭn'drōm) *n. phr.* Neurological disease marked by rigidity and tremors.

Pathogenic (păth"ö-jĕn'ĭk) *adj.* Disease-causing.

Pathology (pa-thŏl'ö-jĭ) *n.* Science treating of diseases, their nature and causes; condition produced by disease.

Peristaltic movements (pĕr'ĭ-stăl'tĭk) *n. phr.* Movements in the muscle walls of the intestinal tract which force the food contents through it.

Phobia (fō'bĭ-a) *n.* Fixed, morbid fear not susceptible of relief by rational explanation.

Phobic reaction (fō'bĭk rë-ăk'shŭn) *n. phr.* Neurosis predominantly characterized by one or more phobias.

Pleasure-pain principle *n. phr.* Principle of learning which holds that behavior culminating in pleasure tends to be learned and retained while behavior culminating in pain tends to be forgotten.

Postural sway *n. phr.* Technique used as an indicator of suggestibility and also as a method for inducing hypnotic trance.

Predisposition (prē"dĭs-pö-zĭsh'un) *n.* Inherited and experiential background of a patient which renders him susceptible to emotional maladjustment or psychiatric illness.

Prognosis (prŏg-nō'sĭs) *n.* Forecast of the course of a disease.

Progressive relaxation *n. phr.* Method of treatment involving the successive relaxing of different muscle groups until the body attains a state of extreme flaccidity.

Projection *n.* Neurotic defense mechanism in which the individual avoids anxiety by imputing to others his own repressed, unconscious impulses which are unacceptable to his conscience or value system.

Projective techniques *n. phr.* Psychological tests designed to present the subject with an unstructured stimulus. In his responses the subject tends to structure the material in terms of his own personality.

Psychiatrist (sī-kī′a-trĭst) *n.* Physician who specializes in the treatment of mental disease.

Psychiatry (sī-kī′a-trĭ) *n.* Branch of medicine dealing with mental disease.

Psychoanalysis (sī″kö-a-năl′ĭ-sĭs) *n.* Theory of mental processes and a method of treating them resting on the principle that abnormal behavior is the result of unconscious motives. It was first advanced by Sigmund Freud.

Psychoanalyst (sī″kö-ăn′a-lĭst) *n.* One who practices psychoanalysis.

Psychodrama (sī″kö-drä′ma) *n.* Method of psychotherapy in which the patient is encouraged to achieve relief from and insight into his problems by reliving them in a controlled dramatic situation.

Psychodynamics (sī″kö-dī-năm′ĭks) *n.* Motivations and mental processes which underlie a normal or abnormal kind of behavior.

Psychogenic (sī″kö-gĕn′ĭk) *adj.* Psychologically caused.

Psychologist (sī-kŏl′ö-jĭst) *n.* One who engages in the study or practice of psychology.

Psychology (sī-kŏl′ö-jĭ) *n.* Science which studies human behavior and mental functioning.

Psychoneurosis (See "Neurosis")

Psychopathology (sī″kö-pa-thŏl′ö-jĭ) *n.* Pathology of mental disorders.

Psychosexual (sī″kö-sĕks′ū-ăl) *adj.* Pertaining to the mental aspects of sex life.

Psychosis (sī-kö′sĭs) *n.* Severe mental disorder involving great derangement of intellectual, perceptive or affective processes. It differs from neurosis in that it involves a retreat from rather than a compromise with reality.

Psychosomatic (sī″kö-sö-măt′ĭk) *adj.* Pertaining to body-mind relationships (used to describe illnesses caused by joint physiological and psychological malfunctioning).

Psychotherapy (sī″kö-thĕr′a-pĭ) *n.* Treatment of personality disorders by psychological methods.

Psychotic (sī-kŏt′ik) *adj.* Pertaining to psychosis.

Rapport (ră-pôrt′) *n.* Intimate or harmonious relationship; relationship of mutual trust.

Rationalization *n.* Neurotic defense mechanism in which the individual avoids anxiety by ascribing acceptable motives to his behavior.

Reactive depression *n. phr.* Neurosis appearing in reaction to a situation which would naturally cause sadness, but of less marked degree and duration.

Regression (rë-grĕsh′ŭn) *n.* 1. Neurotic defense mechanism in which the individual avoids anxiety by returning to thoughts or behavior of an earlier period in his development. 2. Return to an earlier age-level in thought and behavior under hypnotic trance.

Repression (rë-prĕsh′ŭn) *n.* Rejection from consciousness of ideas and impulses that are unacceptable to the conscience or personal value system.

Retroactive inhibition (rĕt″rō-ăk′tĭv ĭn″hĭ-bĭsh′ŭn) *n. phr.* Action of learned material in impairing retention of previously learned material.

Rorschach test (rôr′shäk tĕst) *n. phr.* Psychological projective test in which personality structure and functioning are inferred from the subject's responses to a standardized series of ink blots.

Satisfaction, principle of *n. phr.* Principle of learning which holds that an action resulting in satisfaction to the individual tends to be repeated.

Schizophrenia (skĭz″ö-frēn′ĭ-*a*) *n.* Psychotic disorder manifested by withdrawn manner, intellectual dissociation, and frequently delusions and hallucinations. Since it commonly occurs among younger people, it was originally called dementia praecox, or precocious dementia.

Secondary gain *n. phr.* Advantage derived from being ill. It may continue to maintain an illness after the original cause has been resolved.

Sensory-Motor (sĕn′sö-rĭ-mō′ter) *adj.* Pertaining to reactions involving sense organs and muscular mechanisms, disregarding higher mental functioning.

Shell shock *n.* Term used during the first World War to refer to combat neuroses. It was originally believed that these disabilities were organic reactions to shell explosions.

Somatic (sō-mǎt′ĭk) *adj.* Pertaining to the body.

Somnambulism (sŏm-nǎm′bü-lĭzm) *n.* Hysterical state in which purposeful acts and behavior occur with no subsequent recollection (in psychiatry, a more comprehensive term than "sleepwalking").

Spastic (spǎs′tĭk) *adj.* Pertaining to or affected with spasticity or rigidity in the muscles.

Stress (strĕss) *n.* Action of environmental forces causing pressure on an individual which provokes anxiety within him and may precipitate a failure of adjustment. "Stress" usually refers to those factors which immediately precede a maladjustment.

Structured stimulus (strŭk'chĕrd stĭm'ū-lŭs) *n. phr.* Stimulus accompanied by suggestion of a definite type of response.

Sublimation (sŭb"lĭ-mā'shŭn) *n.* Directing of emotional energies into socially acceptable channels.

Super-Ego (sū'pĕr-ē'gō) *n.* Internalized value system acting as guiding standard to the Ego. It results from the socializing of the individual.

Superficial therapy *n. phr.* Treatment of neurosis which relies on the readjustment of living conditions for its efficacy; contrasted with "depth therapy," in which insight into unconscious dynamics is sought. The word "superficial" does not imply that such treatment is ineffective.

Suppression *n.* Conscious control of unacceptable ideas and impulses.

Symptom *n.* Any apparent evidence of disease; change in patient's condition indicative of some bodily or mental state.

Syndrome (sĭn'drōm) *n.* Group of clinical signs or symptoms which may result from diverse causes (does not necessarily constitute disease entity).

TAT (T-A-T) *n.* Abbreviation for Thematic Apperception Test (q.v.).

Thematic Apperception Test (thē-măt'ĭk ăp"er-sĕp'shŭn tĕst) *n. phr.* Psychological projective test used to reveal underlying motivations in a subject's personality. In it the subject imagines stories about a set of standardized pictures and in so doing reveals much of his own inner dynamic structure.

Therapist (thĕr'a-pĭst) *n.* One who treats disease.

Therapy (thĕr'a-pĭ) *n.* Treatment of disease.

Tic (tĭk) *n.* Intermittent spasmodic or jerky movement of any part of the body.

Tinnitus (tĭn'ĭ-tŭs) *n.* A ringing, whistling, or other sensation of noise which is purely subjective and not caused by external stimulation.

Trance (trăns, träns) *n.* Sleeplike state such as that of deep hypnosis.

Transference (trăns'fer-ĕns) *n.* Displacement of an emotional feeling from the original person who caused it to another, usually the patient's psychoanalyst. The analysis of this reaction constitutes one of the basic approaches in psychoanalytic treatment.

Trauma (trô'ma) *n.* Wound or injury inflicted upon the body or the personality.

Unconscious *n., adj.* N. The whole body of an individual's ideas, affects and motives, potential or operative, which are not able to evoke the phenomenon of consciousness or awareness. (In psychoanalytic theory the unconscious is posited as a part of the mind in which reposes content not accessible to memory.) *Adj.* Not known to the conscious part of the mind.

Vertical exploration *n. phr.* Term used in this book to refer to the technique of tracing etiology and development of any personality trend by studying it at various age levels to which the patient has been regressed under hypnotic trance.

Visceral (vĭs'er-al) *adj.* Pertaining to the viscera or internal organs of the body.

Wechsler-Bellevue test (wĕx'ler bĕl'vū tĕst) *n. phr.* Type of standardized intelligence test designed for adults, used clinically as a method of studying qualitative as well as quantitative functioning of mental ability.

BIBLIOGRAPHY

ALEXANDER, F., and FRENCH, T. M. 1946. *Psychoanalytic therapy.* New York: The Ronald Press Co.

ALPERT, H. S., CARBONE, H. A., and BROOKS, J. T. 1946. Hypnosis as a therapeutic technique in the war neuroses. *Bull. of the U.S. Med. Dept.,* **5,** 315-324.

APPEL, K. E. Psychiatric therapy. In Hunt, J. McV., ed., *Personality and the behavior disorders.* New York: The Ronald Press Co., Ch. 34.

BECK, S. J. 1944. *Rorschach's test.* Vol. I. *Basic processes.* New York: Grune & Stratton, Inc.

———. 1945. *Rorschach's test.* Vol. II. *A variety of personality pictures.* New York: Grune & Stratton, Inc.

BELL, J. E. 1946. *Projective techniques.* New York: Longmans, Green & Co.

BELLAK, L. 1947. *The Bellak TAT Blank.* New York: Psychological Corp.

BERNHEIM, H. 1895. *Suggestive therapeutics.* Translated by C. A. Herter. New York: G. P. Putnam's Sons.

BRAID, J. 1899. *Neurypnology; or, The rationale of nervous sleep, considered in relation with animal magnetism.* London: G. Redway.

BRAMWELL, J. M. 1930. *Hypnotism, its history, practice, and theory.* Philadelphia: J. B. Lippincott Co.

BRENMAN, M., and GILL, M. 1947. *Hypnotherapy.* New York: International Universities Press, Inc.

BRENMAN, M., and REICHARD, S. 1943. Use of the Rorschach test in the prediction of hypnotizability. *Bull. Menninger Clinic,* **7,** 183-187.

BREUER, J., and FREUD, S. 1912. *Studies in hysteria.* Washington: Nervous & Mental Disorder Publishing Co.

CHARCOT, J. M. 1890. *Oeuvres complètes.* Tome IX. *Metallotherapie et hypnotisme.* Paris: Bourneville et E. Brissaud.

COTTON, J. M., SHULACK, N. R., KAPLAN, C., and WATKINS, J. G. 1945. Manual of group psychotherapy. Mimeographed. Daytona Beach, Fla.: Neuropsychiatric Treatment Branch, Welch Convalescent Hospital.

DAVIS, L. W., and HUSBAND, R. W. 1931. A study of hypnotic susceptibility in relation to personality traits. *J. of abn. & soc. Psychology,* **26,** 175-182.

DEUTSCH, F. 1947. Analysis of postural behavior. *Psychoanal. Quart.,* **16:** 195-213.

ELKISCH, P. 1945. Children's drawings in a projective technique. *Psychol. Monogr.,* **58:** No. 1.

ERICKSON, M. H. 1935. A study of an experimental neurosis hypnotically induced in a case of ejaculatio praecox. *British J. of medical Psychol.,* **15:** 34-50.

———. 1937a. The experimental demonstration of unconscious mentation by automatic writing. *Psychoanal. Quart.,* **6:** 513.

———. 1937b. Development of apparent unconsciousness during hypnotic reliving of a traumatic experience. *Arch. Neurol. Psychiat.,* **38:** 1282-1288.

———. 1938. A study of clinical and experimental findings on hypnotic deafness: I. Clinical experimentation and findings. *J. gen. Psychol.,* **19:** 127-150.

———. 1939a. Demonstration of mental mechanisms by hypnosis. *Arch. of Neurol. Psychiat.,* **42:** 367-370.

ERICKSON, M. H. 1939b. Experimental demonstrations of the psychopathology of everyday life. *Psychoanal. Quart.*, **8**: 338-353.

———. 1939c. A study of clinical and experimental findings on hypnotic deafness: II. Experimental findings with a conditioned response technique. *J. gen. Psychol.*, **20**: 61-89.

———. 1939d. The applications of hypnosis to psychiatry. *Med. Rec.*, **150**: 60-65.

———. 1939e. An experimental investigation of the possible anti-social use of hypnosis. *Psychiatry*, **2**: 391-414.

———. 1943a. Hypnotic investigation of psychosomatic phenomena: Psychosomatic interrelationships studied by experimental hypnosis. *Psychosom. Med.*, **5**: 51-58.

———. 1943b. Hypnotic investigation of psychosomatic phenomena: The development of aphasia-like reactions from hypnotically induced amnesias. *Psychosom. Med.*, **5**: 59-66.

———. 1943c. Hypnotic investigation of psychosomatic phenomena: A controlled experimental use of hypnotic regression in the therapy of an acquired food intolerance. *Psychosom. Med.*, **5**: 67-70.

———. 1944a. The method employed to formulate a complex story for the induction of an experimental neurosis in a hypnotic subject. *J. gen. Psychol.*, **31**: 67-84.

———. 1944b. Hypnosis in medicine. *Medical Clinics of North America*, May: 639-652.

———. 1945. Hypnotic techniques for the therapy of acute psychiatric disturbances in war. *Amer. J. Psychiat.*, **101**: 668-672.

——— and KUBIE, L. S. 1938. The use of automatic drawing in the interpretation and relief of a state of acute obsessional depression. *Psychoanal. Quart.*, **7**: 443-466.

——— and ———. 1939. The permanent relief of an obsessional phobia by means of communication with an unsuspected dual personality. *Psychoanal. Quart.*, **8**: 471-509.

——— and ———. 1940. The translation of the cryptic automatic writing of one hypnotic subject by another in a trance-like dissociated state. *Psychoanal. Quart.*, **9**: 51-63.

——— and ———. 1941. The successful treatment of a case of acute hysterical depression by a return under hypnosis to a critical phase of childhood. *Psychoanal. Quart.*, **10**: 583-609.

ESTABROOKS, G. H. 1944. *Hypnotism*. New York: E. P. Dutton & Co., Inc.

FARBER, L. H., and FISHER, C. 1943. An experimental approach to dream psychology through the use of hypnosis. *Psychoanal. Quart.*, **12**: 202-216.

FENICHEL, O. 1945. *The psychoanalytic theory of neuroses*. New York: W. W. Norton & Co., Inc.

FERENCZI, S. 1928. Das Problem der Beendigung der Analysen. *Int. Z. Psycho-Anal.*, **14**: 1.

FINK, H. D. 1943. *Release from nervous tension*. New York: Simon & Schuster, Inc.

FISHER, C. 1943. Hypnosis in treatment of neuroses due to war and to other causes. *War Medicine*, **4**: 565-576.

FREUD, A. 1937. *The ego and mechanisms of defense*. London: Hogarth Press, Ltd.

FREUD, S. 1935. *Autobiography*. Translated by J. Strachey. New York: W. W. Norton & Co., Inc.

———. 1938. *Basic writings*. Translated by A. A. Brill. New York: Modern Library, Inc.

FRIEDLANDER, J. W., and SARBIN, T. R. 1938. The depth of hypnosis. *J. abnorm. soc. Psychol.*, **33**: 453-475.

GRINKER, R. R., and SPIEGEL, J. P. 1944. Brief psychotherapy in war neuroses. *Psychos. Med.,* **6:** 123-131.
—— and ——. 1945. *War neuroses.* Philadelphia: The Blakiston Co.

HOCH, Paul H. (Editor). 1948. *Failures in psychiatric treatment.* New York: Grune & Stratton, Inc.
HULL, C. L. 1933. *Hypnosis and suggestibility.* New York: Appleton-Century-Crofts, Inc.
HUNT, J. McV. 1948. Discussion following Lucille N. Austin, Failures in social casework. In Hoch, P. H., ed., *Failures in psychiatric treatment.* New York: Grune & Stratton, Inc., pp. 216-223.

INBAU, F. E. 1942. *Lie detection and criminal interrogation.* Baltimore: The Williams & Wilkins Co.

JACOBSON, E. 1938. *Progressive relaxation.* Chicago: University of Chicago Press.
JANET, P. 1907. *The major symptoms of hysteria.* New York: The Macmillan Co.
——. 1925. *Psychological healing.* New York: The Macmillan Co.
JENNESS, A. 1944. Hypnotism. In Hunt, J. McV., ed., *Personality and the behavior disorders.* New York: The Ronald Press Co. Ch. 15.
JUNG, C. G. 1918. *Studies in word association.* London: William Heinemann, Ltd.

KANZER, M. G. 1945. The therapeutic use of dreams induced by hypnotic suggestion. *Psychoanal. Quart.,* **14:** 313-335.
KENT, G. H., and ROSANOFF, A. J. 1910. A study of association in insanity. *Amer. J. Insanity,* **67:** 37-96, 317-390.
KLOPFER, B., and KELLEY, D. M. 1942. *The Rorschach technique.* Yonkers: World Book Co.
KOFFKA, K. 1935. *Principles of gestalt psychology.* New York: Harcourt, Brace & Co., Inc.
KUBIE, L. S. 1943. The nature of psychotherapy. *Bull. N. Y. Acad. Med.,* **19:** 183-194.
——. 1943. Use of induced hypnagogic reveries in the recovery of repressed amnesic data. *Bull. Menninger Clinic,* **7:** 5-6, 172-182.
—— and MARGOLIN, S. 1942. A physiological method for the induction of states of partial sleep, and securing free association and early memories in such states. *Trans. Amer. neurol. Ass.,* **68:** 136-139.
—— and ——. 1944. The process of hypnotism and the nature of the hypnotic state. *Amer. J. Psychiat.,* **100:** 611-622.

LE CRON, L. M., and BORDEAUX, J. 1947. *Hypnotism today.* New York: Grune & Stratton, Inc.
LEVIN, M. 1945. Hysteria as a device to prolong hospitalization and evade military duty. *War Medicine,* **8:** 16-17.
LEWIN, K. 1935. *A dynamic theory of personality.* New York: McGraw-Hill Book Co., Inc.
——. 1938. Conceptual representation and measurement of psychological forces. *Contr. psychol. Theor.,* **1:** No. 4. Durham, N. C.: Duke University Press.
LIÉBEAULT, A. 1892. Du sommeil et des états analogues considérés surtout au point de vue de l'action moral sur le physique. Nancy and Paris: 1866. Also Vienna: Deuticke, 1892.
LIEF, A., ed. 1948. *The commonsense psychiatry of Dr. Adolf Meyer.* New York: McGraw-Hill Book Co., Inc.

LINDNER, R. M. 1944. *Rebel without a cause; the hypnoanalysis of a criminal psychopath*. New York: Grune & Stratton, Inc.

MENNINGER, K. A. 1938. *Man against himself*. New York: Harcourt, Brace & Co., Inc.

—— and MENNINGER, J. L. 1942. *Love against hate*. New York: Harcourt, Brace & Co., Inc.

MORENO, J. L. 1946. *Psychodrama*. Vol. I. New York: Beacon House, Inc.

MURRAY, H. A., *et al*. 1938. *Explorations in personality*. New York: Oxford University Press.

——. 1943. *Thematic apperception test manual*. Cambridge, Mass.: Harvard University Press.

OBERNDORF, C. P. 1948. Failures with psychoanalytic therapy. In Hoch, P. H., ed., *Failures in psychiatric treatment*. New York: Grune & Stratton, Inc., Ch. 2.

OVSIANKINA, M. 1928. Die Wiederaufnahme unterbrochener Handlungen. *Psychol. Forsch.*, 11: 302-379.

ROGERS, C. F. 1942. *Counseling and psychotherapy*. Boston: Houghton Mifflin Co.

ROWLAND, L. W. 1939. Will hypnotized persons try to harm themselves or others? *J. abnorm. soc. Psychol.*, 34: 114-117.

SALTER, A. 1941. Three techniques of autohypnosis. *J. gen. Psychol.*, 24: 423-438.

——. 1944. *What is hypnosis?* New York: Richard R. Smith.

SANDLER, S. A. 1945. Camptocormia, a functional condition of the back in neurotic soldiers. *War Medicine*, 8: 36-45.

SARBIN, T. R., and MADOW, L. W. 1942. Predicting the depth of hypnosis by means of the Rorschach test. *Amer. J. Orthopsychiat.*, 12: 268-271.

SCOTT, P. D., and MALLINSON, P. 1944. Hysterical sequelae of injuries. *Brit. med. J.*, Apr. 1: 450-453.

SHAKOW, D., and ROSENZWEIG, S. 1940. The use of the tautophone (verbal summator) as an auditory apperceptive test for the study of personality. *Character & Pers.*, 8: 216-226.

SIMMEL, E. 1944. War neuroses. In Lorand, S., ed., *Psychoanalysis today*. New York: International Universities Press, Inc. Pp. 227-248.

SPIEGEL, H., SHOR, J., and FISHMAN, S. 1945. An hypnotic ablation technique for the study of personality development. *Psychosom. Med.*, 7: 273-278.

STEIN, M. I. 1948. *The thematic apperception test*. Cambridge, Mass.: Addison-Wesley Press, Inc.

STEKEL, W. 1926. *Frigidity in woman*, Vols. I and II. Translated by J. S. Van Teslaar. New York: Liveright Publishing Corporation.

——. 1927. *Impotence in the male*, Vols. I and II. Translated by O. W. Boltz. New York: Liveright Publishing Corporation.

——. 1943. *The interpretation of dreams*, Vols. I and II. Translated by E. Paul and C. Paul. New York: Liveright Publishing Corporation.

——. 1949. Autobiography: VIII. *Amer. J. Psychother.*, 3: 46-73.

SWENSON, E. J. 1941. Retroactive inhibition: a review of the literature. *U. of Minnesota Studies in Education*, No. 1.

TOMKINS, S. S. 1947. *The thematic apperception test*. New York: Grune & Stratton, Inc.

VOGT, O. 1892-93. A contribution to the knowledge of the nature of hypnosis. *Zeitschrift für Hypnotismus*, 3: 277; 4: 32.

WAR DEPARTMENT. 1944. *Occupational therapy*. W.D. Technical Manual, TM 8-291.

WAR DEPARTMENT. 1946. *Nomenclature of psychiatric disorders and reactions.* W.D. Technical Bull. Medical 203. (Reproduced in *J. clinical Psychol.*, 2: 289-296.)

WATKINS, J. G. 1946. The hypnoanalytic location of a lost object. *J. clin. Psychol.*, 2: 390-394.

——. 1947a. The hypnoanalytic treatment of a case of impotence. *J. clin. Psychopath.*, 8: 451-480.

——. 1947b. Antisocial compulsions induced under hypnotic trance. *J. soc. abnor. Psychol.*, 42: 256-259.

——. 1947c. A class in hypnotherapy. *Amer. J. Psychother.*, 1: 436-442.

——. 1949. Poison-pen therapy. *Amer. J. Psychother.*, 3: 410-418.

WELLS, W. R. 1941. Experiments in the hypnotic production of crime. *J. Psychol.*, 11: 63-102.

——. 1944. The hypnotic treatment of the major symptoms of hysteria: a case study. *J. Psychol.*, 17: 269-297.

WETTERSTRAND, O. G. 1902. *Hypnotism and its application to practical medicine.* Translated by H. G. Petersen. New York: G. P. Putnam's Sons.

WHITE, R. W. 1948. *The abnormal personality.* New York: The Ronald Press Co.

WOLBERG, L. R. 1945. *Hypnoanalysis.* New York: Grune & Stratton, Inc.

——. 1948. *Medical hypnosis,* Vols. I and II. New York: Grune & Stratton, Inc.

YASKIN, J. C. 1945. Delayed favorable effects in psychotherapy. *J. nerv. ment. Dis.*, 101: 550-556.

YOUNG, P. C. 1931. A general review of the literature on hypnotism and suggestion. *Psychol. Bull.*, 28: 367-391.

——. 1940. Hypnotic regression—fact or artifact. *J. abnor. soc. Psychol.*, 35: 273-278.

——. 1941. Experimental hypnotism: a review. *Psychol. Bull.*, 38: 92-104.

ZEIGARNIK, B. 1927. Über das Behalten von erledigten und unerledigten Handlungen. *Psychol. Forsch.*, 9: 1-86.

AUTHOR INDEX

SUBJECT INDEX

375